ORAL DIAGNOSIS
AND
TREATMENT PLANNING

Publication Number 856
AMERICAN LECTURE SERIES®

A Monograph in

The BANNERSTONE DIVISION *of*
AMERICAN LECTURES IN DENTISTRY

Edited by

ALVIN F. GARDNER D.D.S., M.S., Ph.D.
*Bureau of Drugs
Food and Drug Administration
Department of Health, Education and Welfare
Washington, D. C.*

No official support or endorsement by the Food and Drug Administration or the Department of Health, Education and Welfare is intended or should be inferred.

Oral Diagnosis

and

Treatment Planning

Edited by

LAWRENCE COHEN, Ph.D., M.D., B.Ch.D., F.D.S.R.C.S.

*Professor and Head, Department of Oral Diagnosis,
University of Illinois
Director of Dental Education,
Illinois Masonic Medical Center
Chicago, Illinois
Consultant in Oral Diagnosis,
Veterans Administration, West Side Hospital
Chicago, Illinois
Consultant in Dental Medicine,
School of Dental Medicine, Southern Illinois University
Edwardsville, Illinois*

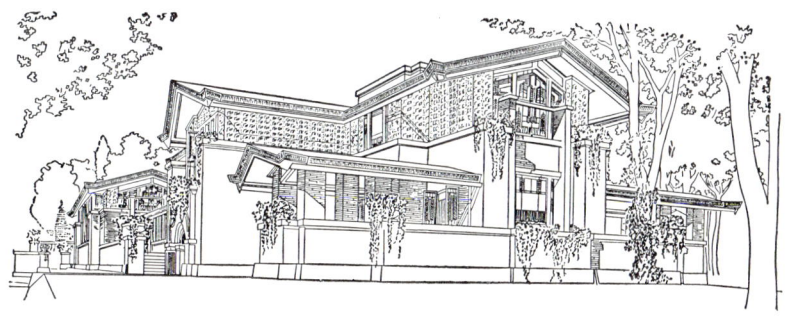

CHARLES C THOMAS • PUBLISHER
Springfield • Illinois • U.S.A.

Published and Distributed Throughout the World by
CHARLES C THOMAS • PUBLISHER
BANNERSTONE HOUSE
301–327 East Lawrence Avenue, Springfield, Illinois, U.S.A.

This book is protected by copyright. No
part of it may be reproduced in any manner
without written permission from the publisher.

© 1973, by CHARLES C THOMAS • PUBLISHER
ISBN 0–398–02568–1
Library of Congress Catalog Card Number: 72–79186

With THOMAS BOOKS *careful attention is given to all details of manufacturing and design. It is the Publisher's desire to present books that are satisfactory as to their physical qualities and artistic possibilities and appropriate for their particular use.* THOMAS BOOKS *will be* **true** *to those laws of quality that assure a good name and good will.*

Printed in the United States of America
K–8

DEDICATION

This book is dedicated to the memory of Edward E. Beveridge (1931–1972) a gifted clinician, researcher and educator.

Contributors

HOWARD ADUSS, D.D.S., *Associate Professor, Center for Craniofacial Anomalies, University of Illinois, Chicago, Illinois.*

ALLEN W. ANDERSON, B.S., D.D.S., M.S., *Associate Professor and Head, Department of Pedodontics, University of Illinois, Chicago, Illinois.*

EDWARD E. BEVERIDGE, D.D.S., M.S.D., F.A.C.D., *Professor and Chairman, Department of Endodontics, University of Southern California, Los Angeles, California.**

RALPH I. BROOKE, B.Ch.D., L.D.S., F.D.S.R.C.S. (Eng.), M.R.C.S. (Eng.), L.R.C.P. (Lond.), *Former University Associate in Oral Medicine, Buffalo General Hospital; Senior Lecturer in Oral Medicine, Leeds University School of Dentistry, Leeds, England; Consultant Dental Surgeon, United Leeds Hospitals, Leeds, England.*

PAUL BURLAKOW, B.S., *Cytotechnician, Department of Oral Diagnosis, University of Illinois, Chicago, Illinois.*

LAWRENCE COHEN, Ph.D., M.D., B.Ch.D., F.D.S.R.C.S. (Eng.), *Professor and Head, Department of Oral Diagnosis, University of Illinois, Chicago, Illinois; Director of Dental Education, Illinois Masonic Medical Center, Chicago, Illinois; Consultant in Oral Diagnosis, Veterans Administration West Side Hospital, Chicago, Illinois; Consultant in Dental Medicine, School of Dental Medicine, Southern Illinois University, Edwardsville, Illinois.*

ALAN J. DRINNAN, M.B., Ch.B., B.D.S., D.D.S., F.D.S.R.C.S. (Eng.), *Professor and Chairman, Department of Oral Medicine, School of Dentistry, State University of New York at Buffalo; Chief, Dental Service, Buffalo General Hospital, Buffalo, New York.*

ARTHUR ELFENBAUM, B.A., D.D.S., *Associate Professor of Oral Diagnosis (Emeritus), University of Illinois, Chicago, Illinois; Professor and Chairman (Emeritus), Department of Oral Diagnosis, Northwestern University Dental School, Chicago, Illinois; Senior Attending Member of the Medical Staff, Section of Oral Diagnosis, Michael Reese Hospital and Medical Center, Chicago, Illinois.*

STUART L. FISCHMAN, D.M.D., F.I.C.D., *Associate Professor, Department of Oral Medicine; Assistant Dean for Academic Development, School of Dentistry, State University of New York at Buffalo.*

RINERT J. GERHARD, B.S., D.D.S., *Former Department Chairman and Associate Professor of Removable Prosthodontics, Loyola University, Maywood, Illinois.*

* Deceased.

STANLEY KENNETT, M.B., B.S. (Lond.), F.D.S.R.C.S. (Eng.), F.A.C.D.S. (Aust.), *Professor, Oral Surgery and Oral Medicine, The University of Manitoba, Winnipeg, Canada; Head, Department of Dentistry and Oral Surgery, The Winnipeg General Hospital, Winnipeg, Canada; Consulting Oral Surgeon to St. Boniface Hospital, Winnipeg, Canada; Oral Surgeon to The Children's Hospital of Winnipeg, Winnipeg, Canada.*

RUSSELL H. LEE, D.D.S., M.S., *Assistant Professor of Removable Prosthodontics, Loyola University, Maywood, Illinois.*

MEMORY ELVIN-LEWIS, B.A., M.S., Ph.D., *Associate Professor and Chairman, Department of Dental Microbiology, Washington University, St. Louis, Missouri.*

WILLIAM F. MALONE, D.D.S., M.S., F.A.C.D., F.I.C.D., *Professor and Chairman of Fixed Prosthodontics and Ceramics, Loyola University, Maywood, Illinois.*

HERMAN MEDAK, D.D.S., M.S., Ph.D., F.A.C.D., F.I.C.D., *Professor of Oral Pathology, Departments of Oral Diagnosis and Preventive Medicine, University of Illinois, Chicago, Illinois; Consultant in Oral Pathology, Veterans Administration West Side Hospital and Illinois Masonic Medical Center, Chicago, Illinois.*

DONALD E. ORE, B.S., D.D.S., M.S., *Clinical Associate Professor of Pedodontics, University of Illinois, Chicago, Illinois.*

JAMES T. OZIMEK, D.D.S., M.S., *Director of D.A.U., Assistant Professor of Fixed Prosthodontics, Loyola University, Maywood, Illinois.*

ZIGMUND C. PORTER, B.S., D.D.S., *Associate Professor of Periodontics, University of Illinois, Chicago, Illinois.*

SAMUEL PRUZANSKY, D.D.S., M.S., *Professor of Dentistry, University of Illinois, Chicago, Illinois; Director, Center for Craniofacial Anomalies, University of Illinois, Chicago, Illinois.*

GORDON R. SEWARD, M.B., B.S., M.D.S., F.D.S.R.C.S. (Eng.), *Professor of Oral Surgery in the University of London, London, England; Head, Department of Oral Surgery, The London Hospital Medical College, Dental School, London, England; Honorary Consultant Oral Surgeon to the London Hospital Group, London, England.*

ROBERT M. SOMMERFELD, D.D.S., M.S., *Assistant Professor of Removable Prosthodontics and Director of the Division of Dentistry for the Handicapped, Loyola University, Maywood, Illinois.*

VINCENT E. URBANEK, B.S., M.A., D.D.S., F.A.C.D., *Professor of Prosthodontics, School of Dentistry, Medical College of Georgia, Augusta, Georgia; Attending Dental Staff, Eugene Talmadge Memorial Hospital, Augusta, Georgia.*

JAMES V. WOODWORTH, M.D., F.A.C.P., *Clinical Associate and Head, Department of Medicine, University of Oregon Dental School, Portland, Oregon; Clinical Instructor in Medicine and Associate Professor of Dentistry, University of Oregon Dental School, Portland, Oregon; Chairman, Department of Medicine, Portland Adventist Hospital, Portland, Oregon.*

Foreword

THE American Lecture Series in Dentistry advances newer knowledge for progress of dental practice. Success in modern dental practice is dependent upon biologic as well as mechanical considerations. The interdependence of dentistry on oral biology is so great that dentists are turning to oral biologists and oral biologists to dentists in order to understand the local and systemic basis of oral disease. The oral biologic processes are currently becoming sound foundations for clinical dentistry resulting in a rather rapid extension of postgraduate instruction. Therefore, each of the books in this series unravels the oral mechanisms and provides the clinical management of many problems which have existed for decades.

The American Lecture Series in Dentistry is charged with a striving ardor of dental wisdom, prepared *de rigueur* by the highly qualified oral *Wissenschaftler*. New insights and *Entscheidungsproblem* are discussed by distinguished dental colleagues. A tradition will be established of offering the dental practitioner comprehensive surveys of recent developments in the various fields of clinical dentistry while presenting self contained independent presentations directed to the general practitioner and specialist. This series is charged with providing the most current concepts in developing the continuing education for the dental practitioner.

The American Lecture Series in Dentistry is based upon the following principles: concern, conviction, competence, commitment and courage. The series will show concern for numerous dental problems, have a conviction that dental problems can be solved, have competence that this series can contribute to their solution, have a commitment of time and energy in the search for answers, and have the courage to take the necessary action to present solutions to various dental problems.

Dentistry is both a science and an art which fulfills a social function. This series will, therefore, encompass clinical, oral biologic and social topics which are most applicable to the general practitioner of dentistry. It is our hope that the efforts of the contributors will assist the dental practitioner in fulfilling his responsibility to his patients through sound judgments, proper technical knowledge and dispatch. The American Lecture Series in Dentistry will serve as extremely practical references to aid the dental practitioner to resolve some of the problems encountered in the practice of dentistry as well as to broaden the horizons of those progressive dentists who desire the postgraduate knowledge and continuing education presented in this series. Contributors will focus attention on those aspects of dental practice causing the general practitioner the greatest concern and difficulty. The contributors of this series will help the practicing dentist to meet the challenges of the various phases of dental practice. Their observations should be beneficial to dentists seeking to attain the best possible treatment for their patients. New oral diagnostic problems, techniques, instrumentation and therapeutic measures are emerging. It is hoped that a tradition will develop whereby the American Lecture Series in Dentistry serves the dental practitioner and dental specialists alike.

Continuing education is dependent upon communicating the newer concepts in dentistry to the dental practitioner. It is hoped that this series will provide the important link of communication and result in better patient care. The continued quest for newer knowledge is the responsibility of the dental practitioner. This series will attempt to put the written current concepts into actual dental practice and therefore combat obsolescence. The editor and publisher are interested in encouraging the correlation of oral biologic principles with the clinical problems encountered by the dental practitioner who will base all his therapy on sound biologic concepts. The undergraduate education of a dental practitioner includes, in part, the development of his knowledge and skills. The continuing education of a dental practitioner includes the further development of his knowledge and skills by means of advanced educational programs which have a profound influence on the services performed by the dental practitioner. This series is predicated on the concept that continuing dental education is no longer confined to a selected few, but rather is a requirement for every present and future member of the dental profession.

There are dramatic changes taking place in dental care which will influence the future of dental practice. The unprecedented growth of scientific knowledge now is being applied to dentistry which is due to create tremendous changes in the art and science of dentistry.

It is not humanly possible to assimilate all of the knowledge in dental school that will be needed for the practice of dentistry. In addition, new knowledge is increasing at a rapid rate. Therefore, the dental practitioner can only keep abreast of the times by showing an initiative for self-learning. It is our hope that the American Lecture Series in Dentistry will stimulate the inquiring mind and provide the dental practitioner with a foundation in basic and new knowledge, skills and attitudes of dentistry upon which he can prepare himself for dental practice in current and future years.

The modern-day dental practitioner is in need of every opportunity possible to extend his knowledge and clinical experience. It is the purpose of the American Lecture Series in Dentistry to represent one kind of continuing education which will be readily available to him. The American Lecture Series in Dentistry places emphasis upon the fact that dental knowledge is not a rigid, fully elaborated system of facts, but rather one that is dynamic and constantly changing as new facets of knowledge are developed into the mosaic pattern of the whole.

Dr. Lawrence Cohen, Professor and Head of the Department of Oral Diagnosis, University of Illinois College of Dentistry, presents the book *Oral Diagnosis and Treatment Planning* which points to fields of interest that are likely to be a major concern to the practicing dentist in his attempt to understand the patient and his oral disease.

The editor and contributors to this book deal with their subject at a very practical level so that this work will profitably be used by the general practitioner of dentistry. The examples presented are numerous and varied, and all of them are set in terms of realistic dental situations so that the dental practitioner should acquire very useful factual information on oral diagnosis and treatment planning.

The remarkable scientific advances which have flourished in the laboratory have been exceedingly well integrated into clinical dentistry by Dr. Cohen and contributors. Oral diagnosis and treatment planning is a widely comprehensive area of dentistry. Its focus, however, is the entire patient, and its effectiveness is in direct proportion to one's skill in recognizing and dynamically meeting the total dental needs of the patient.

This book is extremely well organized and the presentation is clear and enjoyable. This monograph is therefore a unique and welcome guide for those general practitioners who seek to understand the conceptual foundations of oral diagnosis and treatment planning.

Thanks are due to the author-editor and expert contributors of this undated review of oral diagnosis, for sharing with other dental practitioners the knowledge and experience so carefully collected.

ALVIN F. GARDNER

Preface

THE general dental practitioner routinely examines a patient's mouth noting any soft and hard tissue pathology and then formulates a treatment plan with one or more alternatives which he presents to the patient. During the course of the examination the patient frequently asks the dentist for advice concerning the best possible treatment for his particular problem.

Each specialist in the dental field looks at a patient in a different way and his examination brings out certain features which are essential for the formulation of the specialist's treatment plan.

Each contributor to this book was asked to describe what he looked for when examining a patient and the steps he took towards making a diagnosis and evolving a treatment plan. He was also asked to describe some of the modern procedures which he employed in his own practice and the purposes for which they were used. As an example, in the field of oral surgery there are a number of procedures which are employed to improve esthetics and occlusion. The indications and contraindications for these various procedures are important as they enable the oral surgeon to decide the best procedure for the individual patient.

This book is not intended to be a compendium; rather it is hoped that it will provide a new approach to two of the most important aspects of dentistry—diagnosis and treatment planning.

LAWRENCE COHEN

Acknowledgments

During the gestation period of a multiauthored book many people are involved. To mention all would be difficult. However, our thanks are due Mr. William R. Schwartz of the Illustration Studios, University of Illinois for the illustrations in Chapter 13 and to Mr. Alex Domokos, Head of the Photography Section, Faculty of Dentistry, University of Manitoba for the illustrations and photographs in Chapter 19. I should like to thank my friend and former colleague, Dr. Gerald B. Winter, Professor and Head, Department of Childrens' Dentistry, Institute of Dental Surgery, London, for the loan of clinical photographs for Chapter 20. My sincere appreciation to my secretary, Mrs. Dorothy Persico, for all her help in the preparation of the manuscript.

Lawrence Cohen

Contents

	Page
Contributors	vii
Foreword—Alvin F. Gardner	ix
Preface	xiii
Acknowledgments	xv

Chapter

1. THE APPROACH TO DIAGNOSIS—Lawrence Cohen 3
2. THE CASE HISTORY—William F. Malone, Rinert J. Gerhard and James T. Ozimek 6
3. THE IMPORTANCE OF THE MEDICAL HISTORY—James V. Woodworth 8
4. EXAMINATION OF THE ORAL CAVITY—William F. Malone, Rinert J. Gerhard and James T. Ozimek 19
5. DISEASES OF THE ORAL MUCOSA AND SALIVARY GLANDS OF INTEREST TO THE GENERAL DENTAL PRACTITIONER—Herman Medak and Paul Burlakow . 21
6. THE ROLE OF RADIOLOGY IN ORAL DIAGNOSIS—Gordon R. Seward 47
7. DISEASES OF THE JAWS OF INTEREST TO THE GENERAL PRACTITIONER—Ralph I. Brooke, Alan J. Drinnan and Stuart L. Fischman 65
8. HEADACHE AND FACIAL PAIN—Lawrence Cohen 85
9. THE ROLE OF MICROBIOLOGY IN ORAL DIAGNOSIS AND TREATMENT PLANNING—Memory Elvin-Lewis 90
10. THE ROLE OF LABORATORY TESTS IN ORAL DIAGNOSIS—Lawrence Cohen ... 110
11. THE ROLE OF THE ORAL PATHOLOGIST IN ORAL DIAGNOSIS—Herman Medak . 119
12. OCCLUSION AND ITS RELATION TO ORAL DIAGNOSIS AND TREATMENT PLANNING—Vincent E. Urbanek 124
13. ORAL DIAGNOSIS AND TREATMENT PLANNING IN PERIODONTICS—Zigmund C. Porter 141

14. TREATMENT PLANNING FOR RESTORATIVE DENTISTRY—William F. Malone, Rinert J. Gerhart and James T. Ozimek 167

15. ENDODONTIC DIAGNOSIS AND TREATMENT PLANNING—Edward E. Beveridge 186

16. CASE PRESENTATION—William F. Malone, Rinert J. Gerhard and James T. Ozimek 205

17. ORAL DIAGNOSIS AND TREATMENT PLANNING IN REMOVABLE PROSTHODONTICS—Russell H. Lee and Robert M. Sommerfeld 207

18. OTHODONTIC DIAGNOSIS—Howard Aduss and Samuel Pruzansky 219

19. THE ROLE OF THE ORAL SURGEON IN ORAL DIAGNOSIS AND TREATMENT PLANNING—Stanley Kennett 238

20. DIAGNOSIS AND TREATMENT PLANNING FOR THE CHILD—Allen W. Anderson and Donald E. Ore 271

21. DIAGNOSIS AND TREATMENT PLANNING FOR GERIATRIC PATIENTS—Arthur Elfenbaum 299

ORAL DIAGNOSIS
AND
TREATMENT PLANNING

Chapter 1

The Approach To Diagnosis

LAWRENCE COHEN

A PATIENT may visit a dentist for a number of reasons. He may require routine dental treatment or he may have a particular problem such as pain, a swelling or some abnormality such as a white patch on the oral mucosa.

Before examining the patient it is necessary to take a careful history. Many patients when confronted by a sympathetic listener will embroider the narrative and introduce irrelevant material. It is the purpose of the examiner to sift the information and to extract what is relevant. By carefully selecting his questions he is able to steer the patient back to the important details of the history.

The dentist should ask the patient if he requires routine dental treatment or whether he has a specific problem. If he has a specific problem the dentist should ask such general questions as how long has he noticed it; where is it located; is it getting worse or better?

THE PATIENT COMPLAINS OF PAIN

The patient in pain has one desire; to get rid of his pain. He is not concerned with its quality or periodicity. However, there are a number of pain syndromes which have characteristic patterns and which may be diagnosed by a carefully taken history. The following questions should be asked.

What is the character of the pain? Is it sharp, throbbing or dull? Is it localized or diffuse? Is it intermittent or continuous? Is it referred?

How long does the pain last? Seconds, minutes or hours?

Is the pain worse at any particular time of the day? (*See* under acute frontal and maxillary sinusitis.)

What causes the pain? Hot, cold, sweet or sour substances? Is it affected by lying down (*acute pulpitis*) or by mastication (*acute periodontitis*)?

Is the pain relieved by anything? Hot, cold or analgesics? Characteristically the pain of atypical facial neuralgia is not relieved by analgesics (*see* Ch. 8).

Does it prevent the patient from sleeping? Does it awaken him? If it does awaken him during the night, does it do this at a particular time? (*See* under facial migrainous neuralgia.)

THE PATIENT COMPLAINS OF SWELLING

The patient should first be asked how long he has had the swelling.

Is it painful? Swellings associated with acute infections are usually painful, whereas swellings associated with chronic infections such as actinomycosis or tuberculosis are not necessarily painful.

If the swelling appeared recently and is

associated with pain did it occur before or after the pain? If one considers the pulpally involved tooth with an acute periapical abscess, the usual sequence of events is tenderness of the tooth on biting and then continuous aching pain in the jaw. If the condition is left untreated, a painful swelling appears which is associated with the affected tooth.

Is there any precipitating cause? Has the patient had a recent blow or been involved in an automobile accident? or is the swelling allergic in origin? Some patients with angioneurotic edema are sensitive to aspirin and ingestion of this drug may produce swelling of the face.

Is it getting bigger? Neoplasms whether benign or malignant increase in size. The rate of increase in size depends on the character of the tumor; poorly differentiated malignant neoplasms may increase in size very rapidly.

THE GENERAL CLINICAL EXAMINATION

A patient who has severe pain will be distressed and the careful observer will notice alterations in facial expression and in the patient's demeanor. If the patient has been awake the whole night with toothache he appears pale and somewhat distraught. The degree of distress exhibited by a patient to a great extent depends on his ethnic and cultural background and his pain threshold. The patient with atypical facial neuralgia (see Ch. 8) is well nourished and does not appear distressed although she may have had pain for many months or even years.

The physician examines a patient in a definite sequence of inspection, palpation, percussion and auscultation and it is suggested that the dentist adopt this same sequence. Very rarely is it necessary for the dentist to employ auscultation except in testing for crepitus within the temporomandibular joint. For this reason one can replace "auscultation" by "special tests" such as pulp testing, radiographic examination or laboratory tests.

Inspection

During the course of the history-taking the examiner will have noticed any asymmetry or swelling of the face or neck which will suggest an inflammatory swelling or tumor. Protrusion of the eyes (exophthalmos) will suggest *hyperthyroidism*.

Distended neck veins in a patient sitting in the dental chair suggest congestive cardiac failure and this is confirmed if there is pitting edema of the ankles.

Pallor of the skin and mucous membranes suggests *anemia*. The patient with pernicious anemia frequently has a lemon-yellow tint to the skin and oral mucosa. Cyanosis may be the result of cardiac or respiratory disease or *polycythemia*. The jaundiced patient has a yellow tinge to his skin and mucous membranes which may not always be noticeable in artificial light. Patients with *neurofibromatosis* have in addition to the neurofibromata of the skin patches of brownish pigmentation occurring on the neck and back. Some patients with neurofibromatosis have neurofibromata of the oral cavity. *Addison's disease* and *Peutz-Jeghers syndrome* are conditions in which skin and oral melanin pigmentation are found.

Bruising of the legs may be associated with *scurvy* or *thrombocytopenic purpura*. Petechial hemorrhages may be seen in the oral cavity in *purpura* and *infectious mononucleosis*.

Tremor of the hands, particularly at rest, occurs in *Parkinson's disease* (paralysis agitans); the tremor disappears on voluntary movement. In *hyperthyroidism*, there is a fine tremor of the outstretched fingers.

Clubbing of the fingers occurs in *congenital cardiac disease, subacute bacterial endocarditis, chronic suppurative chest conditions* and *carcinoma of the bronchus*. It should, however, be noted that clubbing of the fingers occurs in a proportion of Negro patients in the absence of disease.

Visible cervical lymphadenopathy should make one suspect *syphilis, tuberculosis* or a lymphoma such as *Hodgkin's disease*. A chancre of the lip is usually associated with bilateral, visibly enlarged lymph nodes which usually distinguishes it from herpes labialis.

Palpation

Any swelling should be palpated to determine its size, its situation—whether it is situated in the superficial or deep structures, its shape, its surface; whether it is smooth or lobulated, its consistency; whether it is soft, firm, fluctuant like a cyst, indurated like metastatic lymph nodes or hard like a bone tumor.

No examination is complete without examination of the cervical lymph nodes; metastatic lymph nodes may become fixed to the skin and deeper structures and this denotes a poor prognosis.

Percussion

The teeth are percussed to ascertain if one is tender and this may help to elucidate a diagnostic problem.

Chapter 2

The Case History

WILLIAM F. MALONE, RINERT J. GERHARD AND JAMES T. OZIMEK

DIAGNOSIS

ORAL DIAGNOSIS is the basis for implementation of an effective treatment plan. Unless there is a logical approach with a rational sequence based upon careful evaluation of the clinical needs of the patient, the dental treatment performed will ultimately fail. This is true regardless of the dentist's ability.

A comprehensive diagnosis necessitates the taking of a history together with proper diagnostic aids, the use of which is directly proportional to the complexity of the clinical conditions presented by the patient. Foremost, a diagnosis refers to identification of disease by the observance of signs and symptoms. In other words, it is based upon the deviation from a normal statistical range within a given random sample of patients. Some clinicians have an intuitive skill for diagnosis but a systematic evaluation of clinical symptoms is usually the manner in which most dentists perform their examinations.

There are five basic principles of diagnosis to be followed:

1. *Procurement of essential statistics.* These include such details as sex, age, race and occupation.

2. *Analysis of the chief complaint.* The treatment of a painful clinical situation may be indicated without extensive examination. A thorough, short review of the medical history is, however, always necessary.

3. *Recording of medical and dental history.* One cause of clinical failure is a lack of pertinent information and adequate evaluation of clinical facts which will directly affect the course of treatment. Also if the facts are determined and evaluated but not recorded, they are of little assistance to future treatment planning. The medical and dental histories should complement each other.

4. *General examination and charting of the oral cavity.* A general clinical examination should indicate an overall profile of the patient's oral health. It should include the following: (a) the general appearance of the patient; (b) the condition of the teeth and of the supporting structures; (c) the presence of edentulous areas and their prosthetic replacement; (d) examination of related structures of the oral cavity, the vestibule of the mouth, tongue, palate, frenum attachments, and so forth; and (e) recording specific information directly related to the course of treatment. A complete intraoral examination will incorporate the following information: (1) visual mouth examination, (2) radiographic surveys, (3) mounted diagnostic casts for occlusal analysis, (4) an assessment of soft tissue with periodontal instruments and (5) the use of medical laboratory tests to augment previous data, for example, complete blood count and urinalysis (*see* Ch. 10).

5. *The summary of related facts.* This summary should include the recording of pertinent facts and the patient-doctor agreement following presentation of the treatment plan, together with the estimated fees for a variety of services.

MEDICAL HISTORY

The medical history is usually accomplished in the majority of dental offices by a commercial health questionnaire form which describes the general health profile of the patient (*see* Ch. 3).

DENTAL HISTORY

The primary purpose of the dental history is to inform. The dentist should remember that few patients have had the advantage of a formal dental education. Many patients are uninformed or misinformed of the "why's" and "wherefore's" of dentistry that are basic to the dentist. Since patient cooperation is necessary for attaining and maintaining optimum dental health, it is desirable for the dentist to enlist and encourage cooperation. *An informed patient is more likely to be a cooperative patient.* This concept is commonly referred to as patient education.

The dentist should not only inform during the case review but should allow himself to become informed. By asking questions of the patient and allowing the patient to ask questions of him, he may be able to gain some insight into the patient's interest and attitudes concerning dentistry. This insight is necessary in evaluating the amount of patient cooperation that can be expected and in formulating the best approach in dealing with the dental problem.

CHIEF DENTAL COMPLAINT

Pain or general discomfort is usually the chief complaint of a patient (*see* Ch. 8). An organized approach should be initiated within a limited time available and the following procedures should be carried out:

1. Review the patient's medical and dental history.
2. Procure radiographic examination, hopefully a Panorex survey, if available.
3. The use of percussion and transillumination techniques.
4. Vitality testing of the teeth either by physical or electrical means.
5. Elimination of pain by diagnostic local anesthetic application.

Facts concerning the pain must be obtained from the patient (*see* Ch. 8). Immediate dental pain must be eliminated before the general dental health of the patient is discussed in any length. The patient is not interested at this time in anything but the relief of his symptoms. However, this may be a convenient time to inform the patient of the importance of prompt biannual dental checkups and for the institution of a preventive dentistry program.

Chapter 3

The Importance of the Medical History

JAMES V. WOODWORTH

A COMPREHENSIVE medical history is essential to good treatment planning. Through knowledge of present and past medical problems, current drug usage and known drug allergies, the dentist will reduce the incidence of medical complications, adverse drug action and medical emergencies. A questionnaire is the simplest means of obtaining a medical history.

Many different questionnaires have been prepared for use by the dentist. The questionnaire in the back of this chapter varies from that used by a physician in that whereas it is the physician's responsibility through his training to evaluate and determine from clinical data the general health status of the patient and to initiate medical therapy, it is the dentist's responsibility to be aware of the patient's general health, to know what medications the patient is taking and to be aware of how the health problems and current treatment will affect oral health and modify treatment planning. The dentist in most instances is not expected to sort out clinical data except where they specifically relate to dental problems. If through a questionnaire or through other studies, unexplained signs or symptoms appear or questions arise concerning the general health of the patient or the medications the patient is receiving, the dentist should consult the physician for further assistance.

Much of the questionnaire is directed towards determining which specific illnesses the patient has and the medications he is taking.

Patients tend to forget portions of their medical history during an initial interview. A questionnaire listing common diseases and frequently used medications aids in recall and will aid the dentist in evaluating his patient. The patient should have an adequate time to complete the questionnaire in a quiet and unhurried manner with assistance when necessary from other members of the family. The questionnaire may be submitted for completion on a clipboard at the initial examination. Better still, it may be forwarded to the patient for completion at home prior to his first visit to the office. An adequate explanation should accompany the questionnaire so that the patient understands the need for its thoughtful completion. The questionnaire should be reviewed by the dentist together with the patient so that both interpret the results and the significance thereof in the same manner. The review of the questionnaire affords the dentist an opportunity to establish better rapport with the patient who cannot but note the thoroughness of the dentist and his awareness of the general medical problems that the patient faces.

The questionnaire may indicate the need for further medical evaluation prior to dental therapy. It may provide invaluable assistance to the dentist in the diagnosis of oral lesions that are commonly seen in many systemic diseases such as diabetes, cancer or drug therapy. The questionnaire may forewarn of the presence of rheumatic heart disease requiring prophylactic antibiotic coverage or indicate the presence of an allergic diathesis or a blood dyscrasia. The patient frequently does not connect systemic disease problems with his oral health. The dentist may fail to relate the two unless medical problems are brought out in the initial interview.

The questionnaire should be updated at intervals much as a physician performs an annual examination to reevaluate the health of the patient.

The initial part of the questionnaire relates to the patient's current source of medical care. It provides the dentist with the name of a physician to whom he may turn if an emergency arises, for amplification of the remaining parts of the questionnaire or someone to whom he may refer the patient if he finds evidence of the need for further medical care. If the medical history appears unreliable, if there is a question concerning the medications which the patient is taking or there is need for further information relating to the patient's medical problems, a phone call to the patient's personal physician is likely to provide significant assistance.

DRUGS

In many instances the patient who is seeking dental services is also receiving medical care and taking some type of medication. The questionnaire has been prepared in a manner that relates the use of drugs to areas of systemic disease. Several drugs that warrant special consideration are mentioned repeatedly. Some drugs may indicate to the dentist that a particular disease process is present and forewarn the dentist of a specific problem facing the patient. Certain drugs are particularly prone to produce allergic reactions.

Adverse Drug Interactions

The dentist today faces the problem of protecting his patient from adverse drug interaction. Drug interactions may produce dramatic manifestations such as hemorrhage, hypoglycemic coma or hypertensive crisis. Interactions associated with single and multiple agents can be minimized if the dentist remains abreast of the data concerning the drugs that he uses and their interaction with drugs the patient is taking. Information concerning drug interactions has not been widespread and dissemination of this information as it becomes available is essential. The dentist must protect his patient by prudence in drug choice and discernment during multiple drug therapy.

Penicillin

The use of penicillin may be followed by an immediate anaphylactic reaction that is life-threatening or by a delayed serum sickness reaction that is very uncomfortable. Any history of a previous penicillin reaction should forewarn against the repeated exposure to this family of drugs. The absence of a previous drug reaction does not rule out the possibility of a reaction when its use is repeated and the dentist should be prepared for the treatment of an acute reaction to any drug.[1]

Cortisone

Cortisone is generally used for the treatment of many serious illnesses including allergic diseases such as asthma, life-threatening illnesses such as cancer and disabling diseases such as rheumatoid arthritis. Its use usually signals the presence of a serious illness that is likely to compromise or change a dental program.

If cortisone is being used, it is the dentist's responsibility to determine what precautionary measures should be taken and how the illness for which it is being used will affect the patient's health and life expectancy. This will be amplified in the discussion of endocrine diseases.

CARDIOVASCULAR DISEASE

The various forms of cardiovascular disease are responsible for over half the deaths of people over the age of sixty and are responsible for a great deal of illness in people of younger years. Patients with cardiovascular disease have a decreased ability to stand stress and yet when dental treatment is properly performed, few complications will result. Management of dental problems in patients with cardiovascular disease requires co-operation between physician and dentist. When dental treatment is necessary, the dentist should discuss the problem with the patient's physician and proceed only after there is agreement on the course of action.

Patients, when asked, are likely to know if they have had angina, myocardial infarction, rheumatic fever, congestive heart failure or congenital heart disease. Symptoms of shortness of breath, chest pain with exertion, unexplained fatigue or ankle edema in patients over sixty in the absence of known cardiovascular disease should suggest to the dentist the need for further medical evaluation prior to any major dental treatment.

Prophylaxis for Bacterial Endocarditis

A history of rheumatic fever, congenital heart disease or prosthetic valve replacement indicates the need for antibiotic coverage when scaling or oral surgery is performed. Penicillin given to prevent recurrent rheumatic fever does not provide sufficient coverage to prevent subacute bacterial endocarditis. The appropriate antibiotic is preferably given while the patient is undergoing dental treatment. In addition, the dentist should schedule the patient's treatment in as few consecutive days as possible to avoid repeated courses of antibiotics that are likely to sensitize the patient or to produce a drug reaction.

Arteriosclerotic Heart Disease

The presence of angina pectoris, the history of a myocardial infarction (coronary) or the use of nitroglycerin usually indicates the presence of arteriosclerotic heart disease with compromised circulation to the myocardium. In the presence of arteriosclerotic heart disease the stress of a dental procedure and the fear of pain, blood loss, hypotension or fatigue from long dental procedures can produce angina or a myocardial infarction. The dentist should have nitroglycerin, sedatives, narcotics and oxygen available for administration and he should know the steps to take if the patient develops a myocardial infarction.[1] Those patients who have angina should have short appointments, local anesthesia, appropriate sedation, avoidance of stress and avoidance of dental procedures following large meals. Dental treatment, unless of an emergency nature, should be deferred for at least three months following a myocardial infarction. Care should be taken to prevent excessive bleeding and avoid medications that will depress the blood pressure. The patient who has had a myocardial infarction may be receiving anticoagulant therapy. Many drugs interact with the anticoagulants and in particular salicylates are contraindicated. Barbiturates tend to increase the clotting time in patients taking anticoagulants. Consultation with the patient's physician is indicated whenever oral surgery is performed on such a patient and interruption in a course or adjustment of the dosage of anticoagulant therapy should be made only by the patient's physician.

Hypertension

The history of hypertension is usually associated with the prescription of various drugs to control the hypertension. If reserpine, phenothiazine or antihistamines are being used, the dentist should be aware that their action may be potentiated by the use of analgesics, narcotics, barbiturates, tranquilizers or the use of general anesthesia. Other drugs used in conjunction with sedatives may produce a dangerous hypotension. Dental treatment on the patient who has hypertension should be performed when the patient is at ease, under local anesthesia, preferably without epinephrine and appointments should be short. In most instances the patient's hypertension will be asymptomatic and he will be able to handle moderate stress without difficulty.

Congestive Heart Failure

Congestive heart failure is often associated with rheumatic or congenital heart disease, arteriosclerotic heart disease and hypertensive cardiovascular disease. It is commonly seen in the elderly and it is the manifestation of the inability of the heart to cope with circulatory demands of the body. It is often associated with the retention of fluid and symptoms include dyspnea, edema, fatigue, chest pain, irregular heartbeat and frequently an unexplained cough. When the underlying disease process is controlled with the assistance of **digitalis**, diuretics and antiarrhythmic agents, the patient may become symptom free, ambulatory, and remain relatively well for an extended period of time. The patient's physician should be consulted and therapy be provided as indicated under the general discussion of cardiovascular disease.

The use of digitalis may be associated with nausea, vomiting and anorexia; diuretics, with hyponatremia and hypotension. Certain of the diuretics may produce blood dyscrasias and stomatitis, or both, and the antiarrhythmic agents may produce a leukopenia or hypotension. Patients who have been in congestive heart failure should have short appointments and general anesthesia should be avoided without medical consultation. These patients warrant full dental care since nutrition is important and they may live for an extended period of time once the diagnosis is made and therapy instituted. If a general anesthetic is to be given, these patients should be treated within a hospital environment.

ENDOCRINE DISEASES

Dental care may be affected by such endocrine disorders as pancreatic (including diabetes), thyroid (hypo- or hyper-), adrenal (iatrogenic adrenal insufficiency associated with corticosteroid usage) and ovarian change (menopause). Pituitary (gigantism or acromegaly) and parathyroid (hyperparathyroidism) are only occasionally seen.

Diabetes Mellitus

Although a patient may know that he has diabetes mellitus, he may not be receiving or accepting adequate treatment.

A "yes" answer may explain the presence of gingivitis, sensitive teeth, loss of supporting tissue or the rapid deposition of calculus. Should the dentist note periodontal disease with no history of diabetes, he should feel justified in requesting at least a routine urinalysis or, even better, a blood sugar drawn two hours following a meal. In controlled diabetes there is no characteristic gingival or periodontal lesion; however, the oral tissue may have a lowered resistance to infection. Diabetes should be well controlled when elective oral surgery is undertaken.

Dental therapy should be deferred in the presence of uncontrolled diabetes except when urgent and then only if the patient is receiving medical care. Surgical procedures should be as atraumatic as possible and local anesthesia is preferable to general anesthesia. Antibiotics should be used when appropriate to treat specific infections. The presence of an infection tends to make diabetes worse and the patient may become refractory to the oral hypoglycemic agent so that insulin may be required and hospitalization necessary. If a patient with diabetes is not doing well, medical consultation is indicated as soon as possible. Diet or insulin dosage should not be changed without consulting the patient's physician.

Diseases of the Thyroid Gland

The use of thyroid as a means of increasing the patient's feeling of well-being or to help him lose weight is debatable but frequently used. With an appropriate dosage schedule of thyroid, hypothyroidism will not represent a problem in dental therapy. There will be an increasing number of truly myxedematous patients among those who have received iodine 131 or have undergone thyroid surgery. Untreated or inadequately treated myxedematous patients are unduly sensitive to opiates. Except in an emergency, the patient with hypothyroidism should be restored to euthyroid state before dental treatment is instituted.

Hyperthyroidism, which produces symptoms of weight loss, increased tolerance to cold, excessive perspiration, tremor, nervousness, irritability, tachycardia and sometimes exophthalmos is a contraindication to dental therapy until such time that the hyperthyroidism has been corrected. Treatment of hyperthyroidism is complex and is often a combination of both medical and surgical procedures. Treatment often includes the use of thiouracil drugs. Their use may be followed by parotitis or agranulocytosis predisposing to oral infections or ulceronecrotic lesions. Dental treatment should be withheld in the hyperthyroid until he is euthyroid except in an emergency because of the danger of a thyroid crisis and an abnormal response to drug therapy. If surgery is essential, medical consultation is a necessity.

Diseases of the Adrenal Gland

Primary adrenal disease is not common but many patients are taking cortisone. The prolonged use of corticosteroid therapy may be followed by adrenal insufficiency. The dentist should be forewarned of this possibility and should consult the patient's physician before undertaking any major dental procedure on a patient who is receiving or who has received cortisone. The dentist should be aware of the symptoms of adrenal insufficiency. He should have available hydrocortisone sodium succinate for emergency use prior to undertaking dental treatment. The patient receiving corticosteroid therapy is likely to have adrenal glands unable to respond to stress. The patient's physician is likely to propose a supplemental dose of cortisone for the patient undergoing extensive dental procedures or surgery. Corticosteroids may be given either orally, intramuscularly or intravenously as indicated by the type of procedure and the status of the patient at the time the medication is given.

HEMATOLOGIC DISEASES

Dental problems developing within the field of hematology appear not only as the result of some systemic problem such as pernicious anemia or hemophilia but often follow the use of many drugs for the treatment of various illnesses. Chemotherapeutic agents are used for the treatment of leukemia, cancer and the lymphomas and often result in depression of the bone marrow with associated problems in healing and bleeding. The presence of any bleeding disorder including hemophilia or related problems, the various platelet disorders or the presence of cancer under treatment with chemotherapeutic agents warrants medical consultation before proceeding with treatment of oral lesions.

The presence of lymphoma, leukemia or a blood dyscrasia may shorten the life span and affect the dental treatment program. Therapy may alter the patient's reaction to infection and his response to trauma. The margin of safety that exists between the therapeutic and toxic levels of the chemotherapeutic agent is small and at times nonexistent. The treatment of these diseases and of other malignancies may explain the presence of leukopenia, thrombocytopenia, the presence of stomatitis, petechiae, failure to heal, bleeding bullae and other lesions of the mucous membranes. Certain forms of leukemia are commonly associated with oral lesions. The history of bleeding, especially following extractions, lacerations or minor surgery indicates the need for medical consultation prior to oral surgery.

The Anemias

The use of iron suggests some type of anemia and if the patient is receiving vitamin B_{12} by injection, pernicious anemia should be suspected although it is used for other illnesses. Pernicious anemia, which is a disease of late adult life, has an insidious onset which may be referable to many organ systems including the oral cavity with glossitis and glossopyrosis as an early symptom. Patients with pernicious anemia may complain of difficulty in wearing dentures. Those under treatment are not likely to present problems.

GASTROINTESTINAL DISEASE

The diseases of the gastrointestinal tract beyond the upper portion of the esophagus do not usually affect dental treatment. However, the presence of a peptic ulcer or a hiatus hernia may explain the source of the patient's sour taste, the use of antacids may explain the coating on the tongue or the use of an anticholinergic agent may explain the presence of a dry mouth. The patient with a peptic ulcer should not receive aspirin.

Malignancies of the Gastrointestinal Tract

By asking a few further questions relating to difficulty in swallowing, significant or unexplained weight loss, change in bowel habits or presence of rectal bleeding, the dentist may detect the presence of a malignancy before it becomes apparent to the patient and refer the patient to his physician early enough to afford the patient a chance for cure.

Diseases of the Liver

The presence of jaundice or a history of hepatitis should forewarn the dentist of hepatocellular disease that may represent a hazard to the dentist's health or to subsequent patients if the dentist does not take appropriate safety precautions. Hepatocellular damage may occur secondary to infection, drugs, alcohol or obstruction to the biliary tract. Many drugs are metabolized in the liver and if there is a history of liver disease care must be observed in prescribing various medications including the phenothiazine derivatives and barbiturates. In patients with serious liver disease blood clotting may be delayed because of inadequate production of prothrombin.

Hepatitis

If there is a history of hepatitis in the recent past the dentist should not undertake any treatment of oral lesions without consulting the patient's physician. Under any circumstances care must be taken to avoid self-inoculation with the patient's blood or sputum; disposable needles and syringes should be used and instruments should be autoclaved. Since hepatitis may be transmitted through saliva if the dentist is significantly exposed, he may need a prophylactic dose of gamma globulin.

RESPIRATORY DISEASE

The dentist should avoid doing anything that will reduce the ventilatory exchange in patients who already have compromised pulmonary function. This includes patients with emphysema, asthma, chest injuries and recurrent pulmonary infections. Infections that appear in and about the respiratory tract are often communicable and may threaten the dentist's own health. The presence of infection within the sinuses may explain a toothache and an extraction may be avoided. Antibiotics used in the treatment of respiratory infections may be associated with the development of a candidal infection and, rarely, bone marrow depression.

The presence of asthma or hayfever indicates that the patient has an allergic diathesis and the dentist should be forewarned of the possibility of a drug reaction, particularly to penicillin. In the presence of asthma care should be taken not to depress respiration, excite the patient or use allergenic drugs. The patient with asthma or emphysema may object to a rubber dam. He should be allowed to continue his usual medications. If an attack of asthma occurs during dental therapy relief may be obtained through the use of epinephrine. Barbiturates, narcotics or central nervous system depressants should be used with caution. Drugs that reduce pulmonary secretions such as Pro-Banthine® should be avoided. High concentrations of oxygen should be administered with care. General anesthesia should be given by an anesthesiologist and preferably in a hospital.

Tuberculosis

Tuberculosis which is infectious may may produce oral lesions. Care should be taken to avoid self-contamination. The extent of the disease should be evaluated before undertaking dental treatment requiring close proximity to the patient. Patients with tuberculosis, however, require good nutrition and are not likely to be infectious for an extended period of time once therapy is instituted. They require good dental care.

Malignancies of the Respiratory System

Chronic cough or hoarseness may indicate the presence of a laryngeal carcinoma of which the patient is unaware. Similarly a chronic cough is frequently associated with any disease of the respiratory tract, but in an older individual who smokes, it may be the earliest symptom of a lung cancer. Hemoptysis may arise from any area of the respiratory tract and warrants medical evaluation.

RHEUMATOLOGY

Whenever a patient is being treated actively for a rheumatic disorder, the dentist must be aware of the basic disease, its treatment and the effect of both the disease and the treatment on the general oral health of the patient. Rheumatic problems are most likely to make themselves evident to the dentist in terms of pain in and around the temporomandibular joint. If the patient has rheumatic arthritis and pain in the temporomandibular joint, care must be taken not to overextend the joint during dental treatment. Salicylates will often afford relief, and dental treatment should be adjusted to the time the patient is in remission.

Patients with osteoarthritis, rheumatoid arthritis or gout are likely to be receiving various medications which may produce undesirable side effects. These agents include the corticosteroids, indomethacin, phenylbutazone, gold and aspirin. Their use may result in stomatitis, bone marrow depression, allergic reactions and gastritis.

NEUROLOGIC PROBLEMS

Strokes, facial pain, facial paralysis and epilepsy are all of concern to the dentist.

Stroke

The history of a stroke should forewarn the dentist that the patient's reserve is limited and that precautions will have to be taken to prevent the precipitation of further difficulty. A stroke may occur as the result of thrombosis of a cerebral artery, intracerebral hemorrhage or embolism. In most instances strokes result from thrombosis and forewarn the dentist that cerebral vascular flow is compromised and that he must do nothing to further reduce the cerebral flow and thus precipitate another stroke. The dentist must be prepared to cope with an emergency involving the cerebral vascular system.[1]

A stroke is likely to occur in the elderly arteriosclerotic patient who may have a history of hypertension. A stroke may occur in the dentist's office as the result of stress, drug-induced hypotension or postural hypotension. Patients who have had a stroke may be receiving anticoagulants or medications to control blood pressure. They should have short appointments; bleeding should be kept at a minimum; and medications should be checked against those the patient is taking. Anesthesia should preferably be local. Hypotension should be avoided. The fact that the patient has had a stroke does not indicate that his life will be significantly shortened. Good health is important to the well-being of these patients. The patient's physician should be consulted before undertaking extensive treatment.

Epilepsy

The history of epilepsy should forewarn that convulsive seizures may occur at any time with or without warning. Patients, unless questioned as to whether or not they have epilepsy, are likely to hide this information. The objective of medical treatment is the complete suppression of symptoms by the use of anticonvulsant therapy throughout the life of the patient. Drugs commonly used include phenobarbital, diphenylhydantoin sodium, mephenytoin and trimethadione. Side effects from these medications may include gingival hypertrophy, rashes, bone marrow depression, fever, drowsiness, nausea and ataxia.

The dentist should avoid any action that might precipitate an attack of epilepsy. This includes the use of stimulants such as amphetamines. Appropriate premedication is indicated but because of the danger of oversedation from a combination of the added medicines, the physician should be consulted before therapy is initiated. Medications that the patient currently is taking should not be discontinued. However, if oral lesions are developing secondary to drug usage, the physician may be able to substitute a different medication. General anesthesia may be indicated if extensive procedures are undertaken but again medical consultation is indicated. During an epileptic seizure no specific treatment is necessary except to protect the patient from injury, aspiration or asphyxiation. If a convulsion continues, medical assistance will be needed. In most instances following a convulsion, the patient should not leave the dentist's office without being accompanied by a responsible person.

There are many diseases of the nervous system including multiple sclerosis and other demyelinating diseases. In each instance consultation with the attending physician is important. In most instances good oral hygiene is necessary and simple precautions to avoid stress, hypotension, anoxia or the aspiration of foreign objects should be followed. In each instance the patient's prognosis and needs must be kept in mind.

GENITOURINARY DISEASE

Diseases of the genitourinary tract, although seemingly remote from the oral cavity, may present problems to the dentist. A history of kidney stones may indicate that the patient has hyperparathyroidism and explain the presence of bone changes in the mandible remote from the teeth.

A history of glomerulonephritis or the presence of albumin in the urine suggests compromised renal function. Oral infections may worsen the renal damage. When prescribing drug therapy care should be taken to avoid or adjust dosage of those drugs excreted through the kidney. Certain antibiotics can prove to be particularly dangerous including the tetracyclines, cephaloridine and gentamicin sulfate.

Renal failure is often associated with uremia and may explain the uriniferous smell of the patient's breath and the presence of a stomatitis. Careful attention to oral hygiene and medical consultation is indicated.

More recently renal transplants are being performed with increasing frequency. These patients are likely to be receiving immunosuppressive agents which may depress the bone marrow and other immune protective reactions, making the patient more susceptible to infections. No medicine or treatment should be instituted without medical consultation.

Most diseases in some way affect the oral cavity, the patient's need for dental care and the manner in which it is delivered. Through the use of a questionnaire the dentist can more quickly and thoroughly evaluate the diseases of the patient. He can then examine the patient for any oral manifestations and if necessary modify his treatment plan so that the total health care of the patient is best served.

REFERENCES

1. Woodworth, J. V.: Recognition and treatment of medical emergencies in the dental office. *JADA*, 81:887–893, 1970.

QUESTIONNAIRE FOR ADULT DENTAL PATIENTS

Name_____ Age_____ Sex_____ Date_____
Occupation_____ Birthplace_____ Race_____
Who is your personal physician?_____
Have you been in ill health recently?_____
Have you consulted or been treated by a physician in the last five years?_____
Are you using or have you ever used penicillin or have you ever used any drug or medication to which you have had an unusual reaction: Yes____ No____
List such medications:_____

HAVE YOU EVER HAD, DO YOU HAVE OR HAVE YOU EVER BEEN TREATED FOR ANY OF THE FOLLOWING ILLNESSES, MEDICAL PROBLEMS OR SYMPTOMS:	ARE YOU TAKING OR HAVE YOU TAKEN ANY OF THE MEDICATIONS LISTED:	IF SO, ARE YOU OR HAVE YOU REACTED UNFAVORABLY TO ANY LISTED:
Yes___No___ Heart attack	Yes___No___ Digitalis	Yes___No___
Yes___No___ Heart disease in childhood	Yes___No___ Nitroglycerin	Yes___No___
Yes___No___ Rheumatic heart disease	Yes___No___ Pills to control blood pressure	Yes___No___
Yes___No___ Heart murmur		
Yes___No___ Myocardial infarction	Yes___No___ Anticoagulants-Coumadin® (sometimes referred to as blood thinner)	Yes___No___
Yes___No___ Angina		
Yes___No___ High blood pressure	Yes___No___ Quinidine or other medication for irregular heartbeat	Yes___No___
Yes___No___ Congestive heart failure		
Yes___No___ Shortness of breath		
Yes___No___ Swelling of ankles		
Yes___No___ Chest pain with exertion		
Yes___No___ Heart surgery		
Yes___No___ Diabetes	Yes___No___ Insulin or pill to control diabetes	Yes___No___
Yes___No___ Increased thirst		
Yes___No___ Thyroid disorder	Yes___No___ Thyroid	Yes___No___
Yes___No___ Menopause	Yes___No___ Propylthiouracil—medication to control thyroid activity	Yes___No___
Yes___No___ Pituitary disorder		
Yes___No___ Pregnancy now or in the past	Yes___No___ Cortisone or similar medication	Yes___No___
Yes___No___ Menstrual disorder	Yes___No___ Birth control pills	Yes___No___
Yes___No___ Adrenal disorder	Yes___No___ Hormones	Yes___No___
Yes___No___ Anemia	Yes___No___ Iron	Yes___No___
Yes___No___ Pernicious anemia	Yes___No___ Medicine to treat cancer	Yes___No___
Yes___No___ Leukemia		
Yes___No___ Hodgkin's disease	Yes___No___ Shots to build blood	Yes___No___
Yes___No___ Cancer		
Yes___No___ Blood disorder of any sort	Yes___No___ Any medication for blood disorder	Yes___No___
Yes___No___ Excessive bleeding following a dental extraction or laceration	Yes___No___ B_{12} vitamin	Yes___No___
Yes___No___ Easy bruising		
Yes___No___ Hemophilia		

HAVE YOU EVER HAD, DO YOU HAVE OR HAVE YOU EVER BEEN TREATED FOR ANY OF THE FOLLOWING ILLNESSES, MEDICAL PROBLEMS OR SYMPTOMS:	ARE YOU TAKING OR HAVE YOU TAKEN ANY OF THE MEDICATIONS LISTED:	IF SO, ARE YOU OR HAVE YOU REACTED UNFAVORABLY TO ANY LISTED:
Yes___No___Peptic ulcer	Yes___No___Antacids	Yes___No___
Yes___No___Hiatus hernia	Yes___No___Medicine to calm stomach or anti-spasmodics	Yes___No___
Yes___No___Cancer of stomach or bowel		
Yes___No___Hepatitis or any form of liver disease	Yes___No___Laxatives	Yes___No___
Yes___No___Trouble swallowing	Yes___No___Aspirin	Yes___No___
Yes___No___Recent change in bowel habits or blood in stool		
Yes___No___Recent change in weight either up or down		
Yes___No___Asthma or hayfever	Yes___No___Cigarettes	Yes___No___
Yes___No___Tuberculosis	Yes___No___Cortisone	Yes___No___
Yes___No___Sinus infection	Yes___No___Iodides	Yes___No___
Yes___No___Chronic cough or hoarseness	Yes___No___Medicine either pills or inhalor to make breathing easier	Yes___No___
Yes___No___Pneumonia		
Yes___No___Blood spitting	Yes___No___Antibiotics	Yes___No___
Yes___No___Emphysema		
Yes___No___Cancer of nose, mouth, throat or lung		
Yes___No___Arthritis or rheumatism	Yes___No___Aspirin	Yes___No___
	Yes___No___Cortisone	Yes___No___
Yes___No___Painful or swollen joints	Yes___No___Any medicine to control gout or rheumatism	Yes___No___
Yes___No___Gout		
Yes___No___Bursitis		
Yes___No___Lupus erythematosus		
Yes___No___Epilepsy or convulsive seizures	Yes___No___Dilantin® or any drug to control or prevent convulsions	Yes___No___
Yes___No___Fainting spells		
Yes___No___Recurrent severe headaches	Yes___No___Tranquilizers	Yes___No___
	Yes___No___Sedatives	Yes___No___
Yes___No___Depression	Yes___No___Medicine to control pain	Yes___No___
Yes___No___Nervous breakdown		
Yes___No___Hardening of arteries		
Yes___No___Stroke		
Yes___No___Kidney disorder	Yes___No___Immunosuppressive agents	Yes___No___
Yes___No___Kidney stone		
Yes___No___Albumin in urine	Yes___No___Sulfa drugs	Yes___No___
Yes___No___Glomerulonephritis	Yes___No___Antibiotics	Yes___No___
Yes___No___Kidney transplant		

Chapter 4

Examination of the Oral Cavity

William F. Malone, Rinert J. Gerhard and James T. Ozimek

THE DENTIST should train himself to carry out a routine examination of the oral cavity before he begins to examine the teeth and supporting structures. Particular care must be taken to examine the ventral surface of the tongue and the floor of the mouth to avoid missing an early carcinoma. The tongue should be grasped with gauze and pulled forward so that the whole of the anterior two-thirds can be inspected and palpated. Diseases of the oral mucosa are discussed in Chapter 5.

CHARTING THE ORAL CAVITY

The chart is the dentist's means of recording what is to be done and what existed before he initiated treatment. There are many types of charts or commercial dental forms which record graphically the oral findings. Conventional forms for graphically recording the characteristics of the patient's mouth are essential for the correlation of all the pertinent facts collected by the dentist.

The charting must be organized and recorded as the information is accumulated or the result will be a collection of unrelated facts. It is important to record the existing restorations, the proposed restorations, required occlusal therapy, periodontal disease or associated soft tissue abnormalities. It should also include an estimate of the fee for services rendered. Consultations with other professional personnel and their recommendations are also recorded in the sequences the patient has seen them.

COMPLETING THE DIAGNOSIS RECORD

Treatment of the patients with the dates and the materials used are recorded. The diagnosis of each tooth utilizing the number system starting with the upper right third molar as (#1) to the lower right third molar as (#32). The three-dimensional aspects of the tooth are recorded by segmental circular or square areas and all surfaces are represented in this manner.

Two-Digit System of Designating Teeth

The Federation Dentaire Internationale has suggested a system of tooth designation which lends itself to computerization. According to the Two-Digit System, the first digit indicates the quadrant and the second digit the tooth within the quadrant. Quadrants are allotted the digits 1 through 4 for the permanent and 5 through 8 for the deciduous teeth in a clockwise sequence and starting at the upper right side. Teeth within the same quadrant are allotted the digits 1 through 8 (deciduous teeth: 1 through 5) from the midline backwards. The digits should be pronounced separately; thus, the permanent canines are teeth one-three, two-three, three-three and four-three.

Permanent teeth: (upper right) 18–17–16–15–14–13–12–11; (lower right) 48–47–46–45–44–43–42–41; (upper left) 21–22–23–24–25–26–27–28; (lower left) 31–32–33–34–35–36–37–38.

Deciduous teeth: (upper right) 55–54–53–52–51; (lower right) 85–84–83–82–81; (upper left) 61–62–63–64–65; (lower left) 71–72–73–74–75.

Color Coding

Varying colors are employed to correlate a critical survey of the patient's mouth incorporating radiographs, diagnostic casts and visual information (for example, red for caries, blue for existing restorations).

Periodontal Assessment

The periodontal assessment of the patient is completed with the use of a periodontal explorer. If the tissue pockets are excessive, most recording systems employ a separate chart which is added to the original patient record. The type of tissue and the surgical prognosis are then assessed.

DETERMINATION OF OCCLUSAL RELATIONSHIP

In arriving at a diagnosis the dentist must place emphasis in those areas which merit special attention. Occlusion, which is the key to oral function, has a controversial history, with divergent opinions and conflicting theories. Comprehension of the function of the temporomandibular joint remains singularly elusive, but researchers generally agree that there is an interaction between this joint and the occlusion.

Thorough occlusal analysis is necessary for a complete dental diagnosis when the following conditions exist:

1. Temporomandibular joint problems such as pain, subluxation, clicking and crepitus.

2. Excessive wear (abrasion) of the occlusal surfaces of the teeth.

3. Bruxism and clenching habits.

4. Abnormal relations of two or more teeth.

5. Migration of teeth due to premature loss of teeth.

6. Extensive loss of tooth structure requiring occlusal reconstruction.

Although occlusion is covered in another chapter, there is some latitude for the re-emphasis of certain clinical situations which will assist the dentist during treatment. This will be discussed in detail in Chapter 14.

Chapter 5
Diseases of the Oral Mucosa and Salivary Glands of Interest to the General Dental Practitioner

HERMAN MEDAK AND PAUL BURLAKOW

THE dental practitioner who conducts a thorough, proper and routine examination of the oral cavity of all patients will encounter a variety of pathological conditions. In addition to the common lesions, he will occasionally see rare lesions, and perhaps two or three times in the course of his professional career he will detect a malignancy, hopefully in its early stages, when successful therapeutic intervention will be possible.

It is not essential for the dental practitioner to make definitive diagnoses of rare lesions. It is essential, however, that he recognizes an abnormality or a lesion when present. He must decide whether a condition is trivial and transient, whether drug therapy or minor surgery is indicated or whether to refer the patient for consultation.

There is an understandable tendency for the general practitioner to become careless in the conduct of routine oral examinations. He is primarily concerned with "dental" treatment, and day after day or even month after month without encountering significant abnormalities of the oral mucosa, he may become less thorough in his examination.

It is essential that the practitioner guard against such carelessness. Abnormalities do occur, and early detection can save time, expense and sometimes lives.

The conscientious practitioner should adopt and adhere to a strict and unvarying routine for examining the oral cavity. The practitioner knows proper examination techniques, and he need only develop his own sequence (*see* Ch. 4).

The types of abnormalities to be discussed here may be classified as follows:

1. Congenital and developmental defects.
2. Hypertrophy and hyperplasia.
3. Oral manifestations of dermal lesions.
4. Collagen diseases.
5. Benign soft tissue lesions—(a) epithelial and (b) mesenchymal.
6. Keratotic lesions—(a) keratotic lesions of unknown origin, (b) reversible keratotic lesions and (c) nonreversible keratotic lesions.
7. Potentially malignant lesions.
8. Malignant soft tissue lesions—(a) epithelial, (b) mesenchymal and (c) metastatic to the oral cavity.
9. Lesions of the salivary glands.
10. Oral manifestations of allergic reaction.
11. Oral manifestations of metabolic changes.
12. Oral manifestations of physical injury.
13. Oral manifestations of blood dyscrasias.

It is important for the general dental

practitioner to be aware of the clinical features of these diseases. It is not proposed to discuss histopathology or treatment, but some discussion of etiology is necessary, because oral lesions are sometimes classified by their supposed origin.

CONGENITAL AND DEVELOPMENTAL DEFECTS

Geographic Tongue (Migrating Glossitis)

Geographic tongue is of unknown etiology and has been seen at any age. Clinically, the tongue shows continuously changing patterns of desquamation, giving it a maplike appearance. The desquamated areas appear pink, surrounded by a white hypertrophic band of filiform papillae. Some authors feel that an emotional component may contribute to the lesion (Fig. 5-1).[1-3]

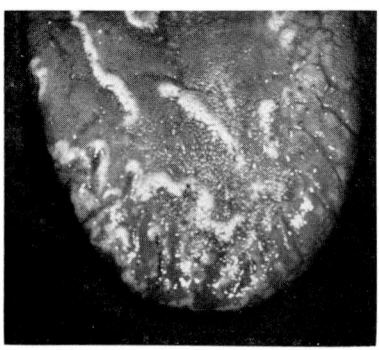

Figure 5-1. Geographic tongue. The desquamated areas appear pink and are surrounded by white margins which represent hypertrophied filiform papillae. This patient was complaining of a sore tongue, a not uncommon symptom associated with geographic tongue. Female, aged 16 years.

Median Rhomboid Glossitis

This condition is considered by some to be of unknown etiology, while others consider it of developmental origin. It is usually first noticed in middle age and occurs more frequently in men. The site of the lesion is always in the center of the posterior portion of the dorsal surface of the tongue. It appears as a depressed or elevated nodular lesion which is roughly diamond, rhomboid or irregularly shaped. In contrast to the surrounding epithelium of the dorsum of the tongue, this area is smooth and devoid of any papillae. It is important to be acquainted with this lesion because the untrained observer may be misled by the appearance of the lesion and seriously consider it to be malignant (Fig. 5-2).[1,2]

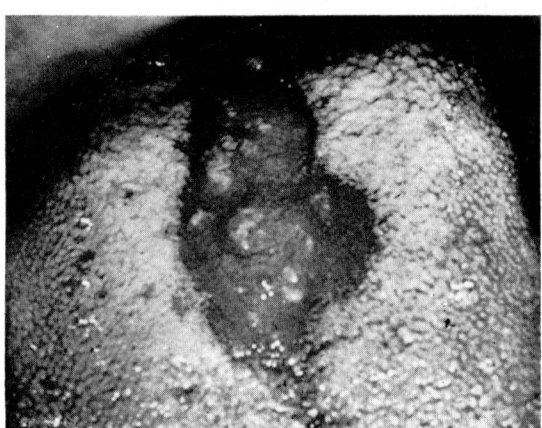

Figure 5-2. Median rhomboid glossitis. The patient had recently noticed the lesion which he thought was cancer. Male, aged 50 years.

HYPERTROPHY AND HYPERPLASIA

Theoretically, hypertrophy refers to an increase in size of individual cells and hyperplasia to an increase in the number of normal cells. Actually, the picture is seldom clear-cut, and both phenomena can be observed in an affected area.

The most common examples of hypertrophy and hyperplasia are associated with

Diseases of the Oral Mucosa and Salivary Glands

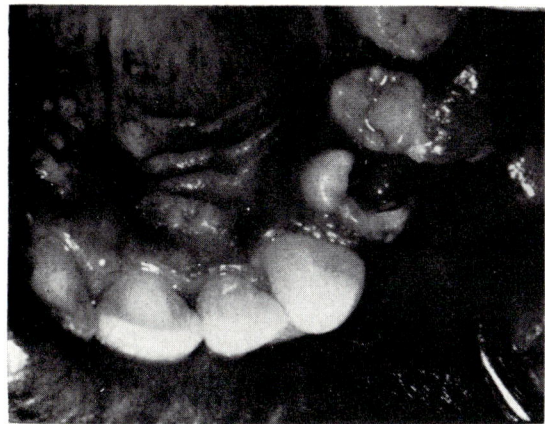

Figure 5-3. Granuloma pyogenicum. The patient was complaining of swelling and soreness between the second right maxillary premolar and the adjacent molar. Note the hyperplastic gingival tissue associated with the carious cavity in the first maxillary premolar. Female, aged 20 years.

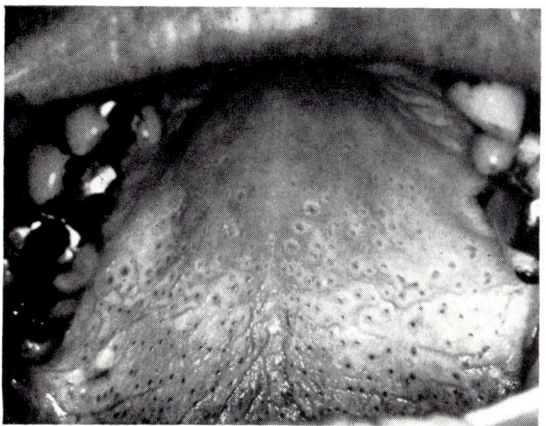

Figure 5-4. Stomatitis nicotina. The affected mucosa has a whitish sheen and the openings of the mucous glands appear as red dots. Male, aged 56 years.

hormonal imbalances occurring during puberty, menstruation, pregnancy or the menopause. Staphylococcal and streptococcal infections may be superimposed.

Clinical symptoms may vary from a mild gingivitis to "tumor" formations. The tissue may be hypersensitive and prone to hemorrhage. Such lesions caused by trauma and infection are classified as *granuloma pyogenicum* and may require surgical excision (Fig. 5-3).[1,2,4]

About 50 percent of women in pregnancy manifest similar symptoms, designated as *pregnancy proliferations*. Similar conditions of different etiology are designated as *pubertal proliferations*.

Epulis Fissuratum (Inflammatory Fibrous Hyperplasia)

Epulis fissuratum occurs in association with ill-fitting dentures which have been worn over extended periods of time. The pressure of the dentures causes first ulceration, then chronic inflammation and hyperplasia of the tissue, which looks like rolls or folds of flabby tissue around the edge of the denture. Since the hyperplastic tissue will not regress, surgical removal is indicated (*see* Ch. 19).[1,2]

Nicotinic Stomatitis

Nicotinic stomatitis is usually the result of severe smoking, especially pipe smoking, which affects the palatal mucosa and palatal glands. The mucosa first becomes red and if the irritation continues turns grayish-white. The openings of the glands

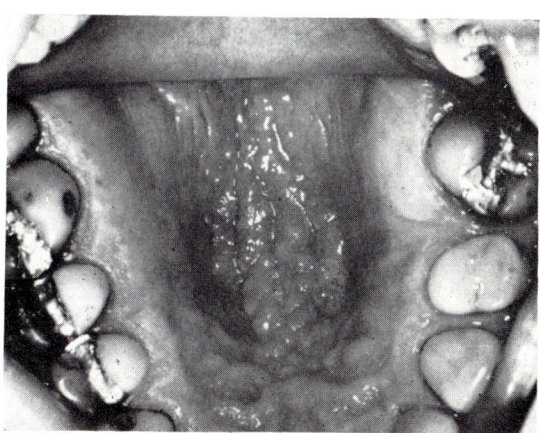

Figure 5-5. Papillary hyperplasia. The patient was wearing an ill-fitting denture replacing two missing maxillary central incisors. Female, aged 38 years.

become occluded, swell up and appear as nodules or papules with a red center (Fig. 5-4).[1,2,5]

Papillary Hyperplasia (Papillomatosis)

Papillary hyperplasia of the palate is usually associated with poorly fitting dentures and poor oral hygiene. Multiple papillary projections less than 4 mm in diameter may cover the hard palate but do not extend beyond the area covered by the dentures.[7] The papillomas rarely ulcerate (Fig. 5-5). Recent reports suggest that papillomatosis of the palate may be due to *Candida albicans* which has penetrated and is growing in the pores of the acrylic denture material. Fungicidal agents will not reverse a well-developed lesion and therefore surgical or abrasive techniques are needed to remove the lesion. A new denture must be constructed and good oral hygiene initiated.[1,2,6,7]

HISTOPATHOLOGIC FEATURES. Histologic examination of excised papillomatous tissue has in rare, long-standing cases shown dyskeratosis and mild dysplasia. Therefore, the possibility of malignant transformation should be kept in mind.

ORAL MANIFESTATIONS OF DERMAL LESIONS

Lichen Planus

Lichen planus is a rather common oral subacute or chronic inflammatory dermatosis of unknown etiology. Lichen planus of the skin is rare. The site of the oral lesions in order of frequency is the buccal mucosa, tongue, lips, gingiva and remaining areas. The lesions are usually symmetrical and are characterized by the presence of a lacy network of white striae. Several clinical forms can be distinguished.

1. The most common form is a reticular type, consisting of grayish-white, lacy lines arranged in a reticular pattern (Fig. 5-6).

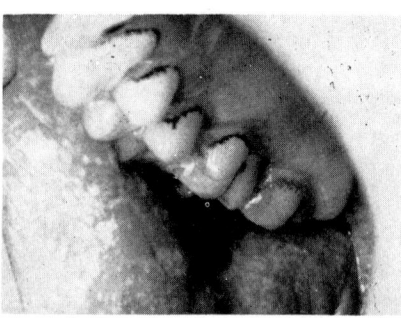

Figure 5-6. Lichen planus, reticular type. Note the pinhead white papules connected by white lines. Male, aged 50 years.

2. In hypertrophic lichen planus, the plaques coalesce and thicken, appearing as well-demarcated, elevated, white lesions with white striae at the periphery.

3. Erosive lichen planus occurs in about 20 percent of cases and is characterized by areas of white plaques and striae alternating with areas of ulceration. Erosive lichen planus starts as such and is not due to transition from another form. This lesion may persist for many years, and several cases of squamous cell carcinoma have been reported in these areas (Fig. 5-7).

4. Bullous lichen planus is rare and usually associated with other forms of this disease. It occurs most often on the tongue and shows vesicles of varying size and shape which rupture, leaving an ulcerated area (Fig. 5-8).

5. Atrophic lichen planus appears clinically as reddening of the oral mucosa, resembling a desquamative gingivitis. White striae can be seen at the periphery.[8-11]

HISTOLOGIC FEATURES. The epithelium usually displays hyperkeratosis or parakeratosis and liquefaction degeneration of the basal layer with invasion of lymphocytes, giving the area a sawtooth appearance. There is a bandlike layer of mononuclear cells beneath the epithelium.

Pemphigus Vulgaris

This is a rare dermatosis involving skin and mucous membranes and is characterized by successive crops of vesicles, bullae and denuded areas. Since in about 50 percent of the cases the initial lesion occurs in the oral cavity, it is important to keep this

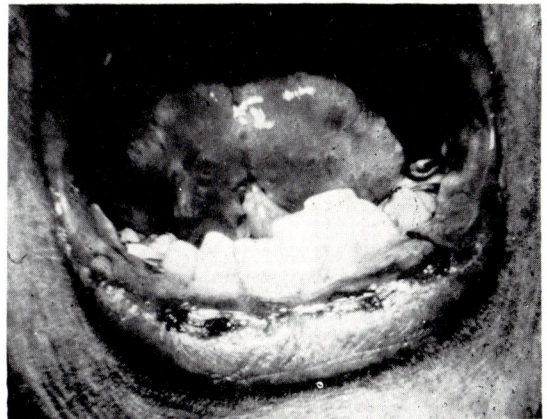

Figure 5-9. Pemphigus vulgaris. The patient presented with a sore mouth of three months duration. The lips and ventral aspect of the tongue show numerous ulcers which represent burst vesicles and bullae. Female, aged 37 years.

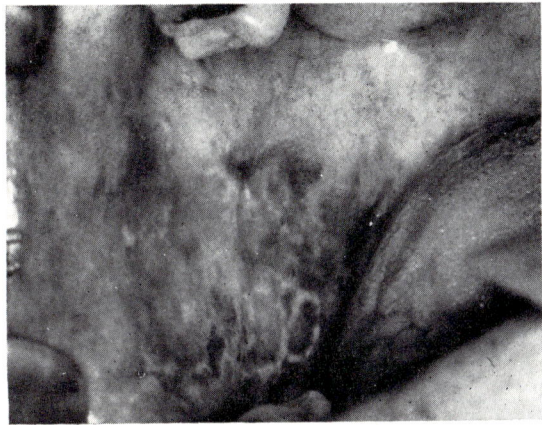

Figure 5-7. Lichen planus, erosive type. There are areas of ulceration which appear red. Note the characteristic white lines at the margins of the lesion which in this case form circles. Female, aged 70 years.

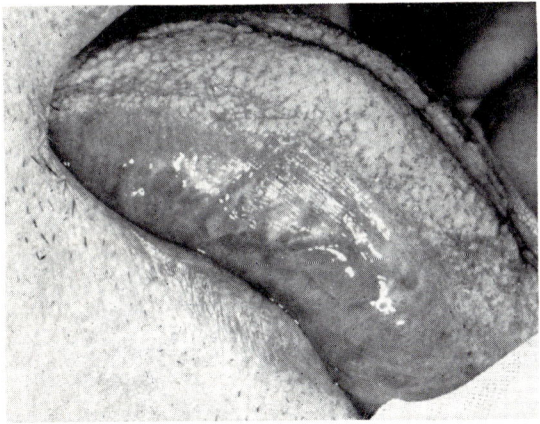

Figure 5-8. Bullous lichen planus. Note the bulla at the margin of the tongue with associated white lines. Male, aged 56 years.

entity in mind whenever an unexplainable large ulcer or bulla of the oral cavity is encountered. Although there is no proof that early diagnosis improves the prognosis, if the disease is recognized in its early stages the patient is spared much discomfort and prolonged remission is possible with corticosteroid treatment.

The initial lesion in the oral cavity appears as a painless vesicle or flaccid bulla which ruptures soon, leaving a raw, denuded surface with ragged edges, which has a tendency to spread. If it is present on the lip, it will expand across the vermillion border. The easy separation of oral epithelium from the submucosa by slight rubbing or trauma is an additional diagnostic feature (Nikolsky's sign). There is usually a poor tendency to heal and secondary infection causes pain, general malaise and debilitation. Sooner or later skin lesions will occur (Fig. 5-9).[12-14,16]

HISTOLOGIC FEATURES. The histology of the oral and skin lesions is identical and is characterized by suprabasal separation of the epithelium due to acantholytic changes. Biopsy as well as cytology is diagnostic for this disease if taken from the early lesion.

Erythema Multiforme

Erythema multiforme may be related to drug reaction, allergic reaction, viral infection or may be idiopathic. It is an acute inflammatory, self-limiting dermatosis involving skin and mucous membranes. Its duration ranges from a few days to several weeks. The clinical manifestations vary and can appear as papules, macules, nodules, vesicles and bullae, leading to an ulcerative hemorrhagic stomatitis. The disease has a tendency to recur, especially during spring and autumn (Fig. 5-10).

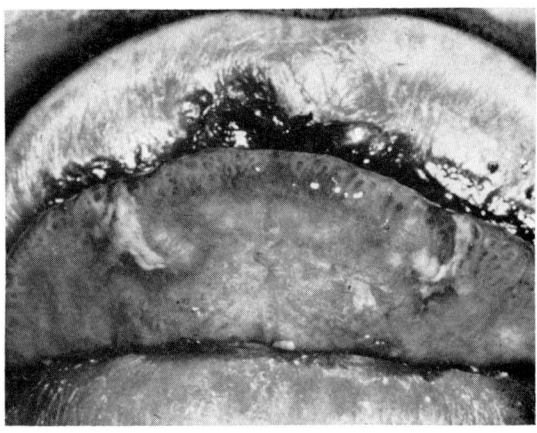

Figure 5-10. Erythema multiforme. Note the blood-encrusted lesions on the upper lip and the ulceration of the ventral aspect of the tongue. Male, aged 29 years.

This disease is self-limiting, but on rare occasions it may result in death; severe pulmonary and kidney complications may be present.[12-14]

The term "mucocutaneous syndromes" is applied to those conditions which involve in addition to the oral cavity, the eyes, genitalia and skin. Stevens-Johnson syndrome is a severe form of erythema multiforme.[15,16]

Behcet's Disease

Behcet's disease is a triple-complex involving the mouth, eyes and genitals. The oral lesions may precede the two other parts of the syndrome by months or years. Usually the oral lesions resemble recurrent aphthae but on occasions may resemble periadenitis mucosa necrotica recurrens and heal by scarring. Neurologic complications may occur and may result in death.[13]

Reiter's Syndrome

Reiter's syndrome is characterized by urethritis, eye lesions and arthritis; when oral lesions do occur they are described as erosions and not true ulcers.[1]

Benign Mucous Membrane Pemphigoid

Benign mucous membrane pemphigoid is a rare, chronic dermatosis which may involve the conjunctiva in addition to the oral mucosa and other mucous membranes. Scarring of the conjunctiva is common (Fig. 5-11 A and B).

Nevi

The term, "nevus," basically means a birthmark and usually refers to colored areas of the skin or mucosa. Even though nevi of the oral mucosa are rare, nonpigmented nevi, pigmented nevi and extremely rarely vascular nevi do occur.[16,18]

Nonpigmented Nevi

This group comprises the white sponge nevus and the basket-weave nevus. The *white sponge nevus* is a hereditary autosomal dominant lesion manifesting itself as white patches in the oral cavity which can be mistaken for *Candida* infections. The mucosa appears thickened or folded, corrugated, soft and spongy. The white patches can sometimes be removed with or without leaving a raw area. The most com-

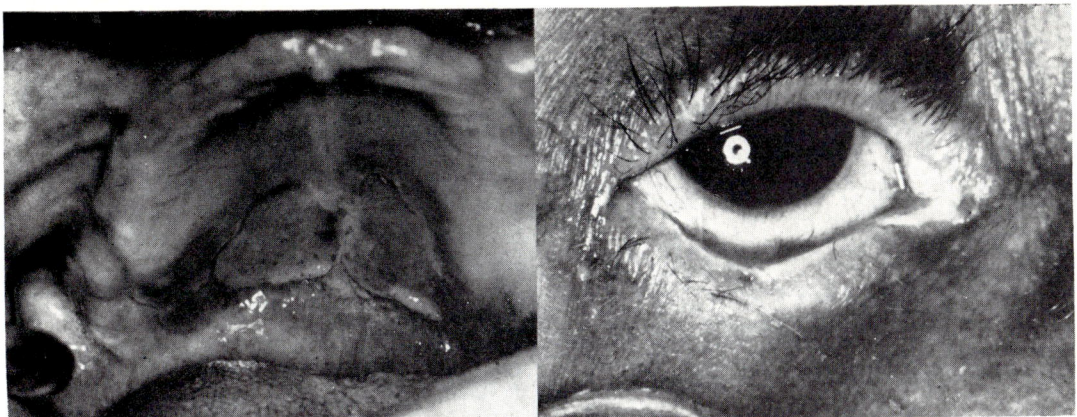

Figure 5-11. Benign mucous membrane pemphigoid. (*Left*) Note the large bulla at the posterior aspect of the hard palate. (*Right*) Note the conjunctival scar which extends from the lower fornix to the corneoscleral junction. Female, aged 56 years.

mon locations is in the buccal mucosa, usually symmetrical, but all areas other than the free gingiva can be affected. There is no sex preference. The lesion is usually present at birth in a mild form and may disappear and reappear and gradually become more pronounced (Fig. 5-12).

HISTOLOGIC FEATURES. The epithelium shows pale-staining superficial cells with a washed-out appearance which is characteristic but not pathognomic. The basket-weave nevus will be discussed in the section on keratotic lesions.[17]

Pigmented Nevi

All three types of pigmented nevi occur in the oral mucosa and appear clinically as a bluish-brown smooth, sessile lesion which varies in color from the normal mucosa.

HISTOLOGIC FEATURES. The three types—intradermal, junctional and compound nevi—are distinguished by the relation of the nevus cells to the epithelium. In the intradermal nevus, the nevus cells are separated from the epithelium by a band of connective tissue; in the junctional nevus, the nevus cells are associated with the epithelium and seem to drop off the epithelial ridges while the compound nevus is a combination of both. Although clinically they cannot be distinguished from each other, junctional nevi are generally considered to be premalignant, compound nevi to a lesser degree and intradermal nevi rarely show malignant transformation. It is therefore essential to remove oral pigmented nevi

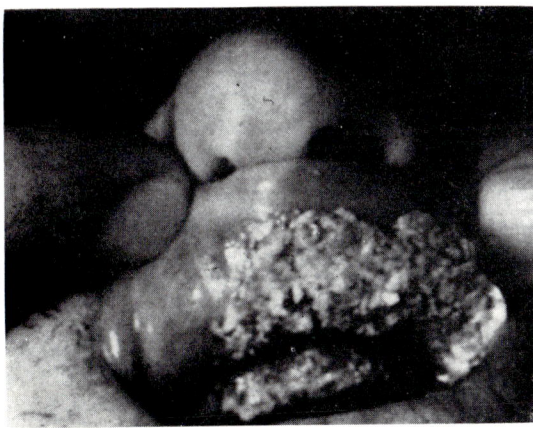

Figure 5-12. White sponge nevus. A white lesion is present on the mucosal aspect of the upper lip. If these lesions are observed over a period of time it is found that at some point desquamation occurs and the affected mucosa appears normal. The cycle is then repeated; this suggests that the lesions may result from a defect in desquamation. Male, aged 18 years.

for histopathologic examination and definitive diagnosis.[18]

Nevus flammeus (*port-wine stain*) will be discussed under soft tissue lesions.

COLLAGEN DISEASES

This is a group of diseases which affect primarily the collagenous connective tissue and include scleroderma, lupus erythematosus, rheumatic fever, periarteritis nodosa and rheumatoid arthritis. They occur most frequently in women of middle age; histologically they demonstrate fibrinoid necrosis. Hypersensitivity may play a part and autoantibodies formed by the patient against his own cells or tissues may be involved.

Rheumatic fever, periarteritis nodosa and rheumatoid arthritis do not show significant oral manifestations. However, the dentist should consult with the patient's physician before initiating any surgical, endodontic or periodontic procedure, since the interaction of systemic manifestations and dental treatment may have adverse effects on the general health of the patient.[1,2]

Lupus Erythematosus

Lupus erythematosus occurs in two forms: (a) chronic discoid lupus erythematosus, affecting cutaneous tissues, and (b) disseminated lupus erythematosus, affecting visceral tissues. The cause of both types is similar and the oral manifestations of both types are similar. Lesions of chronic lupus erythematosus most commonly appear on the face as reddish macules covered by gray or yellow scales. About 25 percent of the patients have oral manifestations which start as erythematous areas which quickly ulcerate. In the disseminated form of the disease, oral lesions tend to be more acute and destructive. The latter usually terminates fatally within eighteen months (Fig. 5-13).[19,20]

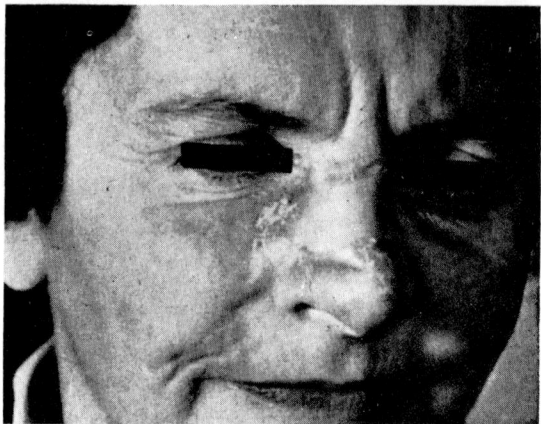

Figure 5-13. Chronic discoid lupus erythematosus. The reddish macules which are covered by yellow scales have a typical butterfly distribution over both cheeks and the bridge of the nose. Female, aged 47 years.

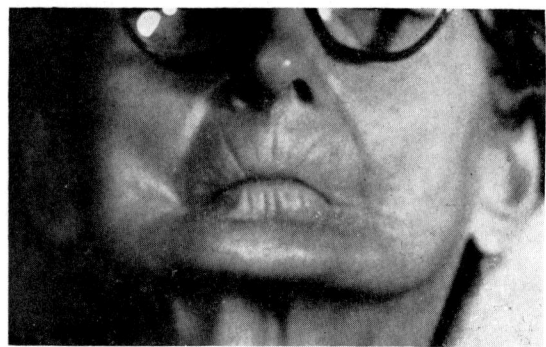

Figure 5-14. Scleroderma. There is diminution in size and opening of the mouth. Female, aged 61 years.

Scleroderma

The affected skin becomes smooth and rigid, erasing the lines of the face. Eventually the skin becomes fixed to the underlying tissues. Routine dental examination may be uncomfortable as the oral cavity diminishes in size and movement is decreased (Fig. 5-14). *Localized sclero-*

derma, referred to as *morphea,* often heals, leaving a depressed area in the skin. Generalized scleroderma is slowly progressive.[12,21]

BENIGN SOFT TISSUE LESIONS

Benign soft tissue lesions in the oral cavity are common—most of them can be removed by simple surgical excision. These benign lesions are characterized by slow, continuous growth and may cause severe discomfort.

The clinician cannot distinguish between the different types of tumors with certainty, with the possible exception of the papilloma. Histopathologic confirmation must be obtained.

Epithelial Benign Soft Tissue Tumors

Papilloma

The papilloma of the oral cavity is one of the most frequent epithelial lesions. Though papillomas in other parts of the body may be potentially malignant, malignant transformation of oral papillomas is extremely rare. It has been suggested that the oral papilloma may be attributed to infection, a virus or irritation. Size, location and color all are extremely variable, but the most common location is the palate. Pain is seldom a feature (Fig. 5-15).

Mesenchymal Benign Soft Tissue Tumors

Fibroma

The fibroma, or fibrous nodule, is also a very common oral lesion and may be composed of firm connective tissue or soft vascular tissue. If the lesion seems to be caused by irritation, it is classified as an *irritation fibroma.* In the absence of a known source of irritation, the lesion is classified as a true neoplasm. At any age it can be found anywhere in the oral cavity. Its size is variable, and it rarely causes discomfort (Fig. 5-16).[1]

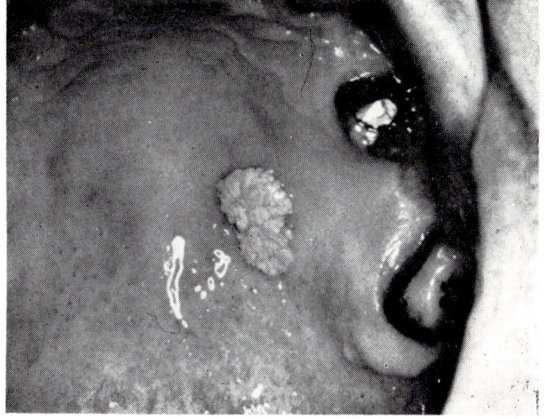

Figure 5-15. Papilloma of hard palate. Note the characteristic "cauliflower" appearance. Male, aged 63 years.

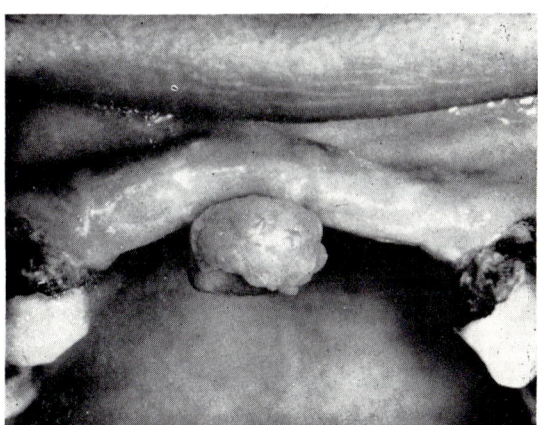

Figure 5-16. Fibroma. Male, aged 45 years.

MYXOFIBROMA. This is a rare variant of the fibroma in which myxomatous and fibrous components are roughly equal.[2]

LIPOMA. The lipoma is a rare tumor consisting of normal adipose tissue. Its most frequent location is the cheek. It occurs mostly in the fourth and fifth decade of life. It is well encapsulated and easily removed (Fig. 5-17).[2]

LIPOFIBROMA. This lesion is also rare. It

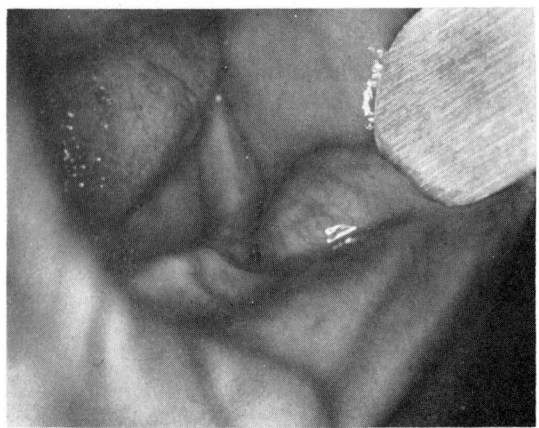

Figure 5-17. Lipoma. This lesion may be confused with the more common soft fibroma. The diagnosis was confirmed histologically. Male, aged 47 years.

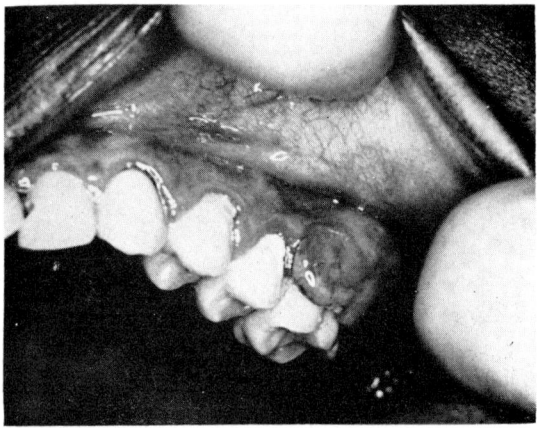

Figure 5-18. Peripheral odontogenic fibroma. The lesion was painful. Note the poor oral hygiene. Female, aged 25 years.

is a lipoma in which the fat is divided into compartments by fibrous tissue. The diagnosis is made histologically.[2]

PERIPHERAL ODONTOGENIC FIBROMA. The peripheral odontogenic fibroma is one of the most important benign soft tissue lesions in the oral cavity, because it is painful and the lesions are difficult to eradicate. The peripheral odontogenic fibroma occurs only on the margin of the gingiva and is attached to the periodontium by a long pedicle. Its appearance is similar to a hyperplastic lesion. If the tumor contains calcified material it may be quite hard and ulcerations are then frequent. Teeth may be pushed out of line by the tumor and there may be considerable pain and bleeding. Extensive surgical excision is required, and sometimes adjacent teeth must be removed as well. Despite the difficulty of complete removal of the tumor and frequent recurrence, no malignant transformations have been reported (Fig. 5-18).

Tumors of Blood Vessels

A group of benign soft tissue lesions which originate from the vascular system can be considered as either true tumors or hamartomas (tumorlike malformations).

HEMANGIOMA. This may occur within the bone or in peripheral locations. Peripherally it may vary widely in size and color, depending in part on whether it is primar-

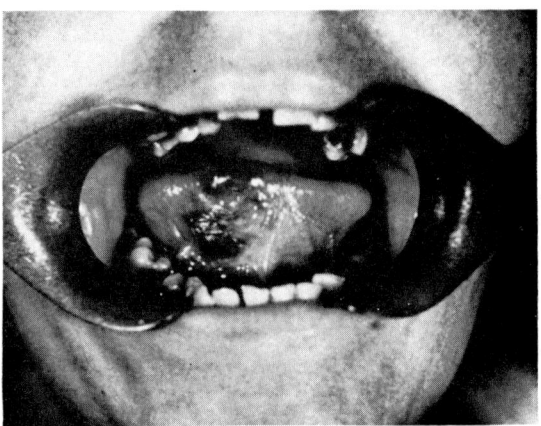

Figure 5-19. Hemangioma of tongue. Occasionally angiomatous malformations of the soft tissues may extend into the bone and result in catastrophic hemorrhage following tooth extraction. Male, aged 45 years.

ily arterial or venous and how near the surface it lies (Fig. 5-19).

HISTOLOGIC FEATURES. Several types of hemangiomas can be distinguished, depending on the presence of capillaries, large cavernous spaces or fibrosis (sclerosing hemangioma).[2]

NEVUS FLAMMEUS (PORT-WINE STAIN). The nevus flammeus is dark purple when on the face, but if the oral mucosa is involved, the lesion is bright red. It involves surface capillaries but nevertheless indicates need for caution in extractions.[1]

HEMANGIOENDOTHELIOMA. This lesion is benign but aggressive and cannot clinically be differentiated from other benign lesions. It is of importance since malignant forms have been reported.[1,2]

Lymphangioma

This is a tumorlike malformation of lymph vessels. It is most often found on the dorsal surface of the tongue and is usually yellowish-brown in color. Ulceration may occur and result in pain.

Tumors of Muscle Tissue Origin

Benign muscle tumors of the oral cavity are rare.[1,2]

GRANULAR CELL MYOBLASTOMA. The granular cell myoblastoma is the most frequently occurring lesion in this group. The severe downgrowth and hyperplasia of the epithelium which covers the lesion has on occasion led to the false diagnosis of epidermoid carcinoma. The lesion is most often found in the tongue. It is a small, firm, elevated growth which seldom causes symptoms. It can be multiple, may occur at any age and is more common in males. Its origin from striated muscle is much debated; some consider it to be of nervous origin (Fig. 5-20).[1,2]

Tumors of Nervous Tissue Origin

Benign tumors arising from the nerve tissue are quite common.

NEUROMA. This lesion is sometimes known as the injury of boxers. It results from overgrowth of Schwann cells and the nerve sheath after the nerve has been severed. It is a hard, painful lesion, consisting of a tangled mass of myelinated nerve tissue.[1,2]

NEUROFIBROMA. The neurofibroma arises in the subcutaneous tissue in association with peripheral nerves. The resultant swelling may be large and the tumor may interfere with mastication or speech.[1,2]

NEUROFIBROMATOSIS. This condition consists of multiple neurofibromas which may

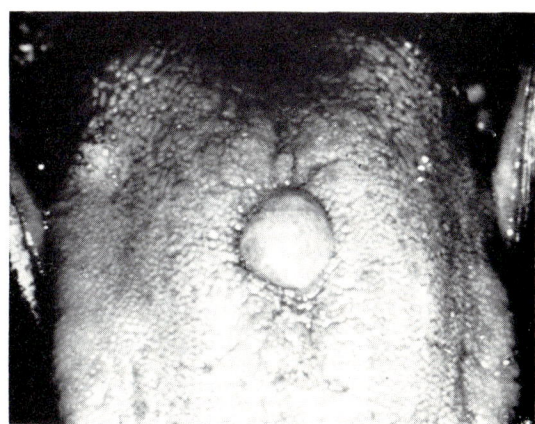

Figure 5-20. Granular cell myoblastoma of tongue. The lesion had been present for three or four months. Male, aged 20 years.

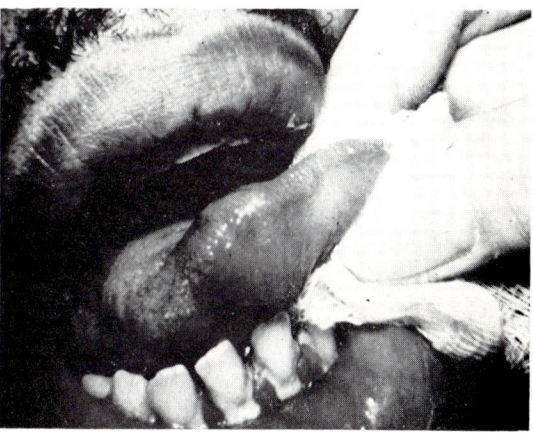

Figure 5-21. Neurofibromatosis. The patient had in addition to this lesion of the tongue neurofibromata of the skin with increased skin pigmentation in the affected areas. The tongue lesion was excised. Male, aged 47 years.

cover the entire skin. Some of them may become extremely large and pendulous. Oral lesions also occur (Fig. 5-21).[1,2,22] A brownish coloration of the skin (café au lait spots) is often seen. This disease shows a predilection for males, starts at about the third decade of life and is easily recognized. About 15 percent of these cases show sarcomatous transformation.

KERATOTIC LESIONS

Keratotic lesions of the oral mucosa are also referred to as *white lesions* or so-called *clinical leukoplakia*. Their etiology may be unknown or may be due to trauma, congenital or environmental factors such as smoking. Though there is much confusion concerning the histopathologic terminology, clinically the different kind of lesions cannot be distinguished. The lesions may be localized or generalized, and may be associated with inflammatory changes. The white color may be due to increased production of keratin, decreased desquamation or both. Though the process of increase of keratin may be essentially the same in normally keratinized and normally nonkeratinized areas, an increase in preexisting keratin is termed "hyperkeratosis" and the presence of keratin in areas normally not keratinized "keratosis." On occasions, the increased thickness of the epithelium itself and edema may give the tissue a white appearance.

The keratotic lesions can be classified as follows: keratotic lesions of unknown etiology, reversible keratotic lesions and nonreversible keratotic lesions.

These lesions cannot clinically be distinguished from each other by appearance or size. The only means of differentiation is histopathological. Let us again emphasize that the term "leukoplakia" is frequently used for a clinical white lesion, while the histopathologic diagnosis of leukoplakia is reserved for the potentially malignant lesion.

Keratotic Lesions of Unknown Etiology

Hairy Tongue

This condition is not uncommon in debilitated patients or in patients who are receiving extensive antibiotic therapy. The lesion occurs on the dorsum of the tongue, anterior to the terminal sulcus, and is characterized by more or less pronounced elongation of the filiform papillae. This may be the result of decreased shedding of the keratin or, according to some authors, the presence of fungi. The lesion may show a great variety of colors, depending on food stains, organisms and medications (Fig. 5-22).

The Reversible Keratotic Lesions

This group of lesions consists of pachyderma oralis, leukoedema, white sponge

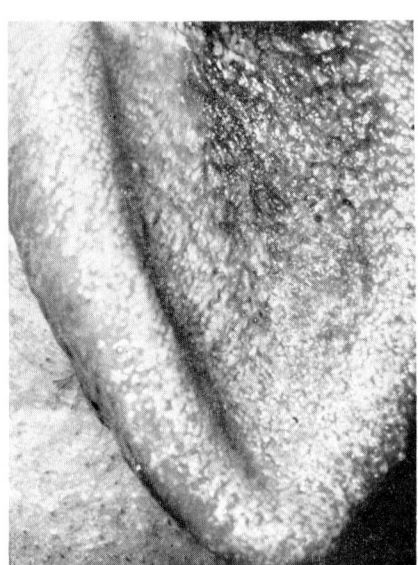

Figure 5-22. Black hairy tongue. The patient had recently completed an antibiotic regimen. Male, aged 56 years.

nevus (see nevi) and so-called mild leukoplakia.

As a rule, after elimination of the irritant, the lesion will sooner or later disappear. Sometimes medication, such as vitamin A, may be helpful in reversing the process.

Pachyderma Oralis (Leukokeratosis, Focal Keratosis, Hyperkeratosis)

This appears as a white irregular lesion usually on the cheek and more commonly in males than in females. The lesions may be elevated or flat; on occasion they may be directly associated with an irritant. Larger lesions may present problems in diagnosis.

Leukoedema

This is a chronic condition of unknown etiology. The oral mucosa appears grayish, transparent in the early stage, and becomes progressively opaque and wrinkled as the lesion becomes older. It usually occurs bilaterally and frequently covers the entire lining mucosa. Leukoedema occurs in over 90 percent of male Negroes and in over 80 percent of female Negroes. It is the only white lesion which disappears on stretching.

"Mild" Leukoplakia

Mild leukoplakia usually starts as a localized reddening due to inflammation and gradually turns into a white patch or plaque which usually occurs locally, single or multiple, and may disappear on discontinuation of the stimulus. The lesion may range from faintly transparent to thick and fissured. This poorly defined entity cannot be clinically distinguished from late pachydermia oralis. However, histopathologically mild leukoplakia shows the presence of dyskeratotic cells in the lower epithelium and some increase in mitotic activity.[1,2,23,24]

Nonreversible Keratotic Lesions

The nonreversible leukoplakia is similar in appearance and distribution to the mild leukoplakia but will not regress or disappear on removal of the cause. The lesion may clinically appear thicker or fissured (Fig. 5-23).

The lesion must be considered as premalignant, although at this time no definite criteria exist to separate it from severe dysplasia and carcinoma *in situ*. Little is known about the time taken by severe leukoplakia to progress through carcinoma *in situ* to invasive carcinoma, nor whether the progression takes place or not.

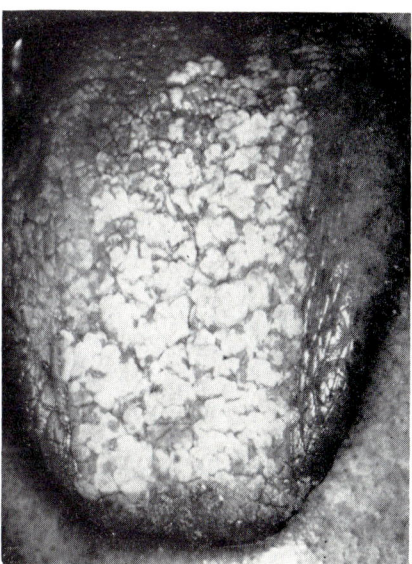

Figure 5-23. Leukoplakia of tongue. There is a danger of malignant change in this nonreversible form of leukoplakia. Some authorities excise the affected epithelium and graft the raw areas. Male, aged 35 years.

HISTOLOGIC FEATURES. Histopathologic examination enables one to distinguish between reversible and nonreversible forms of leukoplakia, as the nonreversible lesion shows dysplasia, individual keratinized cells in the lower layers of the epithelium, some disorientation and increased numbers of mitotic figures.

Candidal Leukoplakia

This form of leukoplakia shows clinically as white and red patches, giving the lesion a speckled appearance. There is evidence that this type of lesion may be associated with progression toward malignancy (Fig. 5-24).

HISTOPATHOLOGIC FEATURES. The white areas are parakeratotic. The dysplastic changes of the epithelium may be severe and difficult to distinguish from carcinoma *in situ*.

Erythroplakia

Erythroplakia is a rare, usually single, elevated velvety, red lesion which can be seen in the oral cavity, most often in the cheek. Occasionally, a few small, white areas can be seen on the lesion.

HISTOPATHOLOGIC FEATURES. The lesion shows epithelial atrophy and histopathologically resembles carcinoma *in situ*. It is considered to progress more rapidly toward invasive carcinoma.[25,26]

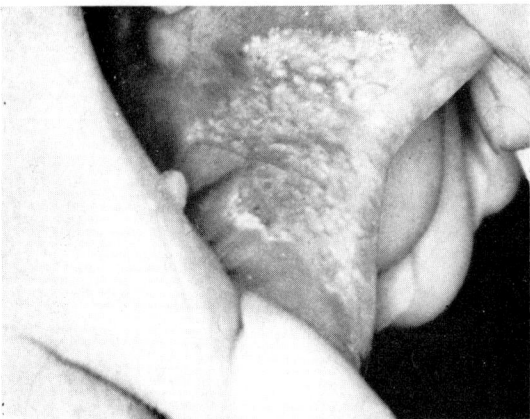

Figure 5-24. Candidal leukoplakia of cheek. *Candida albicans* was isolated from the affected areas. The patient sucked mycostatin lozenges q.i.d. for six weeks and there was slight decrease in size of the lesion. The lesion was excised and the diagnosis confirmed histologically. Male, aged 50 years.

POTENTIALLY MALIGNANT LESIONS

The designation of a lesion as being potentially malignant or precancerous depends partly on clinical experience and statistical data and partly on morphology and histopathology. This term should be used in cases which, if left untreated, may eventually become actual carcinomas.

The following lesions will be considered together as potential sources for malignant transformation, although they have been previously discussed in different chapters:

1. Nonreversible leukoplakia.
2. Erythroplakia (erythroplasia of Queyrat).
3. Solar keratosis of the lip.
4. Submucous fibrosis.
5. Erosive lichen planus.
6. Papillomatosis of the palate.
7. Epulis fissuratum (inflammatory hyperplasia).
8. Oral pigmented nevi.

Some of these lesions, such as nonreversible leukoplakia, erythroplakia and solar keratosis of the lip are thought to have a great tendency for malignant transformation, though there is no definitive time sequence. Therefore these lesions should be excised as promptly as possible. Lesions such as erosive lichen planus may show malignant transformation after many years of acute exacerbation and therefore must be carefully observed, frequently checked by taking exfoliative cytologic smears and biopsied when changes are noted. This particular lesion seems to have a tendency for multifocal malignant transformation.

Submucous fibrosis, which is common in India and Southeast Asia, has a tendency to malignant transformation after the epithelium becomes hyperkeratotic. In lesions such as papillomatosis of the palate and epulis fissuratum, occasional or rare malignant transformations have been reported. These lesions should therefore be excised and the area carefully observed.

Little is reported about malignant transformation of oral pigmented nevi. It has to be assumed that they are potentially malignant, especially junctional nevi, since melanomas of the oral cavity do occur. It is therefore advisable to remove all oral pigmented nevi.

MALIGNANT SOFT TISSUE LESIONS

Malignant soft tissue lesions are rare. It must be stressed, however, that their early recognition may make the difference between the life and death of the patient. They frequently are overlooked in the early stages or may be treated as innocuous for many months, until the symptoms become unmistakable. The five-year survival rate for intraoral carcinoma is low; only carcinoma of the lung and carcinoma of the stomach have lower survival rates. We feel that early recognition would improve the survival rate considerably.[27]

Epithelial Malignant Soft Tissue Tumors

Squamous Cell Carcinoma

The squamous cell carcinoma is the most common form of any malignant tumor in the oral cavity. It may be found on the tongue, buccal mucosa, palate, floor of the mouth, gingiva or lips. The clinical features of the squamous cell carcinoma vary widely. Lesions range in size from a few millimeters to several centimeters. It may occur at any age but is most common in adulthood, and it may occur in any race or in either sex. Growth may be rapid or slow. The tumor may appear initially as a small white patch, a small red area or a diffuse red area, an ulceration, a growth, a fissure or crack, a yellow necrotic area or a swelling. Pain is usually absent or minimal in the early stages but becomes severe in the later stages (Fig. 5-25 and 5-26).[29]

The prognosis depends partially on the location. The posterior portion of the

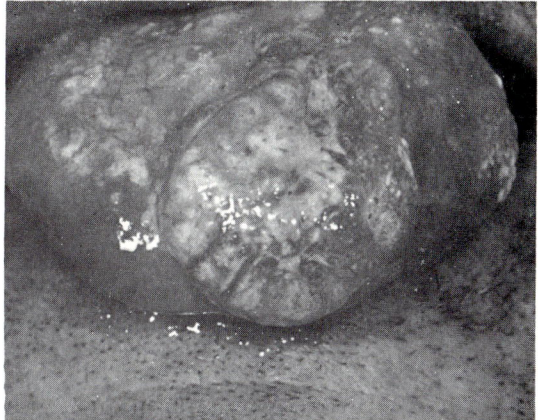

Figure 5-25. Squamous cell carcinoma of tongue. The patient was complaining of a sore tongue. Note the hypertrophic lesion of the tip of tongue and associated leukoplakia of the dorsum. Male, aged 63 years.

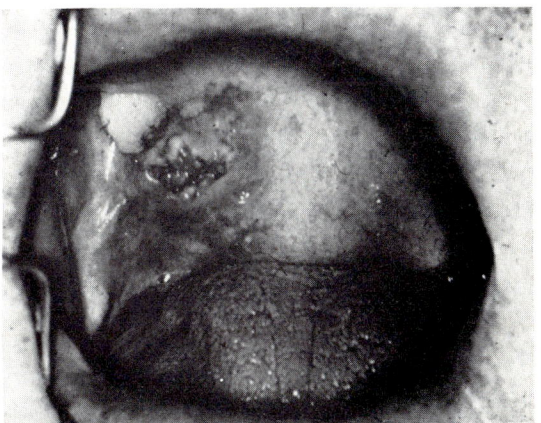

Figure 5-26. Squamous cell carcinoma of hard palate. The patient was complaining of soreness beneath the maxillary denture. Exfoliative cytologic examination of the ulcerated margins of the lesion enabled a rapid diagnosis to be made; a biopsy is, however, still indicated before deciding on the therapy. Male, aged 56 years.

tongue and the floor of the mouth have the gravest prognosis due to early metastases which may be unilateral, bilateral or on the opposite side of the neck. Another factor in the prognosis is the degree of differentiation which can only be estimated by the pathologist. Recurrences of the oral epidermoid carcinoma are common. Epidermoid carcinoma of the lip has the best prognosis. It usually grows slowly, metastasizes infrequently and rarely recurs after adequate treatment.

In the differential diagnosis of squamous cell carcinoma, tuberculosis, syphilis, traumatic lesions, herpetic lesions, periodontitis or other tumors have to be considered.

Basal Cell Carcinoma

The basal cell carcinoma of the face is important since the dentist is in an excellant position for early recognition. It initially appears as a reddish-brown elevation which slowly enlarges and eventually ulcerates. Metastases are uncommon, but widespread destruction of the face, nose and eyes may occur (Fig. 5-27).

Basal cell carcinoma has been linked to

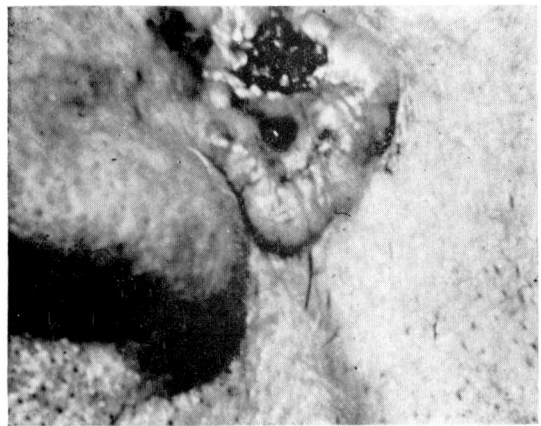

Figure 5-27. Basal carcinoma of face. The lesion lateral to the left ala of the nose was noticed when the patient presented for routine dental examination. Note the rolled edge and the ulcerated center. Male, aged 54 years.

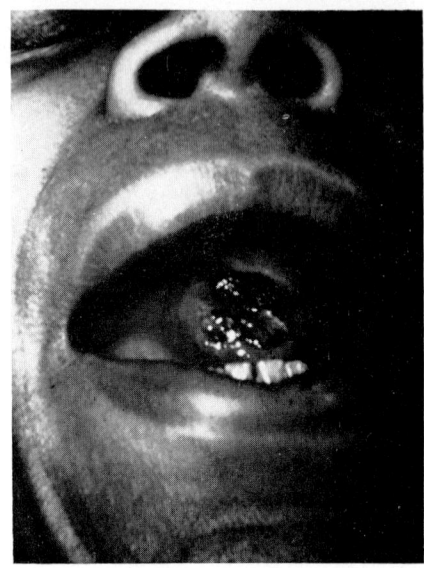

Figure 5-28. Adenocarcinoma of the hard palate. The patient complained of soreness in the upper jaw for some months. The lesion which was situated at the posterior part of the hard palate was ulcerated; the neoplasm had infiltrated the soft palate. A biopsy established the diagnosis. Male, aged 52 years.

excessive exposure to sunlight and to local irritations such as from eyeglasses. The prognosis is good.[1]

Adenocarcinoma

The adenocarcinoma is relatively rare in the oral cavity. It occurs most often on the tongue and is marked by a beefy-red color and a folded or lobulated appearance. Depending on the degree of differentiation it ranges from highly anaplastic to well-differentiated types, which determines the future course of the tumor (Fig. 5-28).[2]

Lymphoepithelioma

The lymphoepithelioma is a highly malignant tumor found chiefly in the nasopharynx. It appears initially as a small, elevated red area that may be ulcerated or eroded. Because of the site it is difficult to visualize. The tumor may be less than 1 mm in diameter. It is painless and may go undetected until after metastasis and has a poor prognosis.

Transitional Cell Carcinoma

The transitional cell carcinoma is also found in the nasopharynx and is highly malignant. This lesion frequently causes sore throat, earache, dysphagia and epistaxis, but the most common symptom is swelling of the lymph nodes.[1,2,28]

The prognosis for both lymphoepithelioma and transitional cell carcinoma is extremely poor, partly due to the high degree of anaplasia, partly because of the inaccessibility of the tumors and the probability of late discovery.

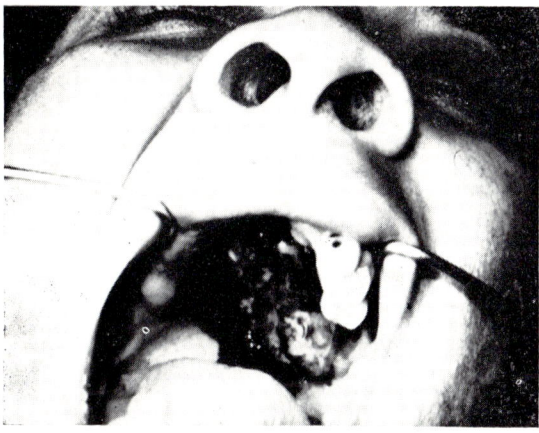

Figure 5-29. Melanoma of the hard palate. The main complaint was discomfort in the palate for some months. Male, aged 42 years.

Melanoma

The melanoma is rare in the oral cavity. It is highly malignant, spreads rapidly and carries an extremely poor prognosis. Initial lesions are elevated and range in color from reddish-brown to black (Fig. 5-29).[32]

Mesenchymal Malignant Soft Tissue Lesions

These lesions are even rarer than epithelial malignant soft tissue lesions and therefore will be mentioned only briefly. They tend to occur at an earlier age than carcinomas and are difficult to find in the early stage due to their deep location and their indistinct outline. Fibrosarcoma, liposarcoma, rhabdomyosarcoma, reticulum cell sarcoma and hemangiopericytoma have been reported. The majority of these are highly malignant and produce early widespread metastases by way of the bloodstream.

Tumors Metastasizing to the Oral Mucosa

Metastases to the oral soft tissues are rarer than metastases to the oral hard tissues but have been reported for any oral location. Any patient with a history of previous malignancy who develops unexplained oral lesions should be biopsied with this possibility in mind. On rare occasions, oral metastases have been found by biopsies of supposedly inocuous lesions before the primary tumor was discovered.[30,31]

LESIONS OF THE SALIVARY GLANDS

Inflammatory Lesions

The major as well as minor salivary glands can show inflammatory changes due to direct infection, metastatic infections or trauma. Swelling of the gland may be parenchymatous, *sialoadenitis,* and follow inflammation or may be due to an obstruction following local irritation and stone formation, *sialolithiasis.* True acute parenchymatous inflammations, which are seen in elderly or debilitated patients, may be the result of organisms spreading along the duct of the gland from the oral cavity. There is rapid swelling associated with elevated temperature and sometimes trismus. In the chronic form the swelling may be intermittent and a discharge may be produced at the opening of the duct. Acute postoperative parotitis is believed to be an ascending infection in debilitated, dehydrated patients (Fig. 5-30).

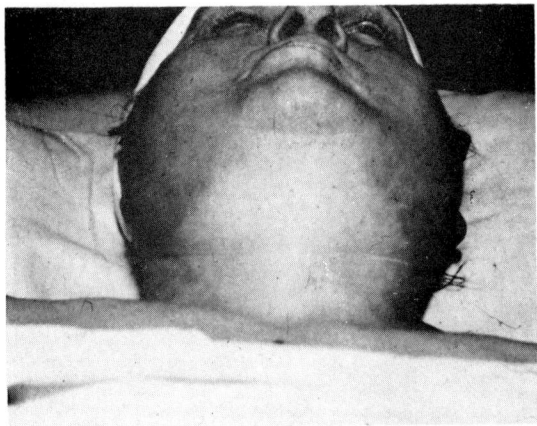

Figure 5-30. Acute parotitis. The patient had been hospitalized for an acute abdominal emergency and had a stormy postoperative period. Note the bilateral parotid swelling in this terminal case. Female, aged 50 years.

Prolonged inflammation or obstruction of major salivary glands will lead to atrophy of the parenchyma and decreased amount of secretion.

Epidemic Parotitis (Mumps)

This is a highly contagious infection of viral origin. It is primarily a disease of childhood and involves most frequently the parotid gland. It is more frequently bilateral, but may be unilateral. Chills, fever and anorexia are common. The dentist should be aware that epidemic parotitis may occur in susceptible adults. The adult form, in contrast to the childhood disease, is a severe disease and may lead to complications such as orchitis and sterility in males.

Granulomatous Infections

Various generalized granulomatous infections such as tuberculosis and actinomycosis may affect the major salivary glands.

Radiation Effects

After extensive oral irradiation, a cessation of secretion of the major and minor salivary glands can be observed, leading to xerostomia, extreme discomfort of the patient and rampant, usually cervical caries of the remaining teeth.

Sjögren's Syndrome

Sjögren's syndrome, which is thought to be an autoimmune disease, occurs predominantly in middle-aged females. The patient complains of a dry mouth (xerostomia) and inability to produce tears (keratoconjunctivitis sicca). Rheumatoid arthritis is found in about one-third of patients with this syndrome.

Tumors of the Salivary Glands

Tumors of the salivary glands may arise from the paired major or the dispersed minor salivary glands and are manifested by swellings covered by normal mucosa. The observant dentist will notice a firm swelling, which does not fluctuate and shows no inflammation. The benign tumors are painless and usually grow slowly. No indication of the type of tumor can be ascertained from the clinical appearance, nor whether it is a benign or malignant variety. A biopsy or excision is always indicated. If a tumor has been in existence for some time and suddenly grows more rapidly, malignant transformation has to be suspected. Since the relative frequency of salivary gland tumors in major and minor salivary glands varies, we will cite mostly the percentage occurrence in the major salivary glands and mention the frequency in minor salivary glands only if indicated.

Pleomorphic Adenoma (Mixed Tumor)

This is the most common tumor of the parotid and other major and minor salivary glands. It comprises about 60 percent of the major salivary gland tumors and about 55 percent of the minor salivary gland tumors. This tumor can occur at any age but is most commonly seen in the third decade of life. If not removed it may become very large and disturbing for the patient. It consists of several different histopathologic types. The rate of recurrence is relatively high and when the tumors recur they show a tendency to become more aggressive. The malignant variety comprises over 6 percent of the major salivary gland tumors and about 2 percent of the minor salivary gland tumors. It is clinically similar to the benign pleomorphic adenoma but may be more nodular, is more fixed, grows rapidly and is painful (Fig. 5-31).[33-35]

Mucoepidermoid Carcinoma

This tumor is next in frequency—about 11 percent—and involves usually the major salivary glands. The majority of these tumors are of low-grade malignancy, do not become large, but do eventually invade and metastasize. They usually occur in the third decade of life and are evenly distributed between the sexes. They do not exhibit any clinically characteristic criteria.

Papillary Cystadenoma Lymphomatosum (Warthin's Tumor)

This tumor comprises about 6 percent of the salivary gland tumors and occurs almost exclusively in the parotid and occasionally in the submaxillary gland. It has a predilection for males, occurs in the fifth decade and usually does not become as large as the pleomorphic adenoma. Clinically it is indistinguishable from the other salivary gland tumors.[35]

Epidermoid Carcinoma

Epidermoid carcinoma accounts for about 4.7 percent of all major salivary gland tumors and about 0.2 percent of the minor salivary gland tumors. This tumor may develop from the epithelial portion of a pleomorphic adenoma or be a primary carcinoma of the ductal elements of the gland; it has a poor prognosis and produces early metastases. Clinically the tumor is poorly outlined, hard, fixed to the underlying structures and grows rapidly. This particular tumor frequently ulcerates and shows more frequently lymphadenopathy than other salivary gland tumors. In the early stages the tumor cannot be definitively distinguished from any other salivary gland tumor, but later by virtue of the ulceration a Papanicolaou smear will aid in the diagnosis.[32,36,37]

Adenoidcystic Carcinoma

This tumor amounts to about 4 percent of the major salivary gland tumors and to

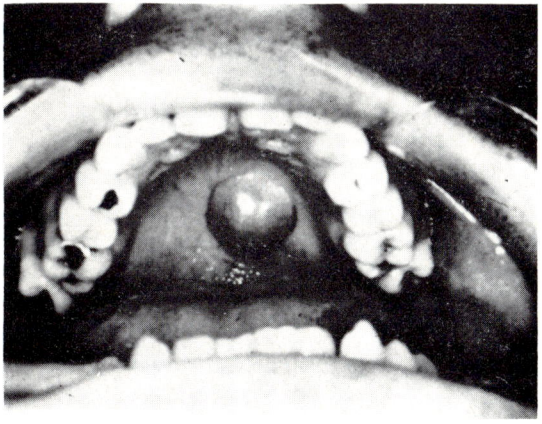

Figure 5-31. Pleomorphic adenoma of hard palate. The lesion was sessile and had been present for about three months. Male, aged 54 years.

about 16 percent of the minor salivary gland tumors. It occurs most frequently in the parotid and may occur at any age but mostly in the fifth to sixth decade of life. Clinically it appears as a nonspecific swelling but may be painful due to invasion of the nerve sheaths.

HISTOPATHOLOGIC FEATURES. The tumor consists of uniform, benign-appearing cells; however, clinically the tumor behaves like a malignant tumor. Even if completely removed, frequent recurrences after five to fifteen years with metastases may be seen.[1,2]

Adenocarcinoma

The adenocarcinomas of the major and minor salivary glands amount to about 4 percent and are the most rapidly growing tumors. Rapid growth and ulceration are the only suggestive features. This tumor is highly malignant and produces early metastases.

The remaining salivary gland tumors, such as *oxyphilic adenoma, canalicular adenoma, sebaceous cell adenoma* and *benign lymphoepithelial lesion* are extremely rare and amount to less than 1 percent of all tumors. Clinically they are also nonspecific and can only be diagnosed by biopsy.[1,2]

ORAL MANIFESTATIONS OF ALLERGIC REACTIONS

The dentist may have to deal with the following four types of allergic reactions: contact allergies, angioneurotic edema, serum sickness and anaphylaxis.

Contact Allergies (Delayed Hypersensitivity)

Contact allergy is due to cellular immunity which may be evoked by surface contact with cosmetics, foods and dental materials. It manifests itself as erythema, vesiculation and pruritus. The causes of this type of sensitivity are difficult to identify and require extensive questioning by the dentist and good observation by the patient. Reddening and burning of the oral mucosa in denture-wearing patients has for a long time been attributed to an allergy to residual monomer. Present thinking tends to attribute this phenomenon to mechanical irritation and moniliasis.

Angioneurotic Edema

Angioneurotic edema is a localized edema without inflammation which usually begins four hours after exposure to the allergen and disappears usually within forty-eight to seventy-two hours. It may occur following injections of procaine and Xylocaine® and after the use of aspirin. All these reactions are transient and are not life-threatening unless they involve the larynx. The reactions of aspirin in the sensitive patient may result in massive angioneurotic edema usually involving the head and face and in asthma, allergic rhinitis or dermatitis. Most patients are aware of this particular sensitivity and it therefore can be easily avoided.

Serum Sickness

Serum sickness is very rare and is seen after injections of penicillin, resulting in a rash, adenopathy, fever, edema, arthralgia and neuritis. Oral administration of penicillin rarely produces this type of reaction.

Anaphylaxis is the most dangerous allergic reaction and is life-threatening. Fortunately it is extremely rare, but it can follow parenteral administration of penicillin. Persons with other types of allergies, such as hayfever or asthma, are more prone to this type of reaction. Skin testing for penicillin hypersensitivity is far from reliable.

The reaction to Dilantin is presumed to involve hypersensitivity though the mechanism is not clear.[1,2]

ORAL MANIFESTATIONS OF METABOLIC DISEASES

The most frequent and significant metabolic disease affecting the oral tissues is *diabetes mellitus.* Diabetes is a disorder of carbohydrate metabolism which occurs in two forms—juvenile diabetes and adult diabetes.

The former is usually controlled by the administration of insulin and the latter by diet. The dental treatment of the controlled diabetic is essentially the same as the treatment of the normal patient, except that extra caution is advised.

The diabetic patient is susceptible to infection, and infection can adversely affect the course of diabetes. It is therefore imperative that diabetics receive excellent dental treatment to aid in the control of the disease. Furthermore, the progress of dental infections in the diabetic can be extremely rapid.

Any unexplained and persistent periodontal abscesses or persistent gingival infections with no apparent cause should lead the dentist to suspect diabetes (Fig. 5-32).

Vitamin Deficiencies

True vitamin deficiencies are rare in America today. They may be encountered in cases of malnutrition. Subclinical vitamin deficiencies are a subject of controversy. Bleeding gums may be treated successfully by giving the patient vitamin C orally, but it has been argued that the ailment was not caused by a clinical vitamin C deficiency.

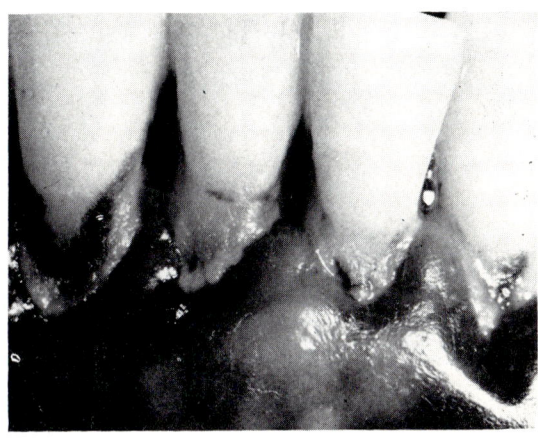

Figure 5-32. Diabetic gingivitis. There had been recent rapid deterioration of the patient's periodontal condition which led to testing of the urine for the presence of glucose and a glucose tolerance test, thereby establishing the diagnosis. Female, aged 27 years.

Vitamin B complex deficiency may result in changes on the lip and tongue at very early stages. *Cheilosis* manifests itself as a dry, vertical cracking of the lip, and the vermillion border outline may fade. Vitamin B complex deficiency may affect new denture wearers and is easily cured by administering vitamins; some authorities recommend postsurgical dietary supplements.[38-40]

ORAL MANIFESTATIONS OF PHYSICAL INJURY

Trauma

Trauma to the soft tissues of the oral cavity is common and usually easy to recognize. Injury from external sources such as acids and caustic agents usually are self-evident. The experienced dentist will recognize traumatic ulcers, trauma due to vigorous brushing of the gingiva and injury

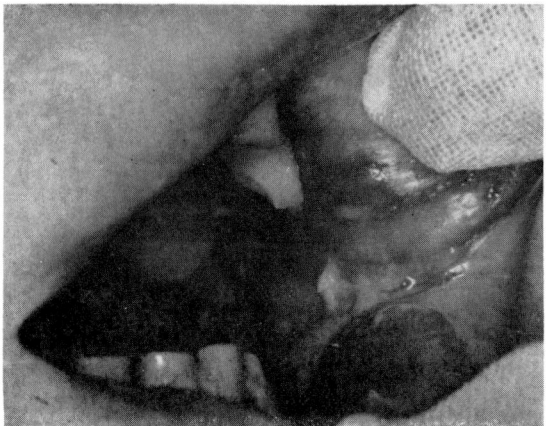

Figure 5-33. Phenol burns. The patient had used an undiluted phenolic mouthwash. Note the areas of desquamated epithelium on the buccal mucosa. Female, aged 29 years.

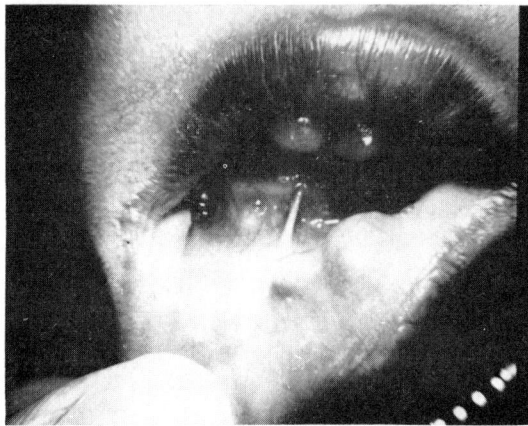

Figure 5-34. Mucocele of the lip. This lesion is bilobed, which is unusual. Female, aged 18 months.

from toothpicks or hard food. Sometimes it is necessary to question the patient about ulcers of the palate and tongue which may be caused by hot sticky food such as pizza, toasted cheese sandwiches or hot coffee or soup. Injury due to extreme *cold* is not of particular significance.

Mandibular local anesthesia may set the stage for self-inflicted trauma of the lower lip—especially in very small children—and great care must be taken in explaining this possibility to parents.

A frequently observed entity is the *aspirin burn*. Many patients who have severe toothaches and do not read instructions will place an aspirin next to the tooth and produce an effective but traumatic counterirritation. Burns by other chemicals do sometimes occur and are sometimes associated with dental procedures. These may involve phenol, silver nitrate, sodium perborate and other chemicals (Fig. 5-33).

Mucocele

The mucocele is the result of trauma leading to rupture of the duct of a minor salivary gland. The continuous secretion of the gland will produce a collection of mucus in the soft tissues surrounded by a wall of granulation or fibrous tissue. This may persist for months or at times burst open, allowing the mucoid material to seep out. The cyst will collapse and the whole process will repeat. These lesions are most common on the lower lip and can be seen in the cheek, tongue and the floor of the mouth but occur rarely on the upper lip (Fig. 5-34).[41]

Ranula

The ranula on the floor of the mouth is a mucocele produced by rupture of one of the ducts of the sublingual gland. It is a

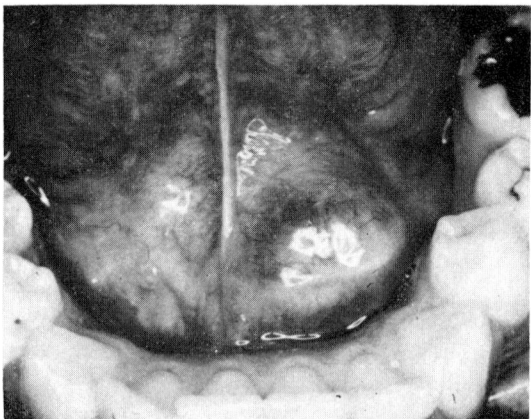

Figure 5-35. Ranula. There is a swelling on the left side of the floor of the mouth lateral to the lingual frenum. Male, aged 35 years.

painless swelling which can reach a considerable size (Fig. 5-35).

Ionizing Radiation

The effect of ionizing radiation on the oral tissues is of importance especially in association with cancer therapy. The oral mucosa is considered to be somewhat more sensitive to radiation than skin. Depending on the amount of radiation an erythema will develop. As the salivary glands cease to secrete two to three weeks after the start of irradiation, xerostomia develops which causes great discomfort and difficulty in swallowing. Changes in taste sensation take place. After extensive irradiation desquamation and slow-healing ulcers may develop which require palliation and good oral hygiene. After termination of the treatment healing will gradually take place and in most cases return of salivation occurs after many months.[1,2]

ORAL MANIFESTATIONS OF BLOOD DYSCRASIAS

It is important for the dentist to recognize any kind of blood dyscrasia in order to protect the patient and himself. Any surgical procedure is hazardous in an anemic patient, who has lowered resistance. A patient with a white blood cell abnormality will have little or no resistance to infection and may show severe periodontal bleeding. Disturbances of the platelets would make almost any procedure extremely dangerous. In general, consultation with the physician for diagnostic purposes or approval of dental procedures is advisable. In the more severe stages of these diseases, hospitalization for certain dental procedures may be desirable.

Anemias

The anemias are the most common disease of the blood-forming organs and are easily suspected by the observant dentist.

The differential diagnosis can only be made by laboratory tests and the patient should be referred to a physician for treatment (see Ch. 10).

Hypochromic (Iron Deficiency) Anemia

The most frequent of the anemias is the iron deficiency anemia, which is caused either by chronic or acute blood loss or nutritional deficiencies. It can occur at any age but is more common in females and older people. The patient presents with pallor of the oral mucosa which is variable in degree. Other symptoms are weakness, palpitations and dyspnea.

Pernicious Anemia

This is primarily a disease of the older female and is caused by vitamin B_{12} deficiency. The untreated patient has a yellowish skin, complains of weakness, atrophy, soreness and burning of the tongue and neurologic symptoms. The dentist can perform a great service for the patient by directing any suspected case to a physician for diagnosis and treatment (Fig. 5-36).

Sickle Cell Anemia

Sickle cell anemia has become increasingly important since it exists in about 2 percent of the black population, while the sickle cell trait is carried by about 8 percent of the population. The anemia as such is difficult to recognize and has no specific oral manifestations, but during periods of anoxia, which may occur under general anesthesia or analgesia, a sickle cell crisis which is life-threatening can develop.

Polycythemia Vera

Polycythemia vera is an abnormal increase of the number of red blood cells in

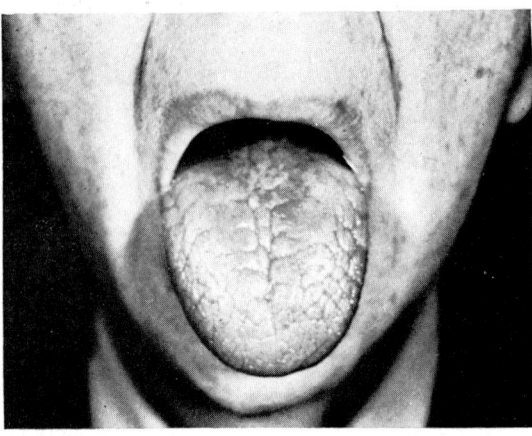

Figure 5-36. Pernicious anemia. The patient complained of a sore tongue. Examination of that organ revealed marked loss of papillae. The diagnosis was confirmed by hematologic examination. Patients with iron deficiency anemia may also have a sore, depapillated tongue. Female, aged 56 years.

the peripheral blood. These patients have periods of headaches and dizziness, flushed appearance of the face and a purplish-red color of the oral mucosa. The gingivae are swollen and bleed easily. Any surgical or gingival procedure is very dangerous since these patients have a tendency to bleed and low resistance to infection. Consultation with the attending physician prior to any extensive dental procedure is imperative (Fig. 5-37).

Leukopenia

Leukopenia is a reduction in the number of white blood cells and may result from damage to the bone marrow or overwhelming infections. Oral lesions are present and are characterized by poor response to any treatment including antibiotics. Due to the seriousness of the condition and the rapid deterioration of the patient, this is rarely seen in the dental office. The same holds true for agranulocytosis, which has multiple foci of ulceration and necrosis and no tendency to heal.

Leukemias

The leukemias are generalized, probably neoplastic proliferations of the white blood cells involving the bone marrow, reticuloendothelial system or lymphoid system, which may occur as acute or chronic forms. The systemic and oral manifestations are more dramatic in the acute forms. The dentist may be the first to suspect this condition, since the early symptoms may be hyperplasia of the gingiva with severe bleeding. Hyperplasia of the gingival tissues is common in subacute and chronic leukemia, and it is advisable to have a laboratory workup whenever an unexplained gingival hyperplasia with bleeding exists (see Ch. 10). Hemorrhages, petechiae or ulcerations of the oral mucosa are frequent symptoms of the further advanced undiagnosed leukemia. The color of the gingivae and the oral mucosa may vary from extreme pallor to deep red depending on the degree of anemia. Severe gingival ulceration may occur, especially in children, due to the decreased resistance to infection. Additional signs are temperature, pallor of the skin, purpuric rash and general malaise. As the disease progresses and the

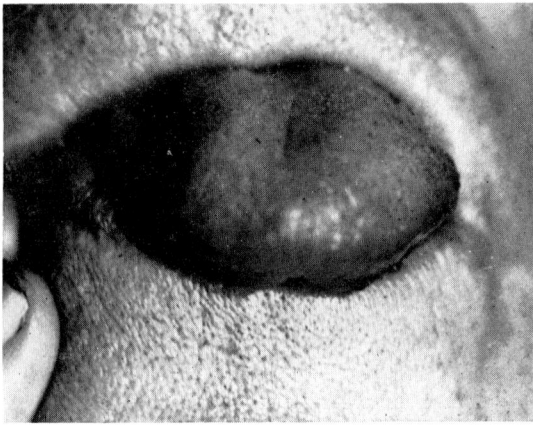

Figure 5-37. Polycythemia vera. Note the purplish-red color of the tongue; the face also had a flushed appearance. Male, aged 65 years.

periodontium becomes involved, the teeth may loosen (Fig. 5-38).

Thrombocytopenic Purpura

Diseases involving the blood platelets are of great importance to the dentist, though they occur rarely. Thrombocytopenic purpura may have many causes but can be recognized by gingival hemorrhages, sometimes even in the absence of skin lesions. The oral mucosa may show petechiae and occasional ecchymoses. This patient will rarely come first to the dentist for diagnosis or treatment (Fig. 5-39).

Hemophilia

Hemophilia, though it is of great interest, is a rare hereditary disease which the general practitioner will not be called upon to treat.[1,2,42-45]

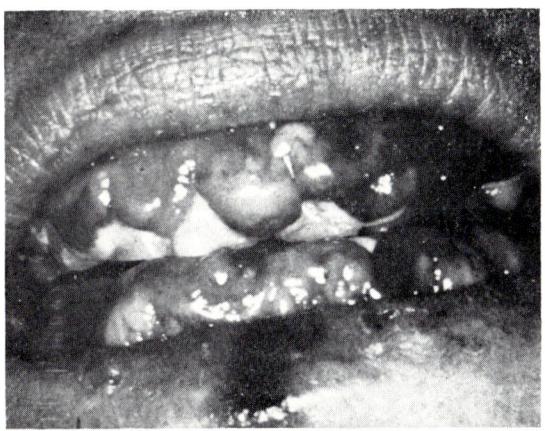

Figure 5-38. Acute myelocytic leukemia. The patient was complaining of a sore mouth and bleeding gingivae of a few weeks' duration. Male, aged 27 years.

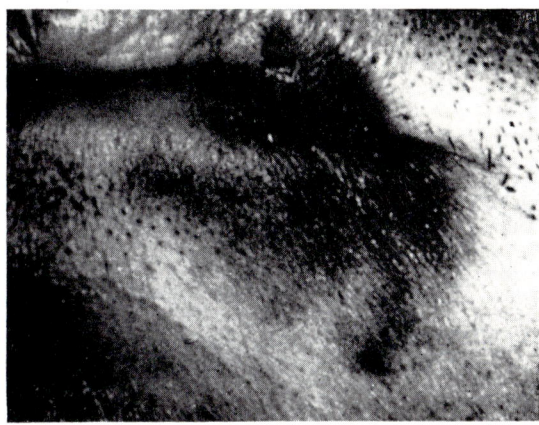

Figure 5-39. Thrombocytopenic purpura. Note the bruising of the lower lip which had occurred spontaneously. Male, aged 35 years.

REFERENCES

1. Tiecke, R. W.: *Oral Pathology*. New York, McGraw-Hill, 1965.
2. Shafer, W. G., Hine, M., and Levy, B. M.: *A Textbook of Oral Pathology*, 2nd ed. Philadelphia, W. B. Saunders Co., 1966.
3. Prinz, H.: Wandering rash of the tongue (geographical tongue). *Dent Cosmos*, 69: 272, 1927.
4. Ziskin, D. E.: Effects of certain hormones on gingival and oral mucous membranes. *JADA*, 25:422, 1938.
5. Lewis, A. B.: Effects of smoking on the oral mucosa. *Oral Surg*, 8:1026, 1955.
6. Kerr, D. A.: Keratotic lesions of the oral cavity. *J Dent Med*, 13:92, 1958.
7. Fisher, A. K., and Rashid, P. J.: Inflammatory papillary hyperplasia of the palatal mucosa. *Oral Surg*, 5:191, 1952.
8. Cauley, E. P., and Kerr, D. A.: Lichen planus. *Oral Surg*, 5:1069, 1952.
9. Darling, A. I., and Crabb, H. S. M.: Lichen planus of the mouth with associated ulceration. *Oral Surg*, 8:47, 1955.
10. Darling, A. I., and Crabb, H. S. M.: Lichen planus. *Oral Surg*, 7:1276, 1954.
11. Andreasen, J. D. et al.: Development of cancer in oral lichen planus. A review of the literature. *Nord Med*, 70:861, 1963.
12. Montgomery, H.: *Dermatopathology*. New York, Hoeber, 1967.
13. Lever, W. F.: *Histopathology of the Skin*, 4th ed. Philadelphia, Lippincott, 1967.
14. Allen, A. C.: *The Skin*, 2nd ed. New York, Grune & Stratton, 1967.
15. Robinson, H. C.: Erythema multiforme. *Arch Derm Syph*, 52:91, 1945.

16. Medak, H., Burlakow, P., McGrew, E. A., Cohen, L., and Tiecke, R.: Cytopathologic study as an aid to the diagnosis of vesicular dermatoses. *Oral Surg*, 32:204, 1971.
17. Cannon, A. B.: White sponge nevus of the mucosa. *Arch Derm Syph*, 31:365, 1935.
18. Cooke, B. E. D.: Leukoplakia buccalis and oral epithelial nevi. A clinical and histological study. *Br J Dermatol*, 68:151, 1956.
19. Mook, W. H., Weiss, R. S., and Bromberg, L. K.: Lupus erythematous disseminatus. *Arch Derm Syph*, 24:787, 1931.
20. Barnes, S. S., Moffatt, T. W., Lane, C. W., and Weiss, R. S.: Study of the lupus erythematous phenomenon. *Arch Derm Syph*, 62:771, 1950.
21. Looby, T. P., and Burket, L. W.: Scleroderma of the face with involvement of the alveolar process. *Am J Orthod Oral Surg*, 28:493, 1942.
22. Ayres, W. W., Delaney, A. J., and Backer, M. H.: Congenital neurofibromatous macroglossia associated in some cases with von Recklinghausen's disease. *Cancer*, 5:721, 1952.
23. Brophy, D., and Lobiz, W. C.: Injury and reinjury to the human epidermis. Epidermal basal cell response. *J Invest Dermatol*, 32:495, 1959.
24. Haenszel, W., Shimkin, M. H., and Miller, H. P.: Tobacco smoking patterns in the United States. *Public Health Monogr*, 45:6, 1956.
25. Clark, R. L., Russell, W. O., and Old, J. S.: Carcinoma in situ. A concept of cancer without invasion. *Postgrad Med*, 18:374, 1955.
26. Boggs, D. R.: The significance of fever and injection in malignant neoplastic disease. *Med Sci*, 14:64, 1963.
27. Ackerman, L. V., and Regato, J. A.: *Cancer Diagnosis Treatment and Prognosis*. St. Louis, C. V. Mosby Co., 1947.
28. Churchill, H. R.: Beiträge zur Klassifizierung der Tumoren des Mundes und seiner Nebenorgan. Inaug. Dissert. Rostock, Carl Hinstorffs Hofbuchdruckerei, 1932.
29. Medak, H., McGrew, E. A., Burlakow, P., and Jans, R. B.: Definitive cytopathologic characteristics of primary oral melanoma. *Oral Surg*, 27:237, 1969.
30. Thoma, K. H.: Tumors of the condyle and temporomandibular joint. *Oral Surg*, 7:1091, 1957.
31. Batsakis, J. G., and Dito, W. R.: Chondrosarcoma of the maxilla. *Arch Otolaryngol*, 75:55, 1962.
32. Medak, H., McGrew, E. A., and Burlakow, P.: Correlation of cell populations in smears and biopsies from the oral cavity. *Acta Cytol (Baltimore)*, 11:279, 1967.
33. Cameron, J. M.: Tumors of salivary tissue. *J Clin Pathol*, 14:232, 1961.
34. Foote, F. W., and Frazell, E. L.: Tumors of the major salivary glands. *Cancer*, 6:1065, 1953.
35. Wheelock, M. C., and Strand, C.: Papillary cystadenoma lymphomatosum. *Surg. Gynecol Obstet*, 98:571, 1954.
36. Cahn, L. R.: Early detection of cancer of the mouth. *Br Dent J*, 111:285, 1961.
37. Englert, R. J., Pasqual, H. N., and Litt, M.: Squamous-cell carcinoma of the lip and tongue. *Oral Surg*, 12:1163, 1959.
38. Spies, T. D. *et al*.: In Duncan, G. G. (Ed.): *Diseases of Metabolism*, 4th ed. Philadelphia, W. B. Saunders Co., 1959, Ch. 6.
39. Stafne, E. C.: Dental roentgenologic manifestations of systemic disease. Endocrine disturbances. *Radiology*, 58:9, 1952.
40. Thoma, K. M., and Goldman, H. M.: *Oral Pathology*, 5th ed. St. Louis, C. V. Mosby Co., 1960.
41. Cohen, L.: Mucoceles of the oral cavity. *Oral Surg*, 19:365, 1963.
42. Burket, L. W.: A histopathologic explanation for the oral lesions in the acute leukemias. *Am J Orthod Oral Surg*, 30:516, 1944.
43. Dameshek, W., and Henstell, H. H.: Diagnosis of polycythemia. *Ann Intern Med*, 224:52, 1941.
44. Dameshek, W.: Familial hemolytic crisis. *N Engl J Med*, 13:1360, 1940.
45. Segal, N. A.: Idiopathic thrombocytopenic purpura. *Oral Surg*, 6:631, 1953.

Chapter 6
The Role of Radiology in Oral Diagnosis

Gordon R. Seward

A RADIOLOGICAL investigation may be used in two ways, as part of an investigation of a specific complaint or as a screening test. As an extension of the second it may be used in epidemiological surveys.

THE SPECIFIC COMPLAINT

The investigation of a specific complaint starts as always with a history and physical examination. On the basis of the information gleaned in this manner one or more provisional diagnoses are reached. These possibilities are tested and explored by selected investigations including a radiological examination.

The radiographic views which are to be taken must be chosen. This is done by considering the possible nature of the pathological process, its site and its size, and by choosing projections which will explore the required region. In dentistry intraoral radiographs are frequently used because of their superior resolution of detail. Several types of intraoral views may be required to demonstrate different aspects of the lesion; for example, a bite-wing radiograph may be taken to reveal a suspected proximal cavity in a maxillary premolar together with a periapical film of the same tooth to confirm the presence of periapical bone destruction and to show the number and shape of the root canals. Where extensive lesions are involved, several periapical films may be required to cover the full length of the affected alveolar process. In such cases further views of the jaws or facial bones should be chosen which will demonstrate, if possible, all the affected area on one film.

Consideration should be given to other factors such as the degree of detail which it is necessary to display. The detail to be seen in the final radiographs is mainly regulated by the type of film or combination of film and screens which is chosen. The likely radiodensity of the part governs the kilovoltage which will be selected and influences the other exposure factors which will be used.

Apart from exploring the radiographic features of the lesion; its size, shape, margin, radiopacity and the reaction of the surrounding tissues and so forth, information should be obtained about its three-dimensional configuration and position. The simplest way to do this is to take radiographs in at least two directions at right angles to one another, three if possible. This routine should be followed for all except the most simple and straightforward conditions. Not only is this necessary to identify accurately the anatomical location of the lesion, but it is only when a three-dimensional mental image of it has been achieved that a proper concept can be formed of its likely morbid anatomy. The additional views from completely different aspects may well show features of the utmost diagnostic importance. An oval zone of bone destruction seen in the mandible in an oblique lateral jaw radiograph is likely to be a cyst, but if an occlusal film demonstrates a polyarcuate outline to the subperiosteal new bone covering the buccal and lingual expansions of the jaw then a giant cell granuloma, or ossifying fibroma are other more likely diagnoses (Figs. 6-6 and 6-7). The exact position of the abnormal structure is, of course, of the greatest importance where there are unerupted teeth or similar objects which require surgical removal.

In some instances a decision must be made whether or not to supplement plain radiography with contrast radiography.

SCREENING TESTS

Screening tests can be very useful but must not be employed without due thought. The percentage yield in terms of positive findings must be balanced against the irradiation of the patient which is involved. The utilization of the personnel and equipment and the cost of the screening test must also be borne in mind. Not only must the yield of unsuspected disease be considered, but the nature and significance of that disease must be evaluated. Progressive processes, like carious cavities, particularly if treatment is more successful in the early stages, are those most often sought by these methods and bite-wing radiographs are probably the most common screening films to be taken in dentistry. An orthodontist will always wish to account for as much as possible of a child's dentition so as to exclude the presence of displaced, supernumerary or unerupted teeth. Other screening examinations are more debatable and vary from patient group to patient group. Radiography should not be used to search for symptomless lesions which are unlikely to give their possessors trouble.

All this, together with the irradiation involved, must be weighed when screening tests are advocated. To take examples from another field it is still valuable to do mass chest radiography in civilized societies even though the yield of tuberculosis cases is falling, because it is beneficial to uncover bronchial carcinoma cases and cardiac deformities, increasing numbers of which can now be treated. By comparison with this it would not be helpful to do full skeletal surveys of elderly people for Paget's disease even though the yield might be of the order of 3 percent since there is no beneficial treatment and many affected persons remain totally unaware of the condition until death.

Following the inspection of the first films either additional plain films or perhaps tomograms or techniques using contrast media may be required.

CRITERIA FOR SUCCESSFUL INTERPRETATION

Diagnostic radiology is fraught with difficulties if the films are not of the best quality. The radiographic technique must be precise, the radiographic apparatus of good quality, the films must be from a reliable manufacturer and should be stored away from chemicals and irradiations. Considerable care should be taken over processing for many films are spoilt by faulty development and fixation.

Examination of the films is also best done under ideal conditions. Gross images can be examined by holding the film up to a window or light, but details can be appreciated only under ideal conditions. The room should be darkened or at least light should not shine directly onto the surface of the film. Modern double-coated films with emulsion on both sides require a fairly bright viewing box. One with a variable intensity of illumination is useful. Masks should be used to prevent light shining out from around the sides of the films for this will dazzle the observer and materially impair his vision. When heavily exposed areas are examined the more lightly exposed areas also should be covered.

A small, cylindrical light of considerable brightness, but with a frosted glass end is also useful for inspecting heavily exposed areas, such as those representing the soft tissues where it is suspected that a calcified body, or a foreign body, of moderate radiopacity is present. Indeed, where the thickness of soft tissues is considerable films should be taken with varying degrees of penetration; for a small exposure with low kilovoltage will clearly display the soft tissues but might not differentiate the object. On the other hand a well-penetrated film at higher kilovoltage may not so clearly show the soft tissues, but the object might be detected with the powerful spotlight.

The use of a magnifying glass to examine the films is mainly a matter of personal preference. Ultrafine grain, single-coated films can be magnified many times and considerable detail brought to light, but the use of such films is confined to morbid anatomical studies and certain special clinical investigations. The amount of irradiation that they require prevents their normal use. Films normally used in current clinical practice are double-coated with a fair thickness of emulsion on a base which may be up to 175 μ thick. When developed the fast emulsion used to conform to current thought on radiation hygiene has a granularity which becomes noticeable at about $\times 3$ magnification. Once the granularity is visible the appreciation of image detail is affected and the appearance of sharpness in the image is lost. Thus most people with normal vision will be able to perceive all that there is to see without the use of a magnifying glass. For those whose near point of distinct vision is receding, however, some magnification is helpful.

A magnifying glass can perform another function. It can concentrate the viewer's attention on a small area and can help in establishing an orderly examination of the films.

THE RADIOGRAPHIC DIAGNOSIS OF CARIES

The bite-wing technique is the method of choice for examining posterior teeth for caries (Figs. 6-2, C, and 6-3, C). The enamel-covered crowns of the posterior teeth are the most dense radiographically of all the human structures and a high kilovoltage is appropriate to investigate them: 70 to 90 kv are required and either one or two films per side. It is reasonable to use a film with a fairly slow emulsion if this is available. Such films have a particular application in this technique since considerable detail must be resolved if the dentist is to be certain of the presence of early lesions. All other aids to a sharp image should be employed: long-cone technique,[1] a narrow beam to reduce scatter and a radiopaque cylindrical collimator to eliminate off-focus irradiation.[2]

RADIOGRAPHIC EXAMINATION OF THE ROOTS AND PERIAPICAL BONE

In the past there has been considerable controversy about the virtues of the two major systems of periapical film technique. Briefly, the parallel film, long-cone technique concentrates on getting the film parallel to the long axis of the teeth and the alveolar process. For anatomical reasons in many parts of the mouth this means an appreciable object-film distance and a minimum anode-object distance of 40 cm (16 inches) is therefore required to ensure geometrical sharpness. Until the advent of modern high-powered, dental x-ray machines, radiography with this technique was quite difficult. More recently the Richard's tube head has been produced.[3] In this machine the tube is at the back of the tube head and 20 cm of the anode-skin distance is absorbed within the tube head so that an extralong suspension arm is no longer necessary and the 40 cm object-film distance can be used with greater ease.

The parallel film technique produces a close approximation to a true lateral projection of the teeth in all parts of the mouth and this facilitates interpretation. On the other hand, film placement is not always easy and in patients with narrow

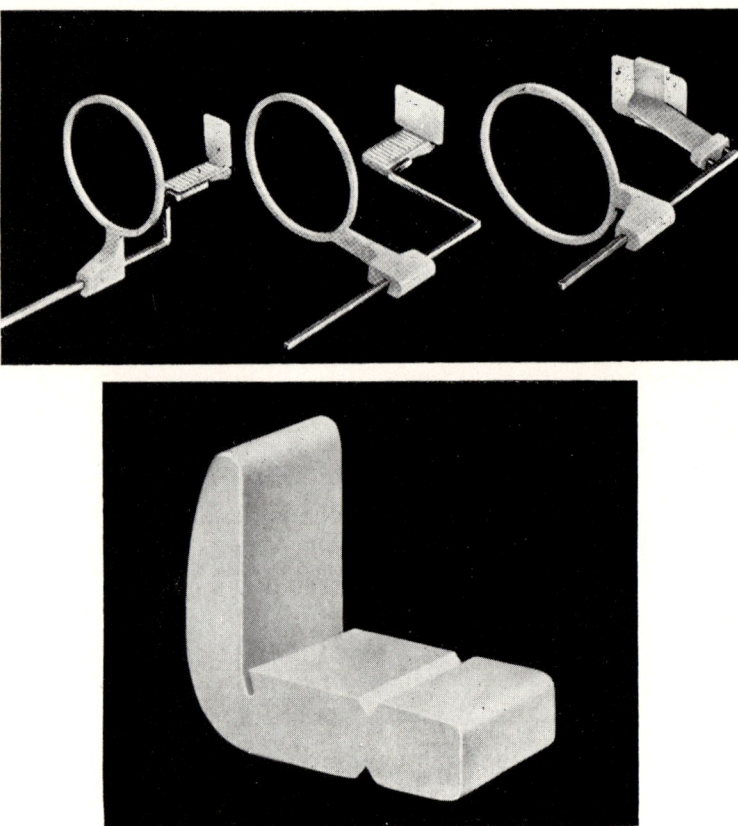

Figure 6-1. (*Above*) Examples of the "Rinn" film holders for long-cone parallel film technique. (*Below*) Stabe film holders which are made in expanded polystyrene by the Delaware Plastics Co. They can be cut or broken to aid positioning in the mouth as indicated in the photograph.

arches correct placement may be impossible. Special film holders such as the "Rinn" or "Stabe" film holders must be used (Fig. 6-1).

The rule of isometry of Ciesynsky technique permits the film to be placed close against the alveolar process and thus permits the use of a short 20 cm (8 inches) anode-object distance. Less powerful and therefore less expensive machines can be used successfully. With the advent of the Richard's tube head some of the mechanical advantages of the short anode-film distance have disappeared, and if this machine is used an even more favorable anode-object, object-film distance ratio can be achieved.

In practice the resulting oblique projection of the roots and alveolar processes does not prove to be a major disadvantage and although it is often the palatal or lingual slope of the tooth apex which is reproduced rather than the true apex this has little effect on ease of interpretation.

There is more noticeable difficulty in reaching a correct conclusion about the state of the crowns of the teeth and periapical films taken of posterior teeth by this technique must be supplemented by bitewing films (Fig. 6-2). On the other hand considerably more periapical bone can be projected down onto the film enabling larger lesions to be examined. While it is reasonable to project such lesions down onto the film when using the parallel film technique by increasing the tube angle, the beam no longer passes perpendicular to both the plane of the teeth and the plane of the film and the advantages of a true lateral projection are lost.

It is, of course, easier to interpret the images of the crowns of the teeth in films taken by the parallel film technique, but where the film has to be placed some distance from the teeth in order to get it parallel to them, the image may not be as sharp as that in a bite-wing film.

RADIOLOGY IN THE DIAGNOSIS OF PERIODONTAL DISEASE

In periodontal disease the height of the alveolar bone is important; the amount of bone which has been lost and the amount that remains. This is most easily appreciated in films taken with a beam which passes parallel to the alveolar crest. Bitewing films therefore are suitable as a screening test for periodontal disease and can be used to investigate early periodontal disease (Fig. 6-3, C). Where more marked bone destruction has occurred it is useful to be able to see the whole length of the root and the supporting bone (Figs. 6-2, B and C). The relative lengths of attached and unsupported root can then be appreciated. Periapical films taken by the parallel film technique are ideal for this purpose (Fig. 6-3, A), but films taken by using the rule of isometry method have their uses (Figs. 6-2, A and 6-3 B). With films taken by the latter method the observer must trace out the buccal and lingual alveolar crests and relate their height to the respective buccal and lingual amelocemental junctions. Indeed, because by this method these two aspects of the socket are not normally superimposed a marked loss of one of them may be more readily detected. It is, of course, important to relate the bone edge to the appropriate amelocemental junction since the buccal bone margin is projected upwards in relation to the tooth in a way which car mask an appreciable degree of bone los (Fig. 6-3, B). Special care must be taken in the upper incisors region to identify the palatal bone edge where this alone may be lost. Both the labial and palatal bone are

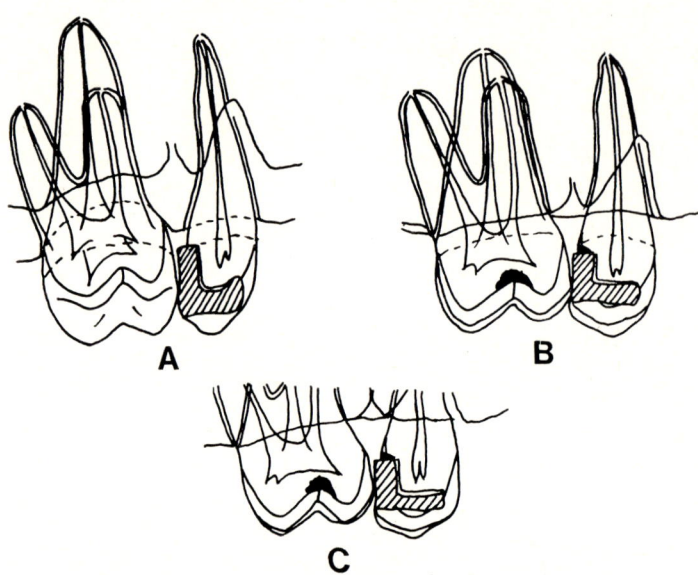

Figure 6-2. The differences between films taken by the rule of isometry, parallel film and bite-wing techniques. (A) The rule of isometry technique periapical film separates the buccal and lingual edges of the alveolar crests and disguises the general degree of bone loss. On the other hand the palatal bone loss is easily appreciated. (B) The parallel film technique periapical gives a better idea of the degree of bone loss and reveals recurrent caries beneath the cervical margin of the distal filling in the premolar. There is slight enlargement of the image. (C) The bite-wing film shows even more clearly the average alveolar bone height but is inadequate for the localized bone loss palatal to the premolar. Again the recurrent caries is clearly seen, as also is a cavity under the buccal fissure in the molar tooth.

reproduced with a similar degree of clarity with the long cone technique facilitating their identification while the palatal edge alone may be more clearly represented where a short anode film distance has been used.

Both rotational tomographic and intraoral x-ray source methods have their application in periodontal disease because a lateral projection of the alveolar process is obtained. Films taken with an intraoral x-ray source have magnified images of reasonable geometrical sharpness and record all parts of the tooth and alveolar process to an equal degree. There is, however, an increasing distortion towards the back of the mouth. Rotational tomographic films on the other hand reproduce one layer in a buccolingual direction more sharply than the rest so they cannot provide so much information about certain aspects of the tooth socket as periapical films. The one great advantage of these techniques is the way the whole length of the alveolar process from end to end is reproduced on one film. Further, and this is particularly true of rotational tomographic films, it is particularly easy to do follow-up films over long intervals of time which can be compared in a meaningful manner.

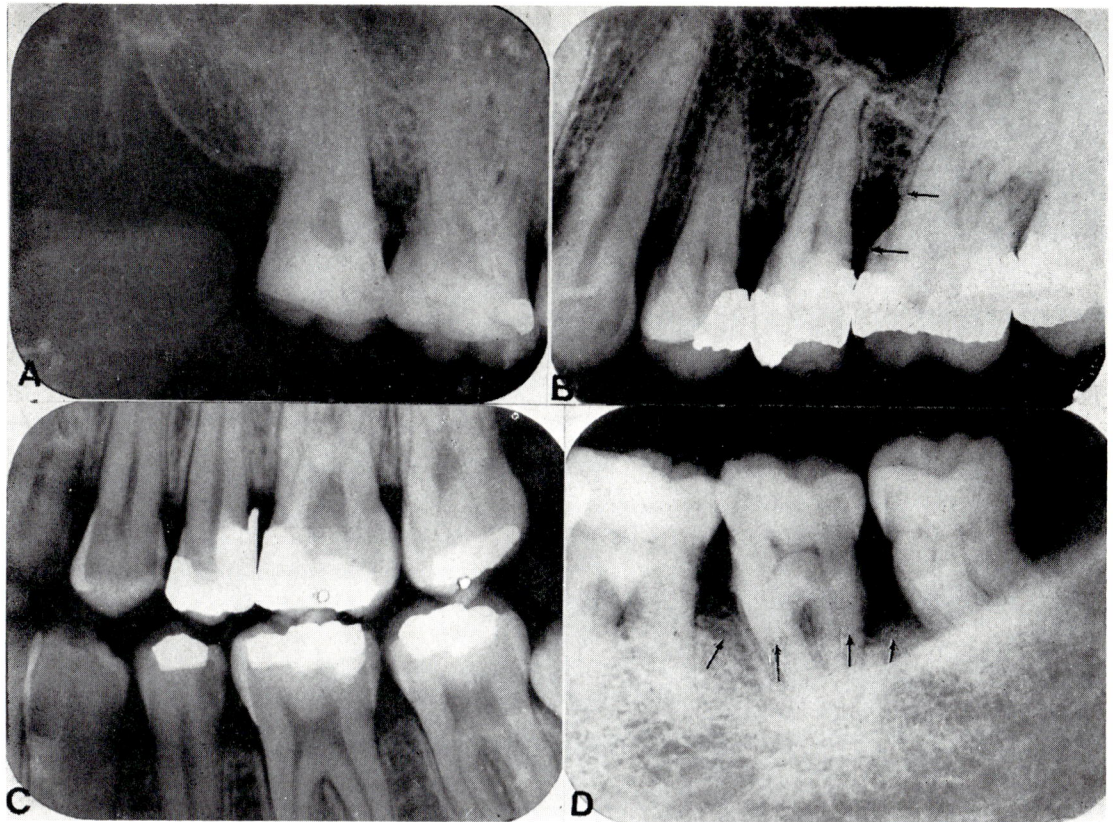

Figure 6-3. (A) Periapical film of upper molar region taken by long-cone parallel film technique. Behind tuberosity is pterygoid hamulus and between tuberosity and base of hamulus, the tubercle of the palatine bone. The coronoid process is seen on the lower left. Observe calculus on necks of teeth. There is some loss of alveolar bone height with "cupping" of alveolar crest distal to last molar and between teeth. There is also some widening of the periodontal membrane mesial to 8 /. (B) Periapical film taken by rule of isometry technique. Although there is a greater degree of bone loss on palatal aspect compared with the buccal, the difference in level of the margins is accentuated by angulation. If buccal margin alone was observed, the loss of alveolar bone height would be overlooked. (C) A bite-wing radiograph in which can be seen a cavity just into dentine distally /3 , a cavity well into dentine /4 , a lined MOD amalgam restoration in /5 with excess amalgam at the cervical margin and an associated loss of interdental bone. There is a sclerotic reaction in the dentine under the filling. A similar reaction is to be seen under the MO restoration in /6 . There is a deep distal cavity in / 5 , calculus mesially / 6 and etched enamel distally in / 6 and mesially in / 7 . / 6 appears to have overerupted and there is widening of the periodontal membrane mesially and at the distal alveolar crest. Cervical radiolucencies are present at the necks of / 4 5 and / 8 is probably mesio-angularly impacted. (D) Periapical film of lower region. A considerable amount of calculus coats the necks of the teeth and there is marked alveolar bone loss including loss of interradicular bone.

LOCALIZATION OF UNERUPTED TEETH

Two basic methods are available for the localization of unerupted teeth or buried foreign bodies: triangulation techniques and views at right angles.

Triangulation uses the same principles that are used in surveying. Observations are made from either end of a baseline and deductions made therefrom about the respective positions of the standing and unerupted teeth. The views at right angles method is like the representation of machine parts or a building by engineering or architectural drawings which involve a plan and elevations. Since information about two dimensions is contained in each film, two films from different directions are the minimum required to provide data about the third dimension.

Three methods have been devised for use in dental radiography which utilize the principle of triangulation; Bosworth's method, Clark's parallax method and stereoscopy (Fig. 6-4). In Bosworth's method the two images are produced by irradiating the same film from positions of the tube at either end of the baseline. The distances between the two images of the various parts which are produced in this manner are measured, and the respective distances of the objects from the film assessed. The greater the gap between the two representations of a particular feature, the greater its distance from the film. Because the application of this technique is not always easy and is open to uncertainty of interpretation it is rarely used.

Clark's parallax method has some similarities to Bosworth's method, but the two images are recorded on separate films. When the films are viewed it is as though the observer were looking at a transparent patient from positions at either end of the baseline formed by the two positions of

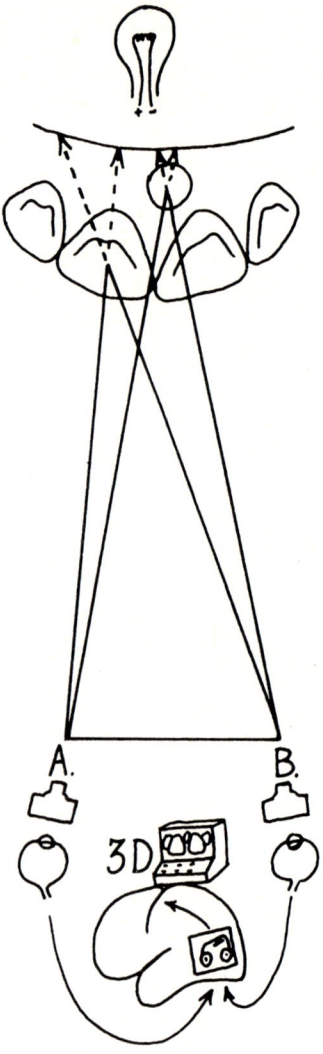

Figure 6-4. The relationship between the localization techniques based on triangulation. By Bosworth's method the images of the central incisor are more widely spaced than those of the supernumerary. By the parallax method, the image of the supernumerary moves to be superimposed on the right central as the tube moves from position B to position A; that is, in the same direction as the tube. Finally, if two radiographs taken from positions A and B are viewed in a stereoscope a three-dimensional image is seen.

the x-ray tube. The relative positions of the objects, as they are represented by the images, are observed; and an assessment made of their respective positions relative to the observer. Because there is a difference in the direction of displacement of the image corresponding to the object being investigated, depending on whether the object is on the film side or the tube side of a reference object, interpretation is less difficult than with Bosworth's method. Objects palatal or lingual to a reference object, which is usually an erupted tooth, appear to move in the same direction as the tube. Those on the buccal or labial aspect appear to move in the opposite direction to the tube. In common with Bosworth's method, however, interpretation proves most difficult just where the maximum care must be exercised; that is, where the two structures are close together. This is because there is then little difference between the images in the two films and virtually no relative movement of its constituent features.

Provided the conditions under which the films are made is sufficiently controlled, both Bosworth's method and the parallax method are capable of precise mathematical interpretation using trigonometric calculations. Such a precise arrangement can be managed with large parts like limbs but is difficult to achieve for the teeth and jaws.

Stereoscopy is a particular application of parallax (Fig. 6-4). The distance between the two positions of the tube is arranged to equal the distance between the two eyes of the radiologist. If, with a suitable viewing device of mirrors or prisms, the image from each film is directed into the appropriate eye the brain causes them to fuse and a three-dimensional image is seen. Parallax then is like viewing a scene first with one eye and then with the other; stereoscopy is like normal vision. The conscious effort of making a parallax assessment is removed since it is performed subconsciously by the radiologist's brain. Like any other observation made in this way, however, the image is subject to optical illusions. Further, the sense of depth is entirely dependent on differences between the two images. Where the distances between the parts is small there may be insufficient differences between the two images to ensure a convincing stereoscopic image.

Because each image is two dimensional, two radiographs taken in directions at right angles to one another will permit the observer to create a three-dimensional mental impression of the subject (Fig. 6-5). What

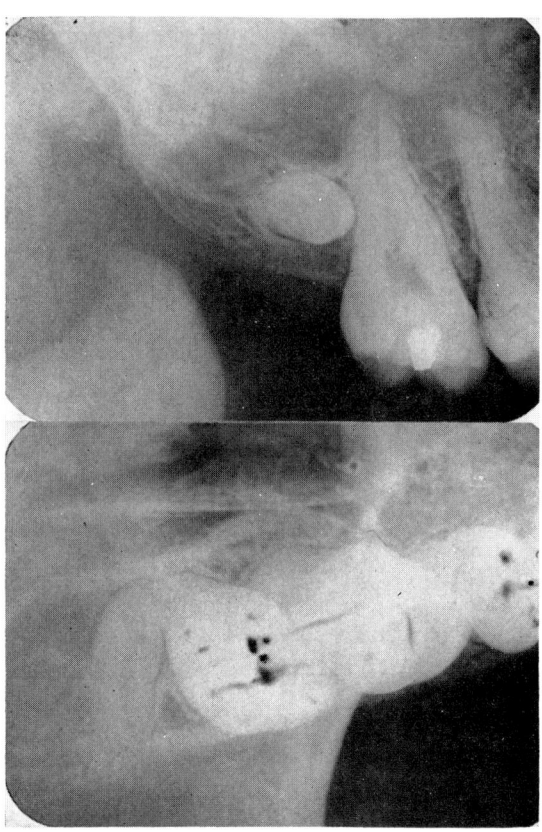

Figure 6-5. Localization by two views at right angles. A periapical film of 8 / reveals a conical tooth end on to the film. An occlusal view shows it to have a single conical root and a palatally directed crown.

almost certainly happens, however, is that the observer first constructs in his mind the view which would result from a film taken in the missing third direction. For example, if he has a plan (occlusal view) and one elevation (a periapical or oblique lateral jaw view) he will visualize in his mind the second elevation (tangential view) before constructing the three-dimensional mental image. Difficulties and errors which arise from the interpretation of films taken in directions at right angles to one another often stem from difficulties and errors in the visualization of the second elevation. Where it is possible to obtain the second elevation radiographically, these difficulties are frequently resolved. An unerupted maxillary canine, for instance, may lie horizontally and immediately over the standing teeth with the tip of the crown labial to one tooth apex and the neck of the tooth palatal to another. A vertex occlusal will show the image of the tooth superimposed on the images of the crowns of the standing teeth. Only a tangential film will demonstrate the crown passing to the labial of the root apices. In the mandible a cyst or an odontoma below the lower incisors can be adequately displayed with periapical, rotated posterior-anterior and occlusal radiographs, particularly if the latter film shows the lower incisors in plan view. Nevertheless a more vivid impression of the situation will be obtained if a tangential view of the chin is also taken.

THE RADIOGRAPHY OF CYSTS, DYSPLASIAS AND NEOPLASMS

Two problems are involved here. The first is to locate the boundaries of the lesion so as to identify its anatomical location. The second is to seek for clues to its morbid anatomy. The question of determining the anatomical location means following a similar routine to that discussed in the preceding section and views at right angles are usually chosen for this purpose. A detailed knowledge of normal radiographic anatomy is, of course, necessary when interpreting these films. Methods for revealing details of the morbid anatomy need further discussion.

Radiographs should be taken from several aspects to reveal the size and shape of the lesion. Where a large lesion is involved, at least one view should be chosen for each aspect which will show the condition in its entirety (Fig. 6-6). For this purpose films taken using one of the rotational tomographic machines such as the Rotograph, Orthopantomogram, Panorex or GE Panoramic system can be very useful. Films taken in this way are also valuable where there are multiple lesions, particularly those affecting the mandible. Not only the size but the number, distribution and arrangement of the lesions can be studied in these films.

To illustrate these points; solid lesions such as ossifying fibromas and giant cell granulomas and slow growing locally invasive lesions like the ameloblastoma tend to cause lateral expansion of the mandible at a comparatively early stage, whereas benign cystic lesions travel through the cancellous bone for a considerable distance before causing lateral expansion. Where there are multiple mandibular fractures and particularly where the jaw is comminuted, a more accurate idea of the number of fragments can be obtained from Panoramic films than when the information has to be put together from a study of several films. The pattern of jaw involvement may likewise help in the differentiation between primary and secondary malignant disease. A rotational tomographic film may show more convincingly whether

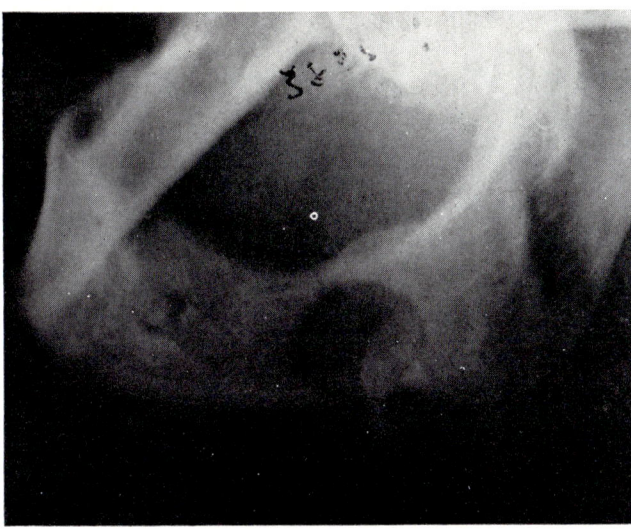

Figure 6-6. A patient with a hemispherical elastic swelling of the buccal aspect of the mandible. An oblique lateral jaw radiograph which shows a circular, circumscribed radiolucency in the mandible. Only the depth of the lesion below the alveolar crest differentiates it from a residual cyst.

the destruction is spreading from a single center or multiple centers.

Further study of the morbid anatomy requires a study of the margins and the intralesional zone on films giving first class resolution of detail (Fig. 6-7). In all ways intraoral views of various types are best for this aspect of diagnosis. Once again it may be necessary to take films from several aspects and periapical films at different vertical or horizontal angles, bite-wing and occlusal views should each be considered as to their likely value (Fig. 6-7). Both in the selection of views and in the interpretation the manner of projection of structures should be considered.

In general, sheets of tissue are shown as linear images only when the x-ray beam passes edgewise on through them. From all other directions there results an overall increase in radiopacity of the part, with or without a margin, but no obvious linear image. Under these circumstances the presence of the sheet of tissue may only become apparent when part is destroyed and a localized increase in radiolucency is seen. This means that cortical bone or the enamel of a tooth produce an intense, white image where the rays pass tangentially to the part but merely an overall increase in radiopacity when viewed from other aspects. A perforation of the cortical plate (Fig. 6-6) or a cavity in the enamel will be seen as a sharply defined dark image. Thin sheets of calcified tissue, like subperiosteal new bone, or the trabeculae of cancellous bone will be visible only when viewed tangentially, since the radiopacity which they exhibit from other aspects is too slight to be appreciated (Fig. 6-7). As a result no increased radiolucency is observed where the continuity of such sheets is interrupted.

Particles depend upon their diameter and their radiodensity for their effect on the image. Small radiodense particles, like tooth substance or metal, may be detectable particularly if the part is not too thick or if they are involved in a zone of bone destruction. They may be displayed more

mellar bone may be picked up when present as a nodule provided it is thicker than the average sheet of cancellous bone.

Both cylindrical and spherical structures produce the maximum effect where the direction of the beam coincides with a diameter. A decreasing radiopacity is recorded as the periphery is approached. Thus with normal exposures the periphery is usually burnt out so that the radiographic image is smaller than the original. The cervical radiolucency is due to this effect (Fig. 6-3, C).

If two views are taken at right angles to one another, sheets of bone, like subperiosteal new bone, which are poorly displayed in one view will be seen as linear images and can be easily studied. The use of fine grain film with suitable adjustments of kilovoltage and exposure may permit small, particulate objects to be visualized where they are external to the original cortex.

As the observer studies the film he must say to himself, What physical form did the part have to produce the images which I see? What shape was it and of what material was it composed? Information from each of the views must be consciously absorbed and mentally synthesized. Apparent discrepancies must be studied until they are resolved, while taking into account the accepted limitations of the method. The questions can then be posed: What type of lesion would look like this? And behave like this? In this particular site? In a patient such as this one? One or more answers will be forthcoming and these possibilities may be tested by yet other diagnostic methods until a firm and convincing diagnosis is reached.

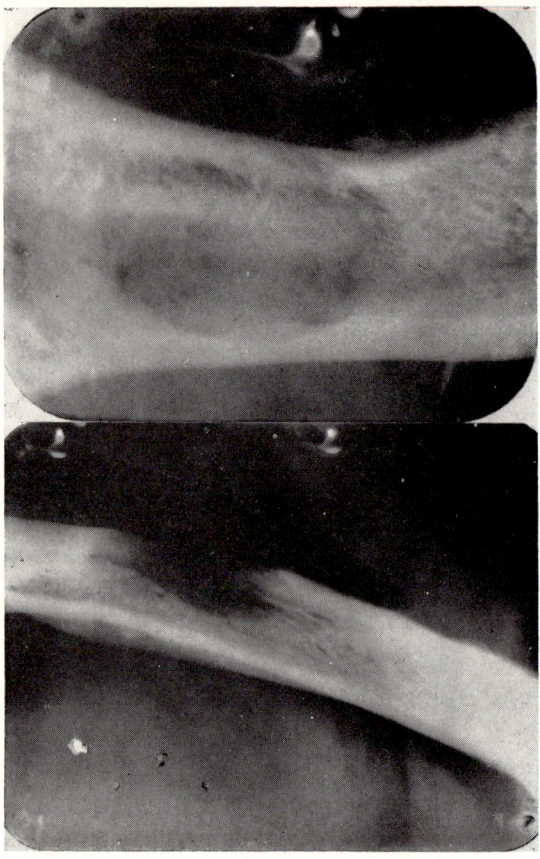

Figure 6-7. The periapical film of the same patient as Figure 6-6 demonstrates rather more medullary trabeculae surviving than would be expected if a cyst occupied this position in the jaw. Below is an occlusal film of the same lesion which now can be seen as an irregular cavity in the bone; an appearance suggestive of a malignant neoplasm. The clear-cut radiolucency seen in the oblique lateral view is now seen to be due to destruction of the buccal cortical plate. A biopsy revealed the lesion to be a myeloma.

clearly if the exposure is suitably adjusted so that their image is not "burnt out." Woven bone is only detectable when present in considerable quantity and scattered individual trabeculae are rarely seen. La-

THE PLACE OF CONTRAST RADIOGRAPHY

Contrast radiography means the establishment of margins in the resulting image by introducing either a radiopaque or a radiolucent substance so that it outlines and contrasts with the image of the surface to be studied. Usually soft tissue surfaces are studied in this way since they are naturally radiolucent. Natural or pathological cavities and tubes are conveniently investigated by this method.

The fluid in a fluid-filled cavity with rigid or semirigid walls can be aspirated. This is done carefully so as not to induce bleeding from the wall of the cavity. Any debris in the cavity is washed out with saline. The soft tissue wall, or lining of the cavity, can then be examined by air-contrast. This technique can be applied with some success to cysts of the maxilla, particularly where they are large enough to involve the antrum and nose (Fig. 6-8). Following aspiration of a liquid-filled cavity the contents can be replaced by a radiopaque contrast liquid.

In practice the technique is not always an easy one. For example, if a strong negative pressure is established within the cavity this may cause pain and bleeding into the cavity. There must always be a second needle penetrating the wall of the lesion so that air can pass in as the fluid is withdrawn. Toller's aspiratory needle is therefore a suitable one to use.[4] Should a blood clot form within the cavity this will produce an indentation in the outline of the contrast material which could be misinterpreted. As a radiopaque contrast medium is introduced it is easy to trap air bubbles, which again can make interpretation uncertain. Finally, the operator must be careful to ensure that the needle is within the cavity when the contrast medium is injected; otherwise it will be forced into the tissues. Once this has happened with an opaque medium the lesion will be obscured and all chance of further radiographic investigation lost. Nonirritant and absorbable media must be chosen where the liquid is to be injected into a cavity such as the temporomandibular joint from which it cannot be easily recovered.

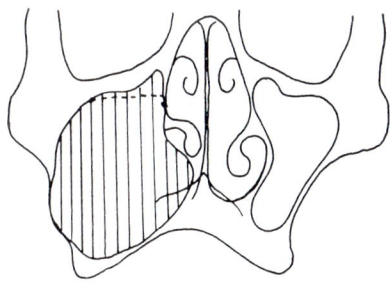
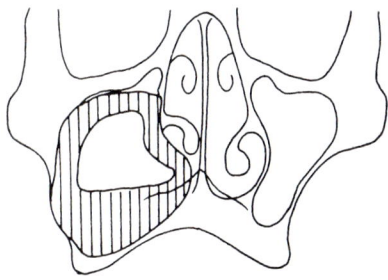

Figure 6-8. (*Top*) An occipitomental radiograph of a large residual cyst of the maxilla. The partition between cyst and antrum is difficult to distinguish in the general radiopacity. (*Below*) Same view after incomplete aspiration. The residual slit of antrum can be distinguished above the cyst, the lining of the cyst is shown up by air contrast and a fluid level established which transgresses normal anatomical boundaries.

Tubes such as the salivary ducts and sinus tracks can be also filled with radiopaque liquids so as to investigate their position, point of origin and the shape of their lumen and so forth. Smears of radiopaque paste applied to the surface of the face, the edges of a cleft palate and the inside of a saucerized surgical cavity may aid the visualization of these parts in relationship to the underlying structures and such methods may be helpful from time to time.

Contrast radiography is not always without risk and should only be employed where a material advance in knowledge of the patient's condition is likely to follow.

SIALOGRAPHY

One application of contrast radiography has particular value in oral diagnosis and this is sialography. Briefly, a radiopaque liquid is injected through the natural orifice and into the duct system of one of the major salivary glands. Either blunt metal cannulae or fine plastic catheters can be used to introduce the contrast medium. There is also a choice of viscous or fluid contrast media. Some contrast media are undoubtedly irritant and should not be used for this purpose.[5] If a fluid contrast medium is chosen it is best to use a plastic catheter, so that reflux of the solution is more easily prevented. Of the viscous media, Lipiodol® is one of the best. Because of its viscous nature it is more difficult to introduce than some, but for the same reason there is ample time for radiography before reflux occurs. Although this material is irritant if injected into the tissues, it is returned after a sufficiently short interval so that no harm comes to the salivary gland. It has good radiopacity and produces clear-cut sialograms. Sialograms will show the proximal dilatations of punctate sialectasis (Fig. 6-9, B). Where this is the result of the primary childhood condition, not only does the sialogram provide definitive diagnostic evidence of the cause of the recurrent inflammatory episodes, but it also seems to cut short the attacks in many cases.

A similar appearance is seen together with large duct changes in a number of conditions which damage the gland and is probably a nonspecific change in these cases. It is seen as a result of irradiation with ionizing radiations, as one of the results of autoimmune disease as in Sjögren's syndrome (Fig. 6-9, C) and after chronic infection.

Damage to the walls of the large ducts

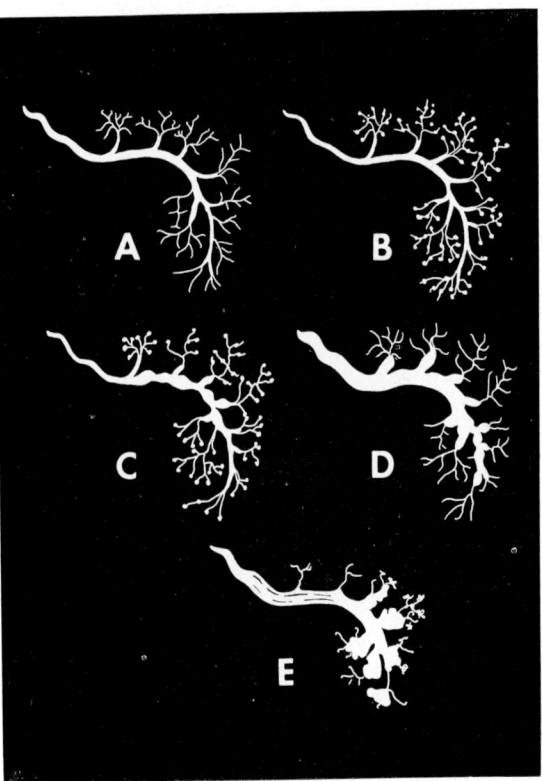

Figure 6-9. Diagrams of appearances seen in sialograms. (A) The normal gland. (B) Primary or childhood sialectasis with the punctuate appearance in the periphery of the gland and *no* changes in the larger ducts. (C) Punctate sialectasis as seen in Sjögren's syndrome and irradiated salivary glands. There is dilatation of the larger ducts as well as the peripheral punctate appearance. (D) Dilation of larger ducts due to relative papillary obstruction in Sjögren's disease. (E) Late Sjögren's disease with epithelial casts in the large duct and irregular abscess cavities in the gland. There is lack of filling of the peripheral ducts.

may produce fibrosis and strictures (Figs. 6-10, A, B and C). Such strictures are seen as a narrowing of the lumen in the sialogram. Dilatation of the duct occurs classically behind an obstruction such as a calculus, or stricture, or where some extensive mass presses on the duct. It can also occur where a mucinous, viscous saliva is being formed as for example in some cases of Sjögren's syndrome (Fig. 6-9, D). Finally dilatation appears to occur as a result of direct damage to the wall of the duct, again in auto-immune disease states.

Neoplastic ulceration of the duct wall produces changes similar to those seen where malignant disease involves other natural channels. There is an irregular outpouching of the duct lumen as revealed by the contrast medium and the outpouching represents the crater of the ulcer (Fig. 6-10, D). Proximally and distally the lumen may be narrowed by the exuberant margins of the lesion. Dilatation may be seen proximal to the ulcer if the neoplasm is rigid and partially obstructs the duct.

Sialography can be valuable in the investigation of salivary calculi. Posterior submandibular and parotid calculi are examined in this way, but care should be taken not to displace the calculus backwards by a vigorous injection. The position relative to the gland of opaque calculi can be established by this method and both the presence and the position of radiolucent calculi can be demonstrated. In some cases the degree of damage which the gland has suffered and which can be estimated from the sialogram influences the operator's choice of treatment.[6]

Provided the duct system is well filled, without excessive reflux and fragmentation of the column of contrast medium a satisfactory diagnostic film will be obtained. Overfilling of the gland tends to obscure the larger intraglandular ducts and is avoided. Where a space-occupying lesion is being investigated, however, the peripheral branches must be sufficiently filled that the outline of the abnormal tissue is delineated (Fig. 6-10, E). With this degree of filling, it is important to avoid excessive injection pressures or the ducts may be ruptured and the contrast fluid

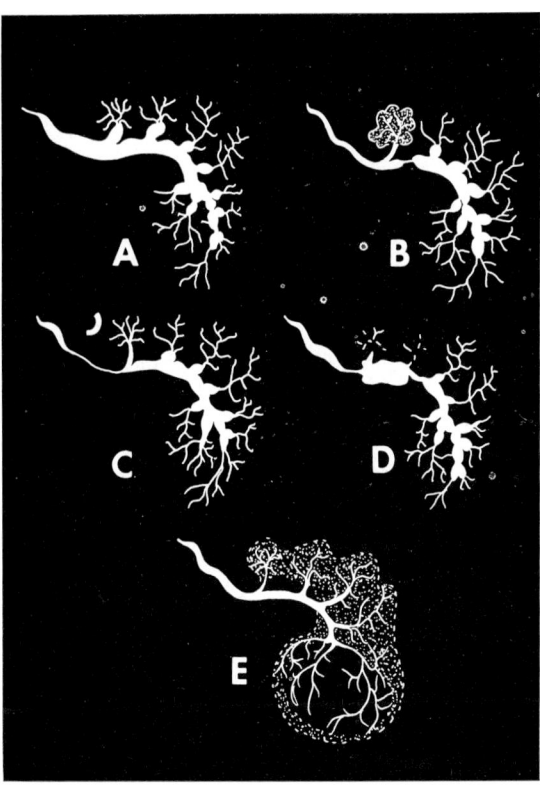

Figure 6-10. Diagrams of appearances seen in sialograms. (A) Papillary obstruction due to a stricture at the papilla. (B) The type of stricture which results from ulceration around a calculus. The gland distal to the stricture has been overfilled as a result of the resistance to the injection. (C) The idiopathic stricture seen where the duct curves around the anterior border of the masseter. (D) A neoplastic ulcer of the duct wall with fragmentary filling of the adjacent involved gland substance. The edges of the ulcer produce a stricture with dilatation of the duct proximally. (E) The "grasping fingers" appearance seen where the ducts curve around a pleomorphic adenoma. The gland is more heavily filled in this type of case so as to outline the periphery of the neoplasm.

escape into the gland capsule. If this happens it will not be returned as the gland empties. It is sometimes difficult to distinguish between a peripherally placed neoplasm and an enlarged lymph node identifying the gland or between the various types of parotid neoplasm, nevertheless valuable information about the size and site of the mass can be obtained by sialography.

THE USE OF SURFACE AND INTERSTITIAL MARKERS

From time to time it is necessary to locate and remove buried roots or foreign bodies from situations where anatomical landmarks provide only a poor or imprecise guide to their position. Artificial landmarks in the form of radiographic markers can be introduced to help in establishing their position. In the case of buried roots, wax or plastic plates with metal shapes embedded therein can be used. These are placed on the patient's ridge before the films are taken and the surgical incision made in the region indicated by the appropriate marker. Alternatively a radiopaque wire or needle may be introduced into the mucosa over, or buccal to, the suspected site of the root. Provided it is securely anchored, the film is developed straightaway and the operation performed immediately this is a satisfactory technique.

Interstitial markers may be used to locate objects buried in the soft tissues such as fractured hypodermic needles. If this method is used care must be taken to have the patient arranged in the operating position. Two or more films are taken in directions at right angles to one another with the patient anaesthetized and on the operating table. The mouth should be propped open, if this is appropriate, so that the patient's position will not be altered between the radiography and the surgery. In practice it may be found that the markers have to be removed to enable the tissues to be separated so that the site of the object can be approached. Despite this, some indication of the depth and direction may be obtained by this means.

CEPHALOMETRIC RADIOLOGY

In cephalometric radiography the patient's head is held in a special device in such a way that it can be repositioned in the same relationship to the film and tube on a subsequent occasion. Ear pieces which fit in the external auditory meati, a nose piece which rests on the root of the nose and a pointer that points to the midpoint of the infraorbital margin are devices which are usually used to effect the orientation of the patient's head. The central ray is commonly arranged to pass through the axis joining the two ear pieces when a lateral skull view is taken. When posterior-anterior or oblique views are used, the beam passes across this axis. Occasionally other centering points are used.

Various measurements may be made on the resulting radiographs and comparisons made between serially taken films. Such films have an obvious place in orthodontics, in oral surgery, especially in relation to the surgery of facial deformity, in prosthetic dentistry to monitor the patient's jaw relationship and facial appearance and as a means of studying facial growth in various diseased states and in anthropological studies.

It is usually necessary to produce a tracing of both hard and soft tissue features.

To reproduce both to an optimum degree on one film involves some difficulty since the radiographic exposures required are different. The problem may be solved in a variety of ways; by the use of relatively high kilovolts, by the insertion of a wedge filter of aluminum between the patient's face and the tube, by the use of a streak of contrast paste on the patient's face and by the double film technique. In the latter technique one of a pair of intensifying screens in a cassette is hinged so that one film may be placed between the screens and the other film outside the screens. Thus two films, one recording bone detail and another recording a soft tissue and bony profile are produced: the two images being superimposable.

RADIOLOGY IN THE DIAGNOSIS OF FACIAL FRACTURES

In this clinical situation the dentist wishes to establish the site or sites of fracture, the direction of the fracture lines in the mandible and the pattern of fracture lines in the maxilla.

Before radiography is undertaken it is important to determine the sites of fracture by clinical means so that a proper plan can be evolved for the examination. Note is also taken of the patient's physical state. While it may be necessary to take films immediately to demonstrate the site of a cranial fracture, or of the chest where there is a suspected collapsed lung or tension pneumothorax, or of the abdomen and pelvis where there may be a ruptured viscus, the same is not true of the jaws.

In the case of a fractured maxilla an occipitomental and a lateral sinuses film at least should be taken.

Standard additional views are posterior-anterior jaws for a central middle third fracture and a 30 degree occipitomental for zygomatic complex fractures. Other views are required to meet special circumstances but are outside the scope of this account.

Suggested views for mandibular fractures are as follows: 1. Lower incisor region—(a) rotated posterior-anterior jaws, (b) mandibular true occlusal, (c) periapical view of incisors and (d) tangential view of chin. 2. Body of mandible—(a) oblique lateral jaw view of body, (b) lateral true occlusal of mandible, (c) posterior-anterior jaws and (d) periapical view of appropriate teeth. 3. Ramus of mandible—(a) oblique lateral jaw view of ramus and (b) posterior-anterior jaws. 4. Condyle neck and condyle—(a) Toller's modified transpharyngeal view [7] and (b) transorbital anterior-posterior.

For the mandible a minimum of two views at right angles is taken of each clinical site of fracture and each suspected site of indirect fracture, not only to provide information about the fractures in three dimensions but also to avoid the diagnostician overlooking a fracture. If the x-ray beam passes through the fracture line oblique to the plane of the fracture and if there is no displacement of the bone ends, then it may be very difficult to detect it in the resulting radiograph. Usually in a view at right angles to the first one the beam will pass through the fracture line and display it clearly. Where the fracture involves the tooth-bearing part of the jaws, periapical films of the appropriate teeth are required so that the closeness of the fracture line to the various teeth can be determined and appropriate action initiated. Fractures of the alveolar process and of the teeth themselves need to be displayed, and periapical films taken with several different horizontal and vertical angulations of the tube may display the injuries more clearly than ones taken in a conventional fashion.

Where limitation of opening of the jaws and swelling of the soft tissues are extreme, the film should be manipulated with a pair of artery forceps.

Diagnostic radiology is both a science and an art. A science to the extent that a systematic study of anatomical specimens and morbid anatomical specimens can demonstrate the way in which particular radiographic appearances arise. An art to the extent that the experienced clinician accumulates many fragments of information which he would find difficult to put into words. Given a film of a difficult case he will appear to know intuitively what the diagnosis is. From his training he will know how to test and confirm this opinion. Such a state of knowledge is only reached after careful and continuous study of many hundreds of films. No film should be considered too "simple" or too "routine" to merit a detailed inspection. Even if no pathological process is to be seen the normal anatomy can be studied. Films of difficult cases should be reviewed as successive pieces of information about the case become available. The radiographic evidence may then be seen in a different light and certain features take on an importance not previously suspected.

The clinician should miss no opportunity to study other practitioners' films and radiographs reproduced in papers and textbooks. He should discuss films of difficult cases or films showing unusual appearances with a number of colleagues to obtain their interpretations. In this way he too will acquire the knowledge which will make his opinion of greater than average value.

REFERENCES

1. Updegrave, W. J.: *Higher fidelity in intraoral roentgenography.* JADA, 62:15, 1961.
2. Seward, G. R.: *Safety precautions in dental radiology.* Proc R Soc Med, 54:801–808, 1961.
3. Richards, A. G.: *New Concepts in dental x-ray machines.* JADA, 73:69, 1966.
4. Toller, P. A.: *Protein substances in odontogenic cyst fluids.* Br Dent J, 128:317, 1970.
5. Lilly, G. E., Cutcher, J. L., and Steiner, M. S.: *Radiopaque contrast medium. Effect on dog salivary gland and subcutaneous tissues.* J Oral Surg, 26:94, 1968.
6. Seward, G. R.: *Anatomic surgery for salivary calculi.* Oral Surg, 25:150,287,525,670,810 and 26:1,137, 1968.
7. Toller, P. A.: *The transpharyngeal radiography for arthritis of the mandibular condyle.* Br J Oral Surg, 7:47, 1969.

Chapter 7

Diseases of the Jaws of Interest to the General Practitioner

RALPH I. BROOKE, ALAN J. DRINNAN AND STUART L. FISCHMAN

It would be impossible in one short chapter to give a comprehensive review of all jaw disease. Our aim will not be to attempt this, nor to usurp the function of any of the excellent texts on oral pathology. It will be to outline the more common dental and nondental lesions which may give rise to symptoms or changes in the clinical and radiographic appearance of the jaws and to mention several rarer lesions which may mimic them.

Where controversy exists a fairly dogmatic approach will be taken, as the writers feel that many contradictory theories with a large number of references make difficult reading. There will thus be some oversimplification, which is felt to be justified if the practitioner is to be given an overall view of the subject.

The jaws are unique. Not only are they prone to the diseases which affect other bones, but in addition they contain teeth and their supporting structures and the upper jaw contains the maxillary sinus, an air-filled space.

When one considers the variety of developmental processes associated with the formation and eruption of the teeth and the formation of the maxillary sinuses, one can see that no other bones are associated with so much pathology. This is borne out by experience in dental practice. Jaw lesions are many and varied and will be discussed under the following headings: (a) odontogenic lesions, (b) inflammatory bone disease, (c) noninflammatory bone disease, (d) fibro-osseous lesions and (e) nonodontogenic neoplasms.

ODONTOGENIC LESIONS

Inflammatory and Cystic

Dental Granuloma

The most common periapical lesion is the dental granuloma. This inflammatory process is almost always the result of pulpal pathology. Irreversible pulpitis results in necrosis or chronic inflammation of the pulp tissues. The inflammatory process extends into the apical periodontal membrane and granulation tissue is formed. The enlarging granulation tissue causes resorption of the surrounding bone. The bone destruction then becomes visible on the radiograph.

On clinical examination, the associated tooth is usually asymptomatic. If the apical periodontal membrane is inflamed, the tooth may be sensitive to percussion. Typically, the tooth will give a nonvital response to the conventional pulp tests such as the electric "vitalometer" and thermal tests (*see* pulp testing in Ch. 15).

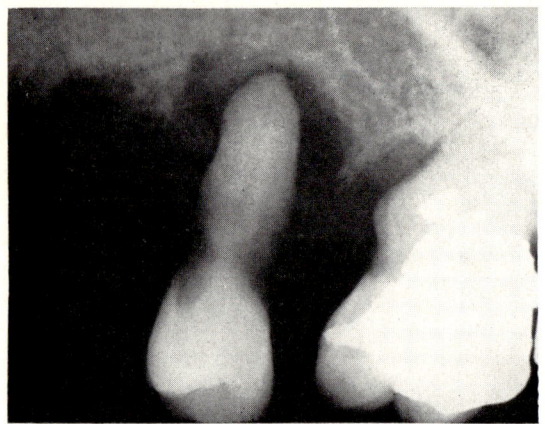

Figure 7-1. Dental granuloma. The patient presented for extraction of teeth prior to the insertion of dentures. Note the periapical radiolucency associated with the maxillary premolar; the tooth was symptomless. Male, aged 50 years.

RADIOGRAPHIC FEATURES. On radiographic examination, a radiolucent area is seen at the apex of the involved tooth. The area may vary in size from a slight increase of the periodontal membrane space to a lesion several millimeters in diameter (Fig. 7-1).

HISTOLOGIC FEATURES. The dental granuloma should not be regarded as a static lesion. It may undergo an acute exacerbation and have the symptomatology and histopathology of an acute apical abscess or the periapical epithelial remnants may be stimulated by the inflammation and proliferate to form a radicular cyst.

TREATMENT. The treatment of the dental granuloma depends on the status of the involved tooth and the remainder of the dentition. The irritant which evoked the change is removed, either by endodontic therapy or extraction of the tooth.

Radicular Cyst

The radicular cyst classically presents as a radiolucent area at the apex of a nonvital tooth. As with the dental granuloma, the involved tooth is usually asymptomatic, although if infected, there may be some tenderness to percussion. A very large cyst may present as a fluctuant alveolar swelling. The clinician may obtain a history of past toothache, followed by relief from pain.

The radicular cyst evolves by the same process as a dental granuloma. As a result of the periapical inflammation, the epithelial cell rests of Malassez are stimulated to proliferate and form a continuous mass of cells. The central portion of this cell mass degenerates to form a cavity lined by epithelium. This cystic cavity may continue to expand and the lesion may reach several centimeters in diameter.

RADIOGRAPHIC FEATURES. The radiographic appearance of the radicular cyst is similar to the granuloma, although the typical cyst is larger in size. The margin may or may not be well demarcated. It should be emphasized that it is not possible to differentiate a radicular cyst from a dental granuloma by radiographic means (Fig. 7-2).

HISTOLOGIC FEATURES. Histologically, the entire spectrum of lesions may be seen ranging from a granuloma with a few cell

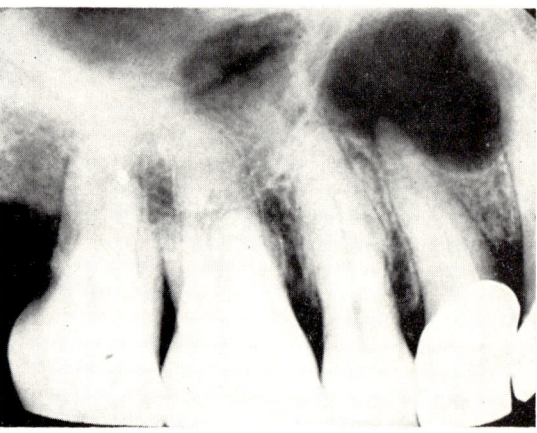

Figure 7-2. Radicular cyst. Note the radiolucency associated with the nonvital maxillary first premolar discovered on routine radiographic examination. Male, aged 47 years.

rests (the "precystic granuloma") to a large cyst with a well-developed lining of stratified squamous epithelium. This process is reversible to a limited extent. Cysts may become secondarily infected resulting in destruction of the epithelial lining and the formation of a granuloma containing pus. Hemorrhage during endodontic therapy may also destroy the epithelial lining which often results in healing of the cyst without curettage.

TREATMENT. The treatment of a radicular cyst is by removal of the irritating or initiating factor and removal of the cyst lining. This may be by extraction of the tooth and apical curettage, by endodontic therapy and periapical curettage, or by endodontic therapy alone. In the last instance, hemorrhage, secondary infection or chemical irritation destroy the cyst lining. In many cases, the choice of therapy depends on the experience of the operator and the status of the remaining dentition.

Residual Cyst

Occasionally, the tooth associated with a radicular cyst is removed, but the cyst is left undisturbed. The lesion may then persist in the jaw for some time, as it is asymptomatic. Residual cysts are generally encountered during routine roentgenographic surveys of clinically edentulous areas (Fig. 7-3).

Apical Scar

In a small number of cases, periapical curettage is not followed by reparative osteogenesis. The resultant apical scar is composed of dense bundles of hyalinized collagen and is, therefore, radiolucent. The lesion is asymptomatic and appears as a well-demarcated radiolucency at the apex of a tooth which has been treated endodontically. The apical scar is asymptomatic and requires no treatment. Routine radio-

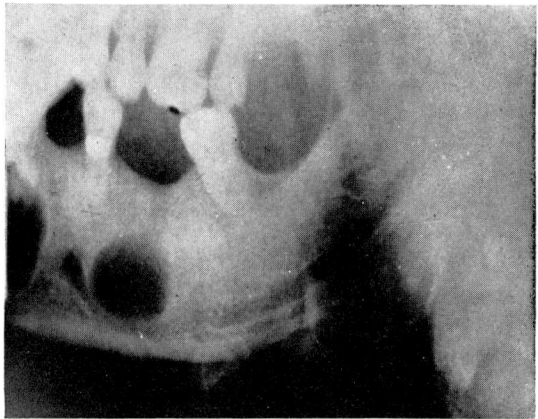

Figure 7-3. Residual cyst. The lesion which is situated in the first mandibular molar region was discovered on routine radiographic examination. Note a further cyst in the mandibular incisor region associated with two nonvital incisors. The patient was involved in an automobile accident seven years previously. Male, aged 42 years.

graphs are necessary at regular intervals to detect any increase in size of the apical translucency; the apical scar does not increase in size.

Dentigerous Cyst

Cysts may also arise from the enamel organ, and the classification of these cysts depends on the presence or absence of a tooth. If a cyst forms from the enamel organ before it has progressed to the stage of recognizable tooth formation it is called a *primordial cyst*. This cyst therefore represents an aborted tooth formation and is always associated with a missing tooth (Fig. 7-4).

If the cyst has formed over the crown of an embedded tooth it is called a *dentigerous cyst*. Three varieties of dentigerous cyst occur: the central, lateral and multilocular, which differ in the relation of the cystic process to the tooth. The central dentigerous cyst forms over the crown of the embedded tooth and may prevent eruption; it is the most common type. The lateral dentigerous cyst is located at the

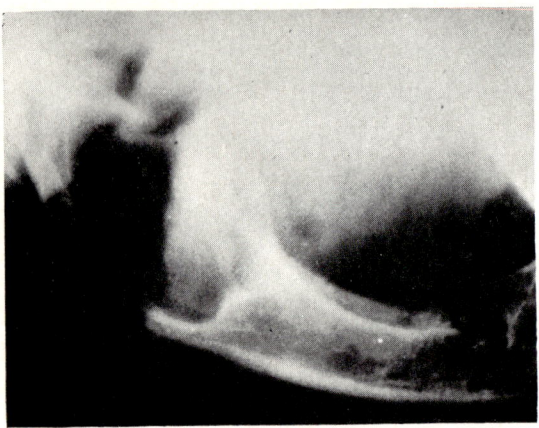

Figure 7-4. Primordial cyst. Note the radiolucency in the ascending ramus. The patient had noticed a swelling in the retromolar area which interfered with the wearing of her denture. Female, aged 45 years.

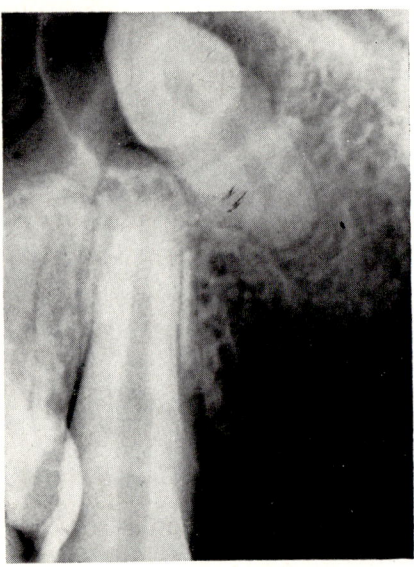

Figure 7-5. Dentigerous cyst. A radiolucency surrounds the crown of a mesiodens. The lesion was discovered on routine radiographic examination. Female, aged 35 years.

side of the affected tooth. The multilocular cyst results from the fusion or coalescence of several smaller cysts to form a many-chambered lesion. It should be noted that the ameloblastoma and central giant cell reparative granuloma may also appear as multiloculated lesions on a radiograph and it is essential to exclude these possibilities.

A dentigerous cyst is frequently asymptomatic and may be discovered on routine radiographic examination. There is commonly expansion of the overlying bone. Ultimately bone resorption occurs and the cyst lies directly beneath the mucosa and may present as a fluctuant mass. Displacement of teeth may occur.

RADIOGRAPHIC FEATURES. The crown of an unerupted tooth is observed in close association with a radiolucent area. As stated above the dentigerous cyst may be unilocular or multiloculated (Fig. 7-5).

TREATMENT. The treatment of the dentigerous cyst usually requires removal of the involved tooth and the entire cyst wall. It is important that the cyst wall be studied in the histopathology laboratory as proliferating odontogenic epithelium is frequently found in the wall or adjacent stroma. Residual epithelial remnants may cause a recurrence of the cyst or may develop into an ameloblastoma. For these reasons, the healing of the area should be followed radiographically at regular intervals. In those cases in which retention of the involved tooth is desirable, marsupialization may be performed and the tooth guided into a normal position in the dental arch. The excised cyst wall should be examined histologically and the patient should be re-examined at regular intervals.

Traumatic Cyst (Solitary Bone Cyst, Hemorrhagic Cyst)

The traumatic cyst is a rare bone lesion and almost invariably occurs in the mandible. The lesion is clinically asymptomatic and is usually detected during routine radiographic examination. The involved teeth are vital.

Of the several theories of its etiology the trauma-hemorrhage theory is mostly accepted. It suggests that following trauma, hemorrhage occurs within the bone leading to resorption of the latter followed by encapsulation and resorption of the clot.

RADIOGRAPHIC FEATURES. The lesion appears as a smoothly outlined radiolucency of varying size; the roots of the molars may give the cyst a scalloped appearance (Fig. 15-16).

TREATMENT. At surgery an empty cavity containing some yellowish fluid is commonly found. Hemorrhage into the cavity is encouraged and the lesion usually heals.

Lingual Mandibular Bone Cavity (Latent Bone Cyst)

This is not a true cyst but a clinically asymptomatic depression of the mandibular bone due to developmental inclusion of glandular tissue.

RADIOGRAPHIC FEATURES. On radiographic examination this lesion presents as a radiolucency situated towards the lower border of the mandible which is not associated with the apices of the teeth. Sialography will confirm the diagnosis (Fig. 7-6).

TREATMENT. None is indicated.

Neoplastic Odontogenic Lesions

The odontogenic tumors are neoplasms which arise from the tissues forming the dental organ. The overwhelming majority of these tumors are benign. Because the dental organ has both epithelial and mesenchymal components, these neoplasms may have the features of either, or both, germ layers. The neoplasm may mimic any stage of tooth development, from proliferating ameloblasts to fully formed teeth.

The classification of odontogenic tumors is of great importance to the oral pathologist but of limited interest to the general practitioner; hence an outline of the classification will be presented, followed by a

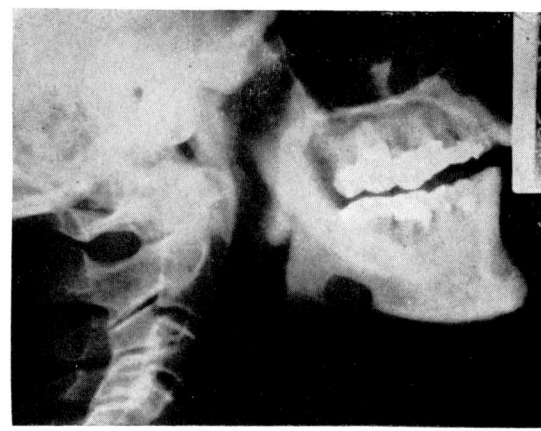

Figure 7-6. Lingual mandibular bone cavity. A radiolucency is present at the lower border of the mandible. The diagnosis was confirmed by sialography. Male, aged 37 years.

discussion of a prototype for each major grouping.

Classification of Odontogenic Tumors

1. *Epithelial odontogenic tumors:* (a) ameloblastoma, (b) adenoameloblastoma and (c) melanoameloblastoma.

2. *Mesenchymal odontogenic tumors:* (a) cementoma, (b) dentinoma, (c) odontogenic fibroma and (d) odontogenic myxoma.

The dentinoma and odontogenic myxoma are rare tumors and will not be discussed. The peripheral odontogenic fibroma is discussed in Chapter 5.

3. *Mixed odontogenic tumors:* (a) ameloblastic fibroma, (b) ameloblastic odontoma and (c) odontoma (complex and composite).

The ameloblastic fibroma and ameloblastic odontoma are exceedingly rare tumors and will not be discussed.

Epithelial Odontogenic Tumors

Ameloblastoma. The ameloblastoma is most common in the second through fifth decade of life and the generally cited average age is thirty-five years. It may be discovered on routine radiographic examination. As noted above, the tumor may arise in the wall of a dentigerous cyst.

On clinical examination, the affected area may appear normal or there may be enlargement of the jaw or displacement of teeth.

RADIOGRAPHIC FEATURES. The ameloblastoma usually presents as a single or multilocular radiolucency. Resorption of the roots of teeth in association with the tumor may occur (Fig. 7-7).

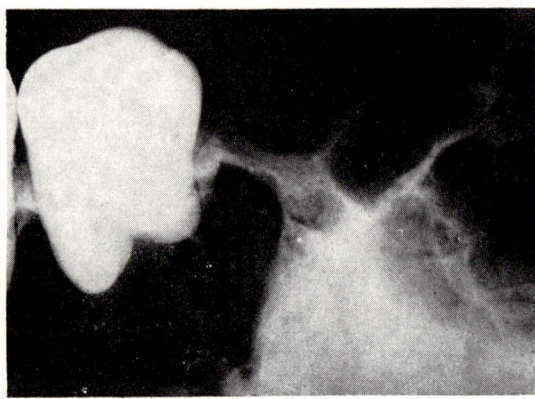

Figure 7-7. Ameloblastoma. Note the multilocular radiolucent lesion which extends into the ascending ramus. There is resorption of the roots of the mandibular second molar. Female, aged 30 years.

HISTOLOGIC FEATURES. The typical tumor is composed of sheets and cords of proliferating odontogenic epithelium, resembling ameloblasts. Islands of tumor cells infiltrate the stroma beyond the surgical and radiographic appearance of the lesion.

TREATMENT. Because the tumor has a tendency to infiltrate, it is, therefore, advisable to perform vigorous curettage or wide excision to prevent a recurrence. Approximately one-third of ameloblastomas recur, and careful postsurgical observation is advisable. Large lesions or extensive recurrences may require a marginal resection of the jaw but only very rarely is a complete resection indicated. Although the tumor is locally aggressive, it should be considered a benign neoplasm.

Adenoameloblastoma. The adenoameloblastoma is found in a much younger age group (usually under twenty years). The tumor does not tend to recur and local excision is usually curative.

Melanoameloblastoma. The melanoameloblastoma is seen in infants and is of disputed origin. The synonyms suggest other theories of histogenesis: retinal anlage tumor, melanotic odontogenic tumor of infancy, progonoma. Conservative surgical excision is the indicated therapy and recurrence is rare.

Mesenchymal Odontogenic Tumors

Cementoma. The cementoma will be discussed only as the prototype of the mesenchymal odontogenic tumors. This neoplasm typically presents at the apices of mandibular anterior teeth. The tumor may be single or multiple.

RADIOGRAPHIC FEATURES. In the initial phase, the tumor is osteolytic and presents as a radiolucency. As cementogenesis takes place, radiopacities are seen within the lesion and eventually the tumor becomes completely calcified. At the final stage, a radiolucent border usually persists around the mass of neoplastic cementum (Fig. 15-12 and 15-13).

TREATMENT. The initial stage of the cementoma resembles a dental granuloma. However, the cementoma is associated with a vital tooth and the astute practitioner should always consider this neoplasm in the differential diagnosis of periapical radiolucencies. Unless the lesion becomes extremely large, no treatment is indicated.

Odontoma (Complex and Composite). The compound or complex odontoma is occasionally considered the "end stage" of odontogenic neoplasia but is more appropriately classified as a hamartoma (tumor-like malformation). Enamel, dentin and cementum are seen in the odontomas. If the calcified masses resemble numerous small teeth, the lesion is called a *compound odontoma;* if the arrangement is more bizarre, it is classified as a *complex odontoma.*

The odontoma is usually asymptomatic but may produce facial asymmetry when of sufficient size and interfere with the eruption of adjacent teeth.

RADIOGRAPHIC FEATURES. Radiographs reveal a well-defined radiopaque mass which may resemble several small teeth. Cyst formation may be associated with the odontoma (Fig. 7-8).

TREATMENT. Excision is the indicated treatment.

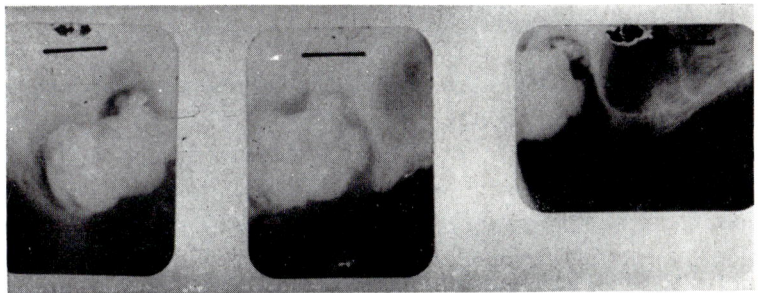

Figure 7-8. Cystic odontoma. Three views of the same lesion which is a complex odontoma associated with a cyst. The patient presented with swelling of the maxilla and inability to wear his denture. Male, aged 57 years.

INFLAMMATORY BONE DISEASE

Dry Socket

This is a well-recognized complication of tooth extraction. The patient returns a day or two following tooth removal with severe pain. On examination, the clot is disintegrating and the socket may be filled with food or other debris. Lower teeth are more frequently affected than upper teeth.

RADIOGRAPHIC FEATURES. This is of little help but will exclude the presence of a fracture or retained roots.

HISTOLOGIC FEATURES. Histologic examination shows the very localized nature of the infection. There is a localized acute osteitis which involves the lamina dura but not the medullary bone.

TREATMENT. The socket is gently irrigated with warm saline and the exposed bone is covered for several days with some bland preparation, for example, zinc oxide and eugenol mixed with gauze. Antibiotics are not usually indicated.

Osteomyelitis

Inflammation of the cortical and medullary bone is termed "osteomyelitis." When the jaws are involved the condition may be localized or spread throughout the bone. Acute, subacute and chronic forms occur and the chronic form may sometimes be sclerosing in nature. The most common cause of osteomyelitis of the jaws is dental infection and with the widespread use of antibiotics to control these infections, it has become much less common in the last two or three decades.

Suppurative Osteomyelitis

In addition to dental infection, jaw fracture (especially if a tooth is retained in the fracture line) or a deep penetrating facial wound may provide a route for invasion of the bone. The organism is rarely blood borne. *Staphylococcus aureus* is the most frequently found pathogen associated with the disease. The mandible is much more frequently involved than the maxilla.

The condition often presents with pain and swelling of the jaws and overlying soft tissue. The patient is frequently feverish and looks and feels unwell. Pus may be draining through skin or mucosal fistulae and may ooze around the teeth. Frequently, there is anesthesia or paresthesia of the lower lip, cervical lymphadenopathy and trismus.

The above is a description of the acute condition. Following the escape of pus, the symptoms are much less noticeable, and the condition enters the subacute phase. Drainage becomes intermittent and small pieces of dead bone, sequestra, may be extruded from the fistulae. The subacute phase lasts for a varying length of time and acute exacerbations may occur or the disease may become chronic. Most of the symptoms will then disappear, though pus continues to ooze from the fistulae. The administration of antibiotics will alter the clinical picture.

RADIOGRAPHIC FEATURES. Radiographic changes are not seen for the first few days but after about one week the bony trabeculae become indistinct. Later, the typical "moth-eaten" appearance is seen and irregular sequestra, separated from the main bony mass, may be recognized. These changes will not be seen unless the disease is allowed to progress. (Fig. 7-9).

HISTOLOGIC FEATURES. The histopathologic appearance is of infiltration of the

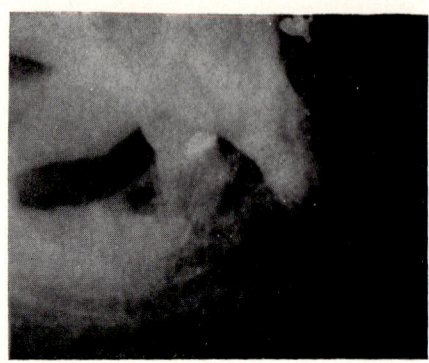

Figure 7-9. Acute suppurative osteomyelitis. The patient presented with pain, swelling and paresthesia of the lip in the distribution of the right mental nerve ten days after extraction of a mandibular first molar. Note the "moth-eaten" appearance of the bone. Treated by sequestrectomy and antibiotics. Female, aged 35 years.

marrow spaces with bacteria and inflammatory cells. The latter are mostly polymorphonuclear leukocytes but there are some lymphocytes and plasma cells. The marrow is being destroyed and the cortical bone is dying. Localized thrombosis occurs and leads to further bone destruction.

TREATMENT. This consists of the administration of antibiotics, drainage of pus and removal of sequestra. The sequelae of osteomyelitis may be unsightly facial scars, pathological fracture or tooth loss. The more serious complications include infected emboli carried to the brain with resultant abscess formation. When the maxilla is involved, cavernous sinus thrombosis may occur.

Chronic Sclerosing Osteomyelitis

This may be focal or diffuse. The focal form or *condensing osteitis* is seen most frequently around the apex of a nonvital lower first molar in the young patient. The disease appears to represent a high resistance of the tissues to mild infection.

RADIOGRAPHIC FEATURES. The condition appears as a sclerotic, radiopaque area

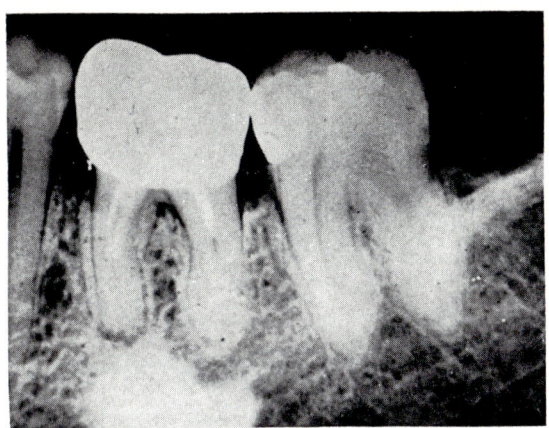

Figure 7-10. Condensing osteitis. There is a radiopacity associated with the roots of an inadequately treated mandibular first molar. Male, aged 50 years.

which remains even after extraction of the tooth (Fig. 7-10).

HISTOPATHOLOGIC FEATURES. The lesion consists of an amorphous mass of bonelike material. The diagnosis is made clinically and treatment is seldom indicated.

The *diffuse* form is seen in older patients. It may be related to decreased blood supply and lowered resistance. It is probably a similar process to the focal form but is more widespread in the bone. The mandibular molar region is frequently involved. The lesion may be symptomless or give rise to a dull, poorly localized pain. There may be draining fistulae.

RADIOGRAPHIC FEATURES. This reveals a diffuse sclerosis with ill-defined margins.

HISTOLOGIC FEATURES. Dense irregular trabeculae are present and the marrow spaces are replaced by fibrous tissue containing an inflammatory infiltrate.

TREATMENT. Extractions should be avoided in the involved region as the sockets are slow to heal and much pain may follow tooth removal. If the patient is asymptomatic, treatment is not usually indicated. Should symptoms occur and persist, antibiotic therapy and occasionally removal of the affected bone may be necessary.

Other Forms of Osteomyelitis

Rarely, tuberculous, syphilitic and actinomycotic osteomyelitis are seen. They will not be discussed here but should always be borne in mind when the differential diagnosis of a bone infection is being considered.

Osteoradionecrosis

This disease may follow irradiation of the oral cavity for treatment of cancer. The irradiated bone becomes relatively avascular and the extraction of teeth (or even the wearing of dentures over the involved region) may result in necrosis of bone.

The main clinical feature is exposed bone and this is accompanied by severe pain. The necrotic bone slowly sequestrates, the disease progresses inexorably and eating becomes difficult, with resultant malnourishment and weight loss (Fig. 7-11).

RADIOGRAPHIC FEATURES. Radiographic changes are similar to those of osteomyelitis and do not often aid diagnosis.

HISTOLOGIC FEATURES. Histologically, there is an obliterative endarteritis with massive death of bone. Inflammatory infiltration is present to a varying extent.

TREATMENT. This is extremely difficult. Supportive measures include attention to the diet.

Preventive Measures

These are most important. In the days when low-voltage x-ray machines were used for irradiation of oral neoplasms, the disease was much more common and full-mouth extractions were advised for patients who were to undergo therapy of this type. Bone absorbs low-voltage radiation much more than soft tissue and extractions

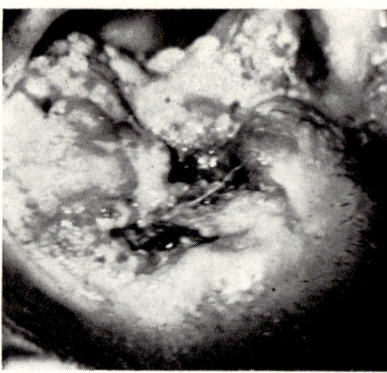

Figure 7-11. Osteoradionecrosis of the mandible. Note the necrotic bone and discharging sinuses in a patient who had received radiotherapy for a squamous cell carcinoma of the floor of the mouth. Male, aged 57 years.

carried out even years later might lead to osteoradionecrosis. Now that high energy x-ray and cobalt and cesium units are used, bone absorption is much the same as that of soft tissue and in addition the irradiated area is better delineated. For this reason, a more conservative approach may be taken.

The decision for the removal of teeth prior to radiation therapy is based upon the following factors: (a) extensive caries, (b) moderate to advanced periodontal involvement, (c) lack of opposing teeth and consequent loss of function and self-cleansing action, (d) partial impaction or incomplete eruption and (e) extensive periapical lesions.

The patient should be taught home-care procedures consisting of (a) brushing, (b) oral lavage and (c) topical fluoride gel in an applicator. These home-care procedures should be carried out during radiotherapy and for the rest of the patient's life.

The fluoride application utilizes (a) plastic carriers, constructed for each individual dental arch (b) fluoride gel,* placed in the carrier and (c) the carrier, placed over the teeth and left in place for five minutes.

Should the extraction of a tooth in an area of irradiated bone become necessary, extreme care should be taken to avoid excessive trauma and an antibiotic cover should be given.

* The fluoride gel used at M. D. Anderson Hospital and Tumor Institute, Houston, Texas, has the following composition

Sodium Fluoride	7.0 gm
Sodium Phosphate, Tribasic	7.0 gm
Sodium Carboxymethylcellulose ether sodium salt	19.6 gm
Citric Acid	3.5 gm
Saccharine Sodium	0.14 gm or 140 mg
Distilled water q.s. to 700 cc	
Add I cc of flavoring to the above (mixed in blender)	
Flavoring:	
Lemon Oil, terpeneless	2 cc
Orange Oil, terpeneless	2 cc
Tween 20	4 cc
Alcohol, Ethyl (95%) q.s. to 40 cc	

NONINFLAMMATORY BONE DISEASE

Giant Cell Lesions

There is a variety of lesions occurring in the jaw bones characterized by the presence of many multinucleated giant cells. There is no clear understanding of the precise nature of the various conditions and numerous attempts have been made to classify them. Lesions which contain giant cells such as osteogenic sarcoma and fibrous dysplasia will be dealt with elsewhere in this chapter. Giant cell reparative granuloma and lesions due to hyperparathyroidism will be mentioned in this section.

Giant Cell Reparative Granuloma

The giant cell reparative granuloma is thought to be formed as a response to injury. It occurs usually in children or young adults. The mandible is more often involved than the maxilla. The lesion may or may not be painful and may present simply as a bulging of the cortical plates.

RADIOGRAPHIC FEATURES. The radiograph shows a radiolucency which may have a smooth or irregular border. The lesion may have a multiloculated appearance (Fig. 7-12).

TREATMENT. The treatment of a reparative granuloma is by curettage following which the area fills with normal bone. When a histologic diagnosis of giant cell tumor or giant cell lesion of the jawbone is made, the serum calcium and phosphorus levels and clinical examination should be made to rule out the possibility of the lesion being a manifestation of hyperparathyroidism.

Hyperparathyroidism

The parathyroid glands are intimately involved in the metabolism of calcium and phosphorus and exert an action not only directly on the bone but also on the renal excretion of inorganic phosphorus. Excess parathyroid hormone results in disturbances in calcium and phosphorus metabolism and changes in the skeleton. In advanced cases of hyperparathyroidism, there may be widespread development of bony radiolucencies and the terms "osteitis fibrosa cystica" or "von Recklinghausen's disease" have been used to describe this condition. Not infrequently, the jawbones are involved, and on occasion, the dentist may be the first to suspect that a patient is suffering from a disorder of the parathyroids.

RADIOGRAPHIC FEATURES. The oral manifestations, which are usually late features of the disease, consist for the most part of radiologic changes. There is a generalized increased radiolucency of the jaws, often with the appearance of discrete "cystlike" radiolucent areas. As a result of increased osteoclastic activity, the trabeculae are thinner and appear lacelike radiographically. The loss of lamina dura around the teeth, a frequently described feature of hyperparathyroidism, is a matter of some dispute and it should be remembered that in many normal mouths the lamina dura is not seen clearly (Fig. 7-13 A, B).

LABORATORY FINDINGS. The diagnosis of hyperparathyroidism cannot be made from x-ray evaluation of the jaws alone. Analyses of the serum and urinary calcium and phosphorus and serum alkaline phosphatase are necessary. The serum calcium is elevated in all cases.

HISTOLOGIC FEATURES. The "cystic areas" show marked osteoclastic and osteoblastic activity with thinning of the cancellous trabeculae, widening of the marrow spaces and fibrosis of the marrow. There are numerous giant cells throughout and often evidence of bleeding. These lesions have been called "brown tumors," the color being due to the presence of blood pigment. They are of similar histologic type to the giant cell lesions discussed above. Occa-

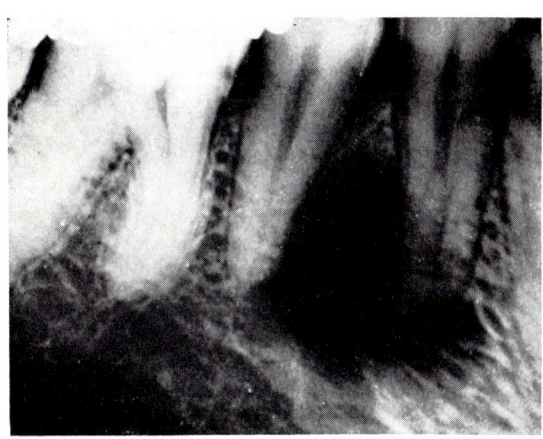

Figure 7-12. Giant cell reparative granuloma. The radiolucent lesion between the mandibular premolars was discovered on routine radiographic examination. Both teeth were vital. The lesion was explored and the diagnosis made histologically. Male, aged 30 years.

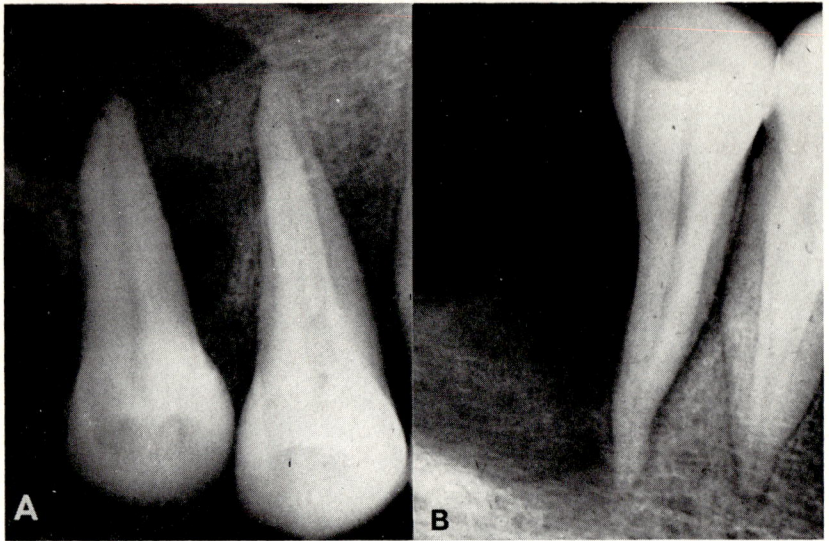

Figure 7-13. Hyperparathyroidism. Note the increased radiolucency and loss of lamina dura in the maxilla (A) and mandible (B). Female, aged 47 years.

sionally peripheral lesions occur and may resemble the peripheral giant cell reparative granuloma.

Histiocytosis X

There is a group of diseases which have been collectively described as histiocytosis X. The group comprises Letterer-Siwe disease, Hand-Schuller-Christian disease and eosinophilic granuloma. In each disease, there is an underlying disorder of the reticulo-endothelial system with the production of many histiocytes. Although relatively uncommon, they are of interest to the dentist because each of the diseases may produce changes in the jawbones. For convenience, the principal features of each will be summarized but it should not be forgotten that there is much overlap between the diseases and the distinction between them is not clear.

Letterer-Siwe Disease

This rare condition occurs most often in children under one year of age. There are generalized lymphadenopathy, splenomegaly, hepatomegaly and blood disorders. There is a widespread histiocytic proliferation throughout the body, particularly in the skin, spleen, liver, lymph nodes and bone. The lesions in the jaws present as multiple radiolucencies and there may be abnormal loosening of the teeth.

Hand-Schuller-Christian Disease

This is a more chronic disease than the aforementioned. It affects children or adults, runs a more prolonged course and the prognosis in any particular case is difficult to determine. There is a proliferation of histiocytes which are laden with lipid. The same organs are involved as in the Letterer-Siwe variant but the most striking feature is the occurrence of bony lesions in the cranium. The jaws may be the site of multiple radiolucencies (Fig. 7-14, A, B, C).

Eosinophilic Granuloma

In this variation of histiocytosis X, there are seldom more than one or two bones involved and often no skin or visceral in-

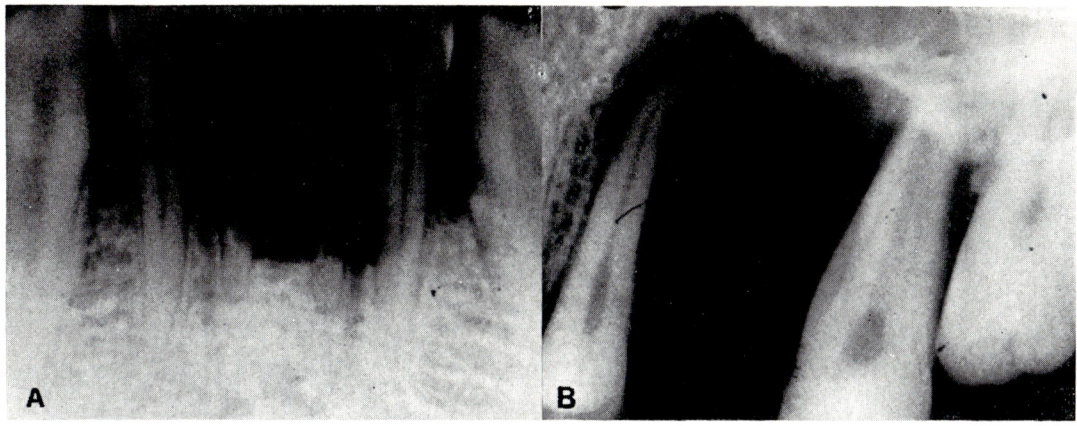

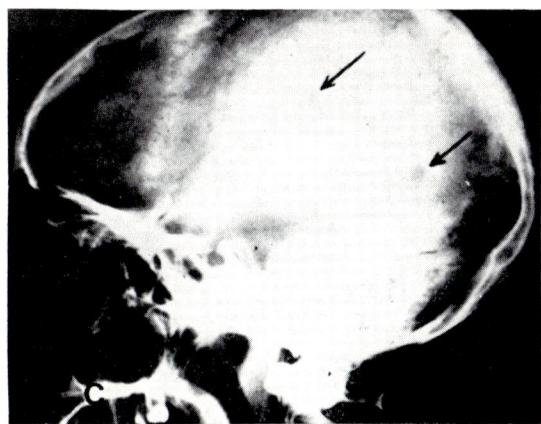

Figure 7-14. Histiocytosis X. Radiolucent areas and bone loss are present in the mandibular incisor region (A) and maxillary first molar area (B). A biopsy of abnormal tissue from the maxilla established the diagnosis. The lateral radiograph of the skull (C) shows two radiolucent areas (arrows). Male, aged 35 years.

volvement. The disease occurs in older children or adults and the prognosis is the best of the three diseases of the group. The cranial bones are often the first to be affected. In the jaw, the disease presents a a well-circumscribed radiolucency which on histologic examination shows histiocytes, plasma cells, lymphocytes and a preponderance of eosinophils.

These three diseases are relatively rare but they should be considered in the differential diagnosis of jaw radiolucencies. The definitive diagnosis is made on clinical, radiographic and histologic grounds.

Multiple Myeloma

This disease occurs in adults and affects males more than females, in the ratio of 3:2. There is widespread bony involve-

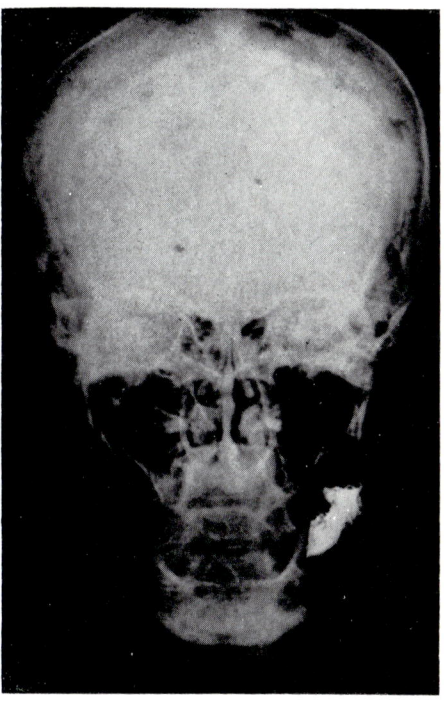

Figure 7-15. Multiple myeloma. Note the radiopaque pack in the left side of the mandible from which tissue had been removed at biopsy. There are multiple radiolucencies in the skull. Bence Jones protein was present in the urine. Male, aged 56 years.

ment characterized by the anaplastic proliferation of plasma cells. The precise relationship between the development of a single tumor mass consisting of plasma cells (solitary plasmocytoma of soft tissue or bone) and the condition of generalized multiple myeloma is not clear. It is believed by many that the single lesion presages the eventual development of multiple myeloma. In addition to the bony lesions, there is hyperglobulinemia with the production of abnormal globulins which can be detected by serum electrophoresis. Bence Jones proteinuria is present in some cases. The jaw lesions present as radiolucencies and there may be such destruction of the cortical bone that the lesions can be felt through a bony surface defect. Occasionally, jaw lesions may be the presenting signs of the disease and the finding of atypical plasma cells in a biopsy specimen from a jaw radiolucency indicates the need for a clinical examination with evaluation of serum proteins and urine (Fig. 7-15).

FIBRO-OSSEOUS LESIONS OF THE JAWS

Controversy still rages as to the true nature and correct classification of fibro-osseous jaw lesions. Several conditions exist in which the normal bony architecture is replaced by fibrous tissue with the deposition of bonelike material.

These changes may differ in their clinical manifestations, histologic and radiographic appearances and need for treatment. For these reasons, it would seem worthwhile to attempt to differentiate them, even though they may be variations of the same condition.

Some of these diseases are seen only in the jaws, others are associated with bony changes or soft tissue lesions in other parts of the body.

Fibrous Dysplasia

This fibro-osseous expansion may occur in one bone (monostotic) or several bones (polyostotic). Most authors accept both diseases as variations of the same process. The polyostotic form is occasionally accompanied by pigmented areas on the skin and mucous membranes and by sexual precocity (Albright's syndrome).

The monostotic form of the disease which involves the jaws, *facial fibrous dysplasia*, will be discussed in some detail.

Females are affected by this disease more frequently than males and the maxilla more often than the mandible. Most cases present below the age of thirty years, but the disease may be seen at any age. In general, the younger the patient, the more severe the condition.

The most common presentation is a gradually enlarging swelling of the jaws, found on routine examination by the dentist or noticed by the patient. Occasionally, noneruption of teeth or movement of teeth with a resultant malocclusion may be the first sign of the disease. Less frequently, it may be heralded by facial pain, infection or jaw fracture.

The enlargement is hard, smooth, ill defined and not tender to palpation. It produces facial deformity which is more obvious in the maxilla than in the mandible (Fig. 7-16, A).

The lesion continues to grow slowly but in most cases no further expansion occurs after the age of thirty. Occasionally, an active lesion is seen in a patient in later life.

LABORATORY FINDINGS. The serum calcium and phosphorus are normal but the serum alkaline phosphatase may be raised.

RADIOGRAPHIC FEATURES. When examined radiologically, changes are seen in the bony contour of the jaws and in the pattern of trabeculae. The border between

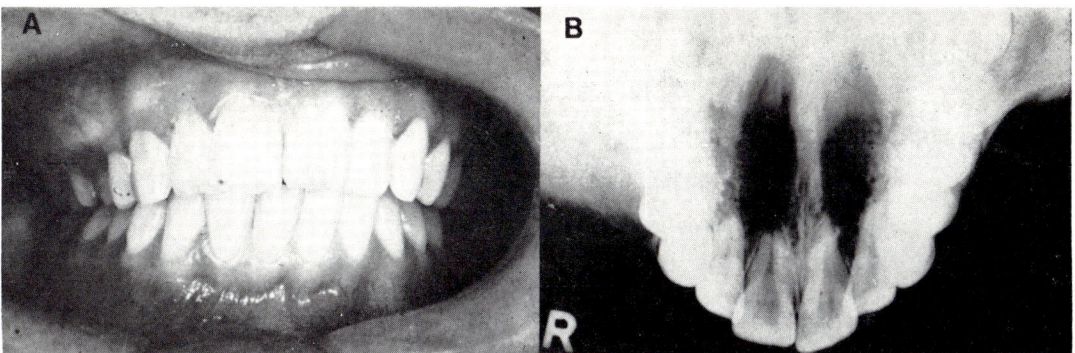

Figure 7-16. Fibrous dysplasia. There is enlargement of the right maxilla distal to the canine (A). The occlusal radiograph (B) shows the "ground glass" appearance of the affected area. Female, aged 19 years.

cortical and medullary bone becomes obliterated early. Changes in the trabecular pattern have been likened to "ground glass," "thumbprints" or "orange peel" but often there is simply an area of radiolucency with an overall mottled effect (Fig. 7-16, B).

HISTOLOGIC FEATURES. On histologic examination, normal bone is seen to be replaced by fibrous tissue which in turn becomes replaced by bonelike tissue. The process may then recommence and be repeated during the active stage of the disease. The trabeculae of the bonelike tissue have an irregular shape and some writers have described the presence of lamellar bone and spherical calcified masses in the lesion. Collections of inflammatory cells may be encountered, especially near areas of hemorrhage.

Following the early phase, in which formation of fibrous tissue and bonelike tissue occurs at a rapid rate, the progress of the disease becomes slower. Expansion of the involved bone ceases and it is thought by many writers that mature bone is eventually deposited in the involved area.

TREATMENT. Treatment is usually directed towards surgical removal of the excess bony tissue to improve appearance or to allow for the construction of dentures.

Radiotherapy is contraindicated and has resulted in malignant change. Rarely, sarcomatous change has occurred in patients who have not undergone irradiation. For this reason, sudden increase in size of the lesion or pain developing in a previously painless lesion should be carefully investigated.

Cherubism

Cherubism is an inherited disease though the occasional sporadic case is reported. The term "cherubism" is usefully descriptive and serves to differentiate the lesion from fibrous dysplasia and giant cell tumor.

The disease manifests itself between two and four years of age. A hard, nontender enlargement is seen bilaterally in the region of the mandibular angle and sometimes the maxillary molar region. As the disease progresses, the facial skin becomes stretched over the swelling with resultant pulling down of the lower eyelids, leading to an upward tilting of the eyes. This combination of deformities gives the so-called cherubic expression to the patient. Submandibular lymphadenopathy often occurs. There may be gross abnormalities of the dentition with disturbance of the occlusion and failure of eruption of teeth.

The disease progresses for about five or six years and usually ceases by the age of sixteen. Regression of the process almost always occurs and there may be no residual signs of the disease in the adult.

The familial nature of this lesion, its predilection for the mandible, the typical facies associated with it and the age of onset help to differentiate cherubism from fibrous dysplasia.

RADIOGRAPHIC FEATURES. Symmetrical radiolucencies occur in the mandibular molar regions. The lesion may have a multilocular cystic appearance or may have the radiographic appearance of fibrous dysplasia. The maxillary lesions are usually more diffuse (Fig. 7-17).

HISTOLOGIC FEATURES. On histologic examination, the lesion is seen to consist of a fibrous tissue stroma in which are seen giant cells in clusters. Scattered areas of hemorrhage are also seen.

TREATMENT. This is a self-limiting disease and more harm than good is done by radical surgery. Removal of teeth in the involved area is advocated by some writers.

Ossifying Fibroma and Fibro-osteoma

These lesions have been variously categorized as true bone neoplasms and a well-circumscribed type of monostotic fibrous dysplasia.

They may present at any age, though the patient is usually over the age of five years. As with other fibro-osseous lesions, ossifying fibroma may present as a smooth, nontender swelling of the jaws, covered with normal-looking mucosa. It may be noticed by the patient or may have interfered with the fit or construction of dentures.

The main feature which differentiates this lesion clinically from fibrous dysplasia is its usually well-defined borders.

RADIOGRAPHIC FEATURES. Radiographically, a well-circumscribed radiolucent defect is seen, in which lie radiopaque masses of varying size. The lesion expands the jaw and a thin rim of radiopaque material may overly the radiolucent area.

HISTOLOGIC FEATURES. The lesion is predominantly fibrous tissue in which are islands of calcified material which may include bone, cementum or amorphous material. When these areas consist of mature bone, the term "fibro-osteoma" is used by some pathologists to describe the lesion.

TREATMENT. Ossifying fibromas may become very large if left untreated and for this reason they are usually removed surgically. With complete removal, they are unlikely to recur.

Paget's Disease

Paget's disease or osteitis deformans is seen more commonly in men and the patients are usually over forty years of age. Bony changes lead to an increase in size of the head, rounded shoulders, sunken chest and bowing of the legs. There may be headache and facial pain. Deafness and blindness may occur as the disease progresses. These effects are caused by encroachment of the proliferating bone onto the cranial nerves as they pass out of the

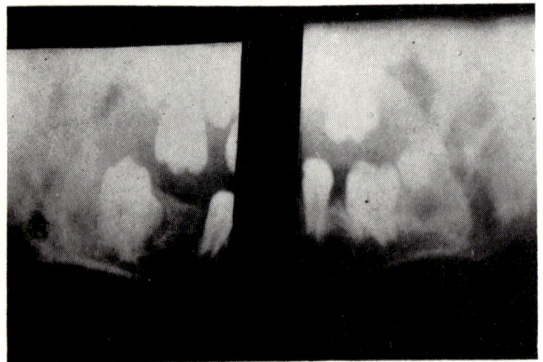

Figure 7-17. Cherubism. There are multilocular radiolucent areas present in both ascending rami. Male, aged 12 years.

skull through their various foramina. The serum alkaline phosphatase level is markedly raised.

The oral changes may be seen early in the disease. The maxilla is commonly involved in the disease process and expansion of the bone, leading to difficulty in insertion of a denture, is a not uncommon presenting symptom (Fig. 7-18).

Other changes involving the oral structures are enlargement of the alveolus and displacement of teeth. Hypercementosis, seen in some cases, is associated with difficulty in the extraction of teeth and failure of the sockets to heal.

RADIOGRAPHIC FEATURES. Typical radiographic findings are a "ground glass" appearance in the early stages and later a "cotton wool" appearance (Fig. 19-7). Variations in the radiographic pattern may be seen in different regions of the same patient.

HISTOLOGIC FEATURES. The pathological process is initially osteoclastic. The resorbed bone is replaced with vascular fibrous tissue, resulting in the "ground glass" appearance of the early lesions. Later, coarse fibrous bone in irregular trabeculae is seen giving rise to a "cotton wool" appearance on the radiograph. As the disease process becomes less active, these trabeculae become thicker and are seen as a mosaic pattern histologically.

TREATMENT. Treatment is symptomatic. Many patients die of heart failure, as the vascular bone acts as an enormous arteriovenous shunt. The most serious complication is that of sarcoma which is a not uncommon cause of the patient's death.

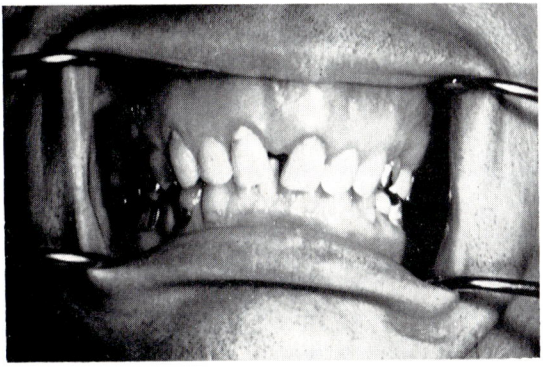

Figure 7-18. Paget's disease. There is enlargement of the labial aspect of the maxilla with displacement of teeth. The patient had noticed increasing protrusion of the upper lip. The alkaline phosphatase level was high. Male, aged 55 years.

NONODONTOGENIC NEOPLASMS

There is a large number of tumor types that may occur in the jaws. They may arise primarily within the jaws from bone or cartilage, or they may develop as metastatic growths from tumors of lung, breast, prostate, thyroid or kidney or as manifestations of generalized neoplastic conditions such as leukemia or Hodgkin's disease. Only the most common tumors will be discussed.

Osteoma

The most common benign tumor of the jaws is an osteoma. It may be confused with excessive bony development either within a bone (enostosis) or jutting out from its surface (exostosis). Osteomas within the jaws produce well-circumscribed radiopaque masses. They are sometimes difficult to distinguish from dense bone produced in an inflammatory process or developing in a malignant neoplasm. The osteoma is slow growing and it may be a long time before any distortion of cortical bone develops (Fig. 7-19). In such cases, an osteoma is likely to be undetected unless seen during radiographic examination of the jaws. Exostoses of the jaw (ex-

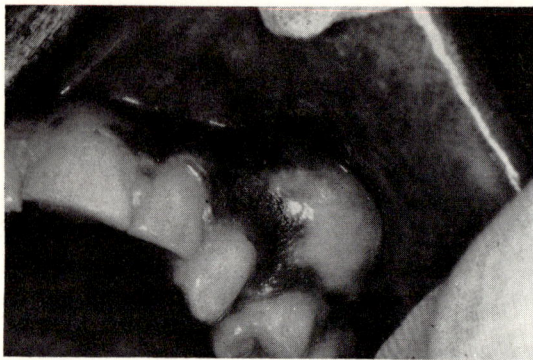

Figure 7-19. Osteoma. The lesion had been present for five months and had increased in size. Female, aged 16 years.

cluding torus palatinus and torus mandibularis) usually are seen as small protuberances on the buccal alveolar bone of the maxilla particularly in the molar area; the mucosa covering them is normal.

TREATMENT. There is no indication for surgical removal of an osteoma, torus palatinus or torus mandibularis unless it interferes with the construction of a prosthetic appliance.

Torus Palatinus

The incidence of some form of torus palatinus in adults has been estimated at about 20 percent. Women are more likely to have a palatine torus than men. The growth presents as a variably shaped midline palatal protuberance. The overlying mucosa is normally unremarkable. The torus consists of either dense compact bone or a compact shell with a cancellous center (see Ch. 19).

RADIOGRAPHIC FEATURES. A torus palatinus is often delineated clearly by a maxillary occlusal radiograph.

Torus Mandibularis

The torus mandibularis occurs in about 5 percent of adults. The condition is usually bilateral and presents as a protuberance on the lingual surface of the mandible in the premolar region. The lesion may be of varying shape and is sometimes multilobular (see Ch. 19).

RADIOGRAPHIC FEATURES. Occasionally, on intraoral radiographic examination, a torus mandibularis appears to resemble an enostosis. Clinical examination usually clarifies the diagnosis.

Osteogenic Sarcoma

This malignant tumor of osseous tissue may show a variety of histologic patterns. In some cases, there is much bone destruction; in others, there is marked osteogenesis. The condition is most frequently seen in young patients and males are affected more than females. Pain and swelling are quite frequently presenting features and if there is nerve involvement, paresthesia may result. Loosening of teeth may occur and for this reason the dentist is often the

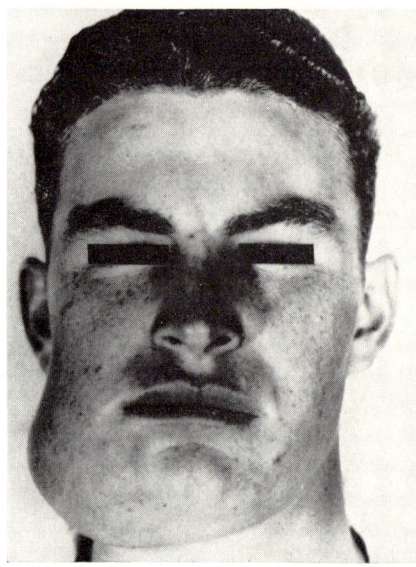

Figure 7-20. Osteogenic sarcoma. The patient presented with a swelling of the mandible which was increasing in size over a period of three months. All the involved teeth were vital. Radiographic examination showed an osteoblastic lesion. Biopsy established the diagnosis. A hemimandibulectomy was performed. Male, aged 27 years.

first person consulted about the disease (Fig. 7-20).

Although an osteogenic sarcoma has the potential for forming bone a rapidly growing tumor may be fleshy and soft.

RADIOGRAPHIC FEATURES. The radiographic features of this disease are variable. In tumors in which there is much osteogenesis, there is an increased radiodensity of the area and a destruction of the normal lamellar pattern of the bone. A "sun ray" appearance of a radiograph results from the irregular spicules of bone projecting outwards from the periphery of a lesion. Osteolytic lesions produce irregular radiolucencies and there is nothing characteristic about these radiographic appearances.

TREATMENT. The treatment of osteogenic sarcoma is by surgical and radiotherapeutic measures. The prognosis is poor and the five-year cure rate is less than 25 percent.

Metastatic Neoplasms and Generalized Neoplastic Conditions

Metastatic growths in the maxilla or mandible may occur from a large variety of primary tumors. Metastases of the jaw are not common, although on occasion a jaw metastasis may be the first overt manifestation of malignant disease. The mandible is more frequently involved than the maxilla and the molar area is the site of predilection. Involvement of periapical bone or nerves will produce loose teeth or paresthesia, respectively.

RADIOGRAPHIC FEATURES. Most of the metastases are osteolytic and appear as irregular radiolucencies. Occasionally, a metastatic osteogenic lesion occurs and in such cases an increased radiopacity of the area results.

DIFFERENTIAL DIAGNOSIS. The possibility of metastatic growth should always be considered in the differential diagnosis and histologic examination of any tissue removed from surgical explorations of bony lesions. Certain of the blood dyscrasias and neoplasms of the lymphoid system also involve the jaws. They may produce signs, symptoms and radiologic changes similar to those described for malignant and metastatic neoplasms.

SUMMARY

Diseases of the jaws may be of local or systemic origin. When confronted with an unusual lesion the practitioner should consider extraoral radiographs in addition to periapical views (see Ch. 6). In some cases a lateral skull view may be necessary to ascertain whether the skull bones are affected (for example, multiple myeloma and histiocytosis X). In conditions involving the jawbones the serum calcium, phosphorus and alkaline phosphatase levels are indicated. To establish a definitive diagnosis a biopsy is essential. However, if the patient is pale (anemia) or plethoric (polycythemia) or if there is evidence of purpura (bleeding into the skin or from mucous membranes) or a history of a bleeding tendency, further tests are necessary before a biopsy is taken. These should include a hemoglobin level, a hematocrit and differential white cell count. In addition the bleeding time, clotting time, partial thromboplastin time and prothrombin time should be ascertained. If these are within normal limits, it is safe to biopsy the lesion without encountering excessive hemorrhage.

On occasions, a lesion may be syphilitic

or secondary to tuberculosis of the lungs. Therefore for completeness the STS (serum test for syphilis) and a chest radiograph are indicated.

REFERENCES

1. Dahlgren, S. E., Lind, P. O., Lindbom, A., and Martensson, R.: Fibrous dysplasia of jaw bones. A clinical, roentgenographic and histopathologic study. *Acta Otolaryngol (Stockh), 68:257,* 1969.
2. Gorlin, R. J., and Goldman, H. M.: *Thoma's Oral Pathology,* 6th ed. St. Louis, Mosby, 1970.
3. Jones, J. C., Lilly, E. S., and Marlette, R. H.: Histiocytosis X. *J Oral Surg, 28(6):* June, 1970.
4. Jones, W. A.: Cherubism. *Oral Surg, 20(5):* 648, 1965.
5. *Oral Care for Oral Cancer Patients.* U. S. Public Health Service Publication No. 1958, 1968.
6. Schmaman, A., Smith, I., and Ackerman, L. V.: Benign fibro-osseous lesions of the mandible and maxilla. *Cancer, 26(2):*303, 1970.
7. Selected papers from conference on surgical pathology of the jaws. *Oral Surg, 28(1):* Jan., 1970.
8. Shafer, W. G., Hine, M. K., and Levy, B. M.: *Textbook of Oral Pathology,* 2nd ed. Philadelphia, Saunders, 1963.

Chapter 8

Headache and Facial Pain

Lawrence Cohen

THE PHYSIOLOGY OF PAIN

RECENTLY a gate control theory of pain has been proposed in which it is postulated that the cortex controls afferent input in terms of its meaning to the individual.[1-3] This theory involves four neural components.

1. *A modulating (gating) spinal cord system.* This system controls the amount of input transmitted from receptors and peripheral fibers through the dorsal horn cells to the ascending fibers in the anterolateral part of the spinal cord.

2. *A sensory discriminative system.* Incoming stimuli are localized in space and time and according to intensity by means of this system.

3. *A motivational-affective (action) system.* This system contributes the quality of unpleasantness and forces the individual to take action aimed at stopping the distress.

4. *A central control (cognitive) system.* This system evaluates and analyzes input in terms of past experience. It regulates response and behavior through inhibiting or facilitating influences on the discriminative and motivational systems.

Receptors and Afferent Fibers

Body sensory function is served by two basic types of receptor organs—free nerve endings and specialized corpuscular regulators. They function by transducing mechanical, thermal and chemical energy into electrical impulses. Free nerve endings are sensitive to all physical modalities, but different endings differ in their sensitivities and thresholds to different stimuli. On the other hand, the corpuscular endings are mainly responsive to various forms of deformation including vibration (pacinian corpuscles).

It is believed that chemical substances formed in tissues in response to injury may increase the sensitivity of some receptors.[4,5] These include histamine from mast cells, 5-hydroxytryptamine (serotonin) from disintegrating platelets, acetylcholine and peptides of the bradykinin group. The kinins have algesic (pain-producing) effects in extremely low concentrations, suggesting that they are special chemical mediators for receptors activated by injury.[5]

The axons serving the receptors differ in size. The larger fibers are the most rapidly conducting and have the lowest threshold. The smallest fibers are the slowest conducting and have the highest threshold.

The surface of the body and the oral mucous membrane have the most extensive innervation. Within skin and mucous membrane are networks of free nerve endings.

Specialized endings, sensitive to pressure and served by large fibers, lie below the epidermis of the palms and soles, in mucocutaneous regions and in the deeper layers of the skin and subcutaneously.

HEADACHE

Pathophysiology of Headache

According to Wolff[6] the following are pain-sensitive structures of the head:

1. The tissues covering the cranium are all more or less sensitive to pain, the arteries being especially so.

2. Of the intracranial structures, the great venous sinuses and their venous tributaries from the surface of the brain, parts of the dura at the base, the dural arteries and the cerebral arteries at the base of the brain, the fifth, the ninth and tenth cranial nerves and the upper three cervical nerves are sensitive to pain.

The fifth cranial nerve is the pathway for pain arising from the pain-sensitive intracranial structures above the tentorium cerebelli. The ninth and tenth cranial nerves and the upper three cervical nerves convey pain impulses from the pain-sensitive intracranial structures below the tentorium cerebelli.

Diagnostic Features of Headaches

Incidence

The vascular headaches of migraine and the headaches from sustained muscular contraction are the most commonly encountered headaches. Headaches are associated with fever and septicemia. These probably rank next in frequency, followed by those due to nasal, paranasal and eye disease. The least common forms of headache are those associated with meningitis and brain tumor.[6]

Intensity

The headaches associated with ruptured intracranial aneurysm, meningitis, fever, migraine and arterial hypertension are the most intense. Ruptured intracranial aneurysm and meningitis are accompanied by a stiff neck which is diagnostic.

The intensity of headaches associated with brain tumors, diseases of the paranasal sinuses and eye disease is usually not severe.

Quality of Headache

The headaches of migraine, fever and those associated with arterial hypertension are characteristically throbbing in quality. The headache resulting from muscle spasm is frequently described by the patient as viselike or like a tight band around the head. The headache of brain tumor and of meningitis is usually of a steady aching quality.

Site

The vascular headaches of the migraine type are most frequently situated in the temporal region, although they may occur anywhere in the head and face. Pain associated with diseases of the eye or sinuses at its onset most frequently occurs in the front of the head; subsequently, if it is associated with secondary muscle contraction, the pain may be situated in the back of the head and neck.

Duration of Headache

The usual migrainous headache lasts about twenty-four hours. Characteristically in migraine there is complete freedom from headache between attacks. Muscle contraction headaches which are associated with tension and anxiety may persist for weeks or months.

Time of Day

Headaches associated with migraine and hypertension frequently awaken the patient in the early hours of the morning. The headache associated with nasal and paranasal disease usually occurs in the morning and improves in the late afternoon. Headache associated with eye disease tends to occur towards the evening.

FACIAL PAIN

Pain in the face may be due to the following causes: *

Note: This list was modified from Cohen, L.: *A Synopsis of Medicine in Dentistry*. Philadelphia, Lea & Febiger, 1972, by kind permission of Lea & Febiger.

1. Dental disease—(a) pulpal, (b) periodontal and (c) gingival.
2. Temporomandibular joint dysfunction.
3. Diseases of the ear, nose and throat—(a) acute sinusitis, (b) otitis media and (c) neoplasms of the sinuses.
4. Diseases of the eye—(a) corneal ulceration and (b) iritis.
5. Neuralgia—(a) primary (no obvious gross pathology): (1) paroxysmal trigeminal neuralgia (tic douloreux), (2) facial (periodic) migrainous neuralgia and (3) atypical facial neuralgia. (b) Secondary or symptomatic (nerve involved by growth, scar, injury or infection).

Dental Disease

This is one of the most common causes of facial pain and occasionally it may prove difficult to pinpoint the cause. Pain of pulpal and periodontal origin characteristically does not cross the midline.

Pain of periodontal origin is relatively easy to diagnose as the affected tooth is sensitive to biting pressure and will be painful on percussion. Food impaction on occasion will cause pain in the teeth on either side of the wedge of food. Periodontal pain is felt initially in the affected tooth or teeth but later secondary muscle contraction may cause pain over the ascending ramus radiating into the opposing jaw.

Hyperemia of the pulp and acute pulpitis cause a throbbing pain in the tooth which is synchronous with the heartbeat and worse in a recumbent position than when the patient is standing. The pain radiates along the affected jaw and into the opposing jaw. Subsequently secondary muscle contraction will superimpose a dull ache over the throbbing pulpitic pain.

Chronic pulpitis may cause difficulty as it produces a dull ache which may be difficult to localize (*see* Chapter 15).

The symptoms of *acute periodontal abscess* vary with the site. If the abscess is situated at the apex of the tooth, the affected tooth which is nonvital will be sensitive on percussing parallel to its longitudinal axis. A *lateral periodontal abscess* usually results in a tender swelling over the lateral aspect of the root and the tooth is not necessarily tender on percussing in its long axis. In addition the tooth is usually vital as the infection occurs via the periodontal membrane and not through the root canal.

Acute gingivitis characteristically causes pain all round the mouth.

Osteomyelitis of the mandible will cause pain in the mandible and anesthesia or paresthesia in the distribution of the mental nerve and this combination of pain and anesthesia or paresthesia is characteristic.

An acutely abscessed mandibular premolar will result in all the characteristics of an acute infection, redness, heat, pain, swelling and loss of function which in this case is difficulty in chewing. If the mental nerve is bathed in pus from the adjacent abscess, the patient may complain of numbness or paresthesia of the lip and this condition must be differentiated from acute osteomyelitis.

Cellulitis of the head and neck may be associated with carious or periodontally involved teeth. The condition which is a nonsuppurative diffuse spreading inflammation is usually associated with highly virulent strains of streptococci and other organisms. The patient complains of severe pain and the temperature is usually raised. Clinical examination reveals a tender, indurated lesion and the overlying skin is reddened. Should fluctuation be present indicating that suppuration has occurred, the lesion is then termed an "abscess."

Pericoronitis or inflammation of the soft tissue around an erupting tooth is more commonly associated with the mandibular third molar. The patient complains of pain and difficulty in opening his jaws due to muscle spasm; the temperature is often raised.

Temporomandibular Joint Dysfunction *

Diseases of the Ear, Nose and Throat

In *acute maxillary sinusitis* there is a dull aching pain which is felt below the eye and in the maxillary teeth and may also be referred above the eye. *Frontal sinusitis* will cause pain in the forehead, above the eyebrow. In *ethmoidal sinusitis*, the pain is medial and deep to the eye. In acute frontal and maxillary sinusitis the pain usually occurs one or two hours after rising and becomes less severe in the evening.

Chronic sinusitis gives rise to a chronic nasal discharge and not facial pain.

Infection of the middle ear results in severe pain which is felt in the ear.

Malignant disease of the paranasal sinuses may give rise to pain, anesthesia or a bloody nasal discharge. There may be associated cervical lymphadenopathy.

Diseases of the Eye

In diseases of the eye, pain is felt mainly in the area supplied by the ophthalmic division of the trigeminal nerve.

Corneal ulceration may result from trauma or infection. In this condition the conjunctival vessels are injected and there are pain, photophobia, lacrimation and spasm of the eyelids.

The patient with *iritis* will complain of pain, photophobia, lacrimation and interference with vision. Because of changes in the iris, the pupil is contracted and reacts sluggishly to light.

Neuralgia

Neuralgia is pain along the course of a nerve. It may conveniently be divided into primary types where there is no obvious pathology and secondary or symptomatic types where the nerve is involved by a neoplasm, a scar or an infection. Of the primary types the most important are paroxysmal trigeminal neuralgia, facial or periodic migrainous neuralgia, and atypical facial neuralgia.

Paroxysmal Trigeminal Neuralgia (Tic Douloreux)

This condition usually occurs over the age of thirty years and affects females more than males. The right side of the face is more commonly affected than the left and the second and third divisions of the trigeminal nerve are more commonly affected than the first. The pain is severe and paroxysmal and lasts only for a few seconds but the actual bout may last for several hours with varying intervals of freedom from pain between attacks. A "trigger area" may be present which when touched may

---

* See Chapter 12.

precipitate an attack but this is not always the case.

Facial (Periodic) Migrainous Neuralgia

This has also been termed "sphenopalatine neuralgia," "vidian neuralgia," "histamine cephalalgia," "cluster headache" and "alarm clock headache." Males between the ages of twenty and forty years are more commonly affected. The pain which is felt in and around an eye is sudden in onset and extremely severe. The paroxysms often occur during the early hours of the morning and will awaken the patient from his sleep at the same time each day. There is often redness of the affected eye with increased lacrimation and the nostril on the same side may feel blocked. The patient may have the pain every night for several weeks, then a period of remission.

Atypical Facial Neuralgia

This form of neuralgia is frequently associated with depression. It usually occurs in young or middle-aged women who complain of a dull, aching pain in the maxilla which at first is unilateral but may become bilateral. The pain is continuous but does not interfere with sleeping and may last for months or years. Analgesics do not relieve the pain but tranquilizers frequently do.

It is not proposed to discuss the treatment of headache and facial pain which have been dealt with by this author elsewhere.[7]

REFERENCES

1. Melzack, R., and Wall, P. D.: Pain mechanisms. A new theory. *Science, 150*:971, 1965.
2. Casey, K. L., and Melzack, R.: Neural mechanisms of pain: A conceptual model. In Way, E. L. (Ed.): *New Concepts of Pain.* Philadelphia, F. A. Davis, 1967.
3. Melzack, R., and Wall, P. D.: Gate control theory of pain. In Soulairac, A., Cahn, J., and Charpentier, J. (Eds.): *Pain.* New York, Academic Press, 1968.
4. Keele, C. A., and Armstrong, D.: *Substances Producing Pain and Itch.* Baltimore, Williams & Wilkins, 1964.
5. Lim, R. K. S.: Pharmacological viewpoint of pain and analgesia. In Way, E. L. (Ed.): *New Concepts of Pain.* Philadelphia, F. A. Davis, 1967.
6. Wolff, H. G.: Headache. In MacBryde, C. M., and Blacklow, R. S. (Eds.): *Signs and Symptoms: Applied Pathologic Physiology and Clinical Interpretation.* Philadelphia, J. B. Lippincott, 1970.
7. Cohen, L.: *A Synopsis of Medicine in Dentistry.* Philadelphia, Lea & Febiger, 1972.

Chapter 9

The Role of Microbiology in Oral Diagnosis and Treatment Planning

MEMORY ELVIN—LEWIS

PERIODONTAL DISEASE

DESPITE the intensive search for a microbial agent as the cause of periodontal disease, no single organism or group of organisms has been directly implicated. An understanding of the results of this research will enable the practising dentist better to appreciate the reasons for the treatment planning adopted by the periodontist.[53]

Chronic marginal gingivitis may result from a variety of predisposing factors which induce plaque and calculus formation above and below the gingival margin. These conditions may be created by poor oral hygiene, open tooth contact, defective restorations, malocclusions and nonfunctional teeth.[3,74] Inflammation of the affected gingival tissue leads to ulceration of the epithelial lining of the gingival sulcus and periodontal pocket formation.[4] Systemic disease and lowered tissue resistance may influence the progress of the lesion and the disease very likely becomes more acute when systemic factors are superimposed over local factors. Furthermore, nutritional deficiencies and psychological disturbances impair collagen biosynthesis by reducing regeneration of gingival fibers, periodontal membrane fibers and the collagenous matrix of alveolar bone and cementum.[9,14,72,92,94]

ETIOLOGY. Of all the factors which may cause gingival irritation, gingival inflammation related to periodontal disease is clearly associated with the presence of oral microorganisms and their products. Plaque accumulation appears to be the predisposing factor to periodontal diseases whereas calculus accumulations do not on their own affect periodontal tissue but do provide a protective nidus where bacteria can accumulate.[3,5,23,30,44,45,70,85] High plaque pH promotes both calculus formation and periodontal disease whereas low plaque pH promotes caries. The plaque-producing organisms such as *Streptococcus mutans* and *Actinomycoses viscosis* are relatively benign whereas other organisms found within plaque may be overt pathogens or produce toxins, enzymes and endotoxins which directly or indirectly produce tissue inflammation and destruction.[18,35,75,76,86]

Various studies have indicated that there is no single biological agent or even group which is consistently associated with periodontal disease. In this instance, the ability of *A. viscosis* to produce subgingival plaque in the absence of dietary sucrose may account for its more frequent isolation from periodontal diseased tissue than *S. mutans* which preferentially produces plaque on the coronal and interproximal surfaces. Under experimental conditions this organism has the potential to induce gingival pathology and alveolar bone loss.[34]

Protozoa such as *Entamoeba gingivalis* and *Trichomonas tenax* have also been associated with periodontal disease. They are found alone or together in both the healthy or diseased mouth and increase significantly during infection. It is not known whether they contribute to periodontal inflammation or whether this increase is a direct result of the bacteria and other substances on which they feed.[63]

Mycoplasma salivarium may also reside in plaque and occurs in the gingival sulcus of a significantly higher number of individuals with diseased rather than normal gingiva.[15,26]

Indirectly, the organisms mentioned above and their metabolites can induce inflammation by eliciting certain host responses and immunologic phenomena.[11,62,68,72,91] Recent research has indicated that animals will develop antibodies to organisms introduced through the gingival sulcus. These antibodies are first found in the lymph nodes draining the affected area and if contact is prolonged may also be elicited by plasma cells in the lesion itself.[11,32,33,66]

Even under normal conditions, antibodies to the oral flora can be found in the peripheral circulation.[32] In periodontal disease, precipitating antibodies to *Bacteroides melaninogenicus* and fusobacteria have been found; however, a better correlation to the severity of the disease was demonstrated by the increase in titer of *A. naeslundii* when inflammation increased from localized gingivitis to periodontitis.[33,34]

Normal numbers of polymorphonuclear leukocytes in the healthy gingival crevice contribute to its well-being for when neutropenia develops severe gingivitis or stomatitis occurs. On the other hand, when the gingiva becomes inflamed, and their numbers increase, their phagocytic ability imposes a detrimental effect. Few are seen ingesting bacteria, but in phagocytosing insoluble immune complexes they release, in addition to lysosomes, a vascular permeability factor which contributed significantly to severe inflammatory reactions.[57-59]

Histamine is released from platelets agglutinated by antigen-antibody complexes, by mast cells undergoing degranulation by lysosomal action or by inflammation factors which promote the change of histidine to histamine. This may lead both to a localized anaphylactoid reaction by causing local tissue fixation of antibody and to increased vascular permeability. It has also been postulated that endotoxin combining with histamine can contribute to bone resorption by inhibiting the protein synthesis necessary for turnover and therefore depleting the protein matrix of bone.[57-59]

DENTAL CARIES

In order to understand the current status of caries activity tests and the use of topical fluorides in the prevention of caries, it is necessary to review recent caries research and the results of clinical trials.

The Disease

Caries, a disease caused by bacteria, is a slow and progressive infection of the calcified structures of the teeth. It results in the decalcification of the mineral components of the enamel and dentin and dissolution of the organic matrix.

The lesions most frequently develop in the pits, fissures and occlusal surfaces of the teeth and in the non–self-cleansing areas such as the interproximal surfaces. The buccal, labial and the lingual surfaces are less frequently affected. In certain types of periodontal disease the carious lesion may also begin in the cementum, as it is exposed by the downward recession of the periodontal membrane and gingiva from the cemento-enamel junction rather than during periodontal pocket formation.[16,72,92]

EPIDEMIOLOGY. Although dental caries may be found within any age group, race or sex, it is generally considered a disease of childhood as its incidence significantly decreases thereafter.[2,40] As the presence of potentially cariogenic organisms is universal and their acquisition from other caries-infected individuals no doubt occurs early in life, the predisposition to caries depends upon certain host and environmental factors.[83] These factors may be genetically determined and are directly related to biochemical defects of the tooth, structural defects of the teeth, buffering capacity and possibly immunological deficiencies of the saliva.[16,78] Caries is significantly lower among populations whose diet contains large amounts of natural foods and in these instances may be as low as 15 percent. In contrast the incidence may increase up to 95 percent where diets contain high amounts of refined foods and particularly large amounts of sucrose. Therefore, the importance of diet cannot be underestimated, for as refined foods are introduced into diets so the caries rate increases. In this instance, the caries rate has increased from 15 to 50 percent within the last three decades in Accra, Ghana, alone.[13] The reasons why some individuals, even on high cariogenic diets, remain caries-free are, on the other hand, yet to be fully determined.

ETIOLOGY. Recent studies using animal models and to a lesser degree man have shown that caries is an infectious and transmissible disease.[90] Certain organisms isolated from carious lesions can produce the disease in susceptible, experimental animals in conjunction with high carbohydrate diets. The cariogenicity of these organisms is directly related to their ability to adhere to teeth, produce plaque, produce acids which decalcify the enamel and proteolytic enzymes which break down its organic matrix.[38,71] Another feature not shared by caries-inactive species is their ability to produce abundant and stable forms of amylopectin.[34,36,42]

It is now well recognized that certain types of oral streptococci as well as other species of *Lactobacillus*, diptheroids, *Actinomyces*, *Rothia*, and *Nocardia* are potentially cariogenic (Fig. 9-1). In this respect, cariogenic streptococci vary in their ability to produce caries in animals and can be identified from noncariogenic types by their cultural, biochemical, physiological and antigenic characteristics. Epidemiological studies have shown that these types predominate in carious lesions and in mouths with a high caries rate. They produce extracellular dextrans, levans or mutans in the presence of sucrose, glucose and other carbohydrates and by forming sticky envelopes around themselves adhere to the tooth surfaces. These polysaccharides also combine with components of saliva to form insoluble precipitates which are absorbed on hydroxyapatite. By using stored intracellular polysaccharides, some of these types may also survive in the absence of extracellular carbohydrates.[22,35,49]

Although smooth surface caries is dependent upon plaque formation, caries may develop in the depths of occlusal fissures because of mechanical impactions of food and bacteria. It is noteworthy that although cariogenic streptococci can initiate plaque formation they cannot survive as the pH of the plaque decreases. As the pH decreases, organisms such as lactobacilli predominate and their isolation in high numbers under highly cariogenic circum-

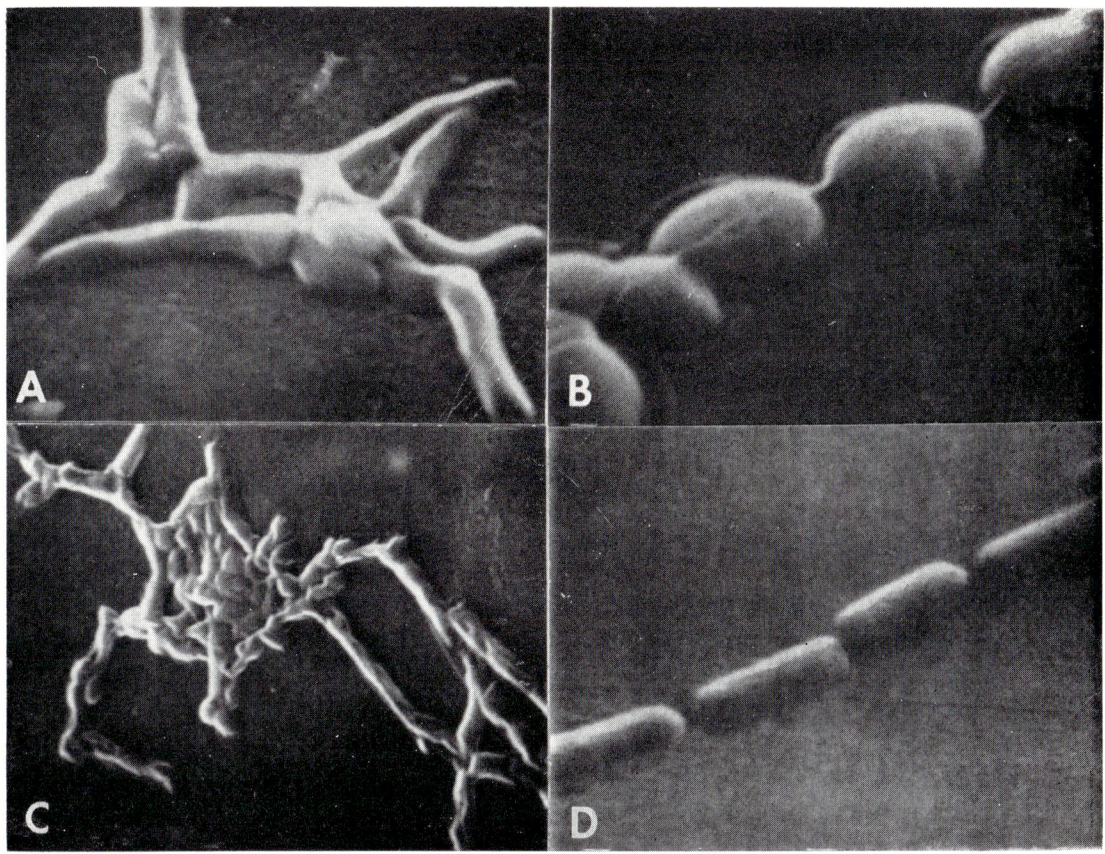

Figure 9-1. Scanning electron micrographs of representative cariogenic microorganisms. (A) *Rothia dentocariosa.* (B) *Streptococcus mutans.* (C) *Actinomyces israelii.* (D) *Lactobacillus acidophilus.*

stances is a direct reflection of this acidogenic environment. To assume, however, that a high *Lactobacillus* count indicates the presence of active caries is presumptuous as high counts have been found among complete denture wearers. Thus, when plaque-forming sites are increased, such as by the fitting of orthodontic bands or dentures, the *Lactobacillus* count greatly increases. Conversely, when plaque-forming areas are reduced, as when oral hygiene is increased and all carious lesions and leaky restorations are restored, the *Lactobacillus* count falls.[77] On the other hand, the mechanism associated with *A. viscosis* infection resulting in root caries and alveolar bone loss differs as plaque formation occurs subgingivally at early stages and is not dependent upon dietary sucrose.[35]

LABORATORY DIAGNOSIS. Although Snyder-type tests and the *Lactobacillus* count are only of relative value in determining caries activity, they are indispensable in preventive dentistry as indicators that preventive therapy is successful[77] (*see* Ch. 20). Tests relying on the acidogenic potential of organisms in carious lesions or stimulated saliva are, at the most, rough estimates of caries activity as yeast such as the *Candida* species, with no known cariogenicity, may also preferentially proliferate in low pH environments and produce false positive reading in the Snyder or its modification, the Alban test.[1,16] In our laboratory, the reliability of these types of tests can be significantly increased if these yeasts are eliminated by the addition of a fungal inhibitor to the media. When modified, this type of acidogenic test is not only inexpensive and reliable but can demonstrate most effectively the state of oral hygiene to the patient.

PREVENTION AND CONTROL. A significant reduction in the amount of caries is evident among populations using water supplies providing 0.5 ppm or more of fluoride. On an individual basis this reduction is not the same for all tooth surfaces but is directly related to the amount of fluoride deposited in the enamel. In this respect, caries is highest in fissures adjacent to occlusal surfaces particularly in the molars and bicuspids where the concentration of fluoride is lowest. As fluoride acts by reducing demineralization, both the number and severity of enamel and dentin lesions can be reduced by topical applications of fluoride in varnish, gels or dentifrices. It also regulates acid-base metabolism 5.0 or below. This effectively inhibits the formation of acid and storage of polysaccharide resulting in more rapid return of the pH to baseline levels. Currently, the selection of fluoride formulation, concentration and treatment is largely empirical. However, a new technique for tooth biopsy should establish the relationship between fluoride levels within enamel and the deeper layers of the tooth. This information should provide a sound therapeutic rationale for the use of topical fluoride within various fluoride areas.[17,44,67,89]

Epidemiological and laboratory findings also support the view that among other trace elements boron, molybdenum and strontium either alone or in conjunction with one another or fluoride have caries inhibiting properties.[43,48,92] On the other hand, high concentrations of certain heavy metals in the environment, such as lead, zinc and cadmium, tend to delay tooth eruption and enhance caries rates among exposed populations.[19,55]

Since persuading patients to alter their dietary habits is virtually impossible, other means of reducing the rate of caries rather than using carbohydrate restrictive diets are currently being investigated. At most, these diets are of limited value, for although their austere conditions can reduce the proportion of cariogenic organisms such as S. mutans in the oral flora, once a normal diet is reestablished their numbers return to prediet levels or higher. A more feasible solution to caries control is to add certain caries prohibitive substances to the human diet or into mouth washes or topical solutions. In this respect, a wide variety of inorganic and organic phosphates have been found to reduce the caries-inducing effect of sucrose when added to either experimental cariogenic diets, chewing gum or breakfast cereal.[12] Other studies indicate that low molecular weight polymers used in sweetening agents can prevent cariogenic streptococci from producing their high molecular weight insoluble polymers required for plaque formation.[35] Certain antibiotics, not useful against systemic disease nor absorbable through the oral mucosa or the gastrointestinal tract, have been incorporated into mouthwashes and found capable of reducing calculus, dental plaque and gingivitis.[29,36,88] In addition, chlorhexidine, when incorporated into mouthwashes or applied topically produces a long-term plaque-inhibiting effect by being released during times when chlorhexidine concentrations are low.[20,52,54,73] On the other hand, although the enzyme dextranase upon topical application could remove gelatinous plaque in experimental animals, it did not prove practical as a caries deterrent in human studies.[35,61]

Caries is essentially a disease of children and the incidence decreases significantly as adulthood approaches (see Ch. 20). The reasons for this are unclear, yet increasing immunity to cariogenic organisms may be a factor.[10] Animal experiments have indicated the practicability of significantly reducing caries by immunization against specific cariogenic organisms or their enzyme dextran-sucrase and it is expected that these studies will be extended in the near future.[35]

Despite all the research into caries and caries prevention it must be emphasized that on a large scale the most effective caries control measure presently available is the fluoridation of the water supplies.[47]

PULP AND PERIAPICAL INFECTIONS

Infection of the pulp may result from extension of carious lesions or by exposure of dental tubules through trauma or dental procedures. Organisms may also directly invade lateral and accessory canals or apical foramina from periodontal pockets. Whenever pulpal inflammation results from various stimuli such as cavity preparation, chemicals, heat and cold, the localization of blood-borne microorganisms is more likely to occur.[31] These organisms may arise from a transient bacteremia, systemic infection, septicemia or through lymphatics draining gingival, periodontal and pulpal areas.[63,72]

The onset of the infection may be acute or insidious and involve all or only a portion of the pulp. A definitive diagnosis of the pulpal condition can only be made histologically; polymorphonuclear leukocytes predominate in acute pulpitis and lymphocytes and plasma cells in chronic pulpitis. In children, chronic hyperplastic pulpitis resulting from the formation of a mass of tissue extending from the pulp chamber of the involved tooth may also occur.[63]

In some cases if the pulpal condition is not treated periapical disease may result. The rate of tissue involvement is dependent upon such factors as anatomic relationships, host resistance and numbers and virulence of the invading microorganisms. As the disease progresses root resorption and granuloma development may become evident. Leading from the granuloma a fistulous tract may arise which drains intraorally anywhere to the buccal, labial, lingual or palatal surface, or extraorally to the face. In addition, an associated cellulitis and osteomyelitis may occur.[16]

LABORATORY DIAGNOSIS. Although root canal culture is a helpful means of determining the involvement of microorganisms in pulpitis, those isolated may also be unrelated to the disease gaining access to the wound through a break in aseptic technique or leaky sealants. Initially, positive cultures are more likely to occur whenever periapical rarefaction is evident or whenever the pulp is necrotic. Chance contamination due to dental procedures becomes less frequent as the case progresses, and usually the canal can be considered "sterile" if two consecutive cultures yield no growth.

Most microorganisms found in root canal cultures can be isolated using such routine endodontic culture media as thioglycollate media enriched with 5% yeast extract. Those which are not readily isolated by this method may often be visualized at the time of sampling by examining a paperpoint in wet mount under phase-contrast microscopy. Only about 10 to 15 percent of cultures examined contain mixtures of microorganisms and in most cases are readily separated in subculture. Whenever infection persists, antibiotic sensitivity testing of the isolates by the Kirby-Bauer method is considered the best way of discerning which antibiotic to use. Most cultures yield organisms normally found in the oral cavity and those associated with carious lesions. The aerobic and facultatively anaerobic streptococci belonging to the poorly classified viridans-cariogenic complex and the enterococci (Group D) are those most frequently isolated with other streptococci including S. *sanguis* and S. *pyogenes* occuring more rarely. Other organisms, such as micrococci, staphylococci, lactobacilli, diphtheroids, *Actinomyces*, *Bacteroides*, enterobacteria and yeasts have on occasion been isolated alone or in various combinations as have oral *Mycoplasma* and bacterial L-forms. The presence of these organisms and their associated toxins and by-products all contribute to symptoms of pain and inflammation found in such an involved tooth.[63]

Intracanal medicaments and sterilization procedures may include one or a mixture of such substances as eugenol, formocresol, beechwood cresote, cresatin, paramonochlorphenol and various broad-spectrum antibiotics. The assumption that certain organisms are always sensitive to particular drugs should be avoided and in persistent root canal infections, whenever antibiotics are included in the treatment regimen, the determination of the inciting organisms and their antibiotic sensitivity should be considered a routine procedure.[46]

If an abscess is incised, a sample of the pus should be taken with a sterile swab and forwarded in appropriate transport media as quickly as possible to the laboratory for determination of the responsible organisms and their antibiotic sensitivities.

TREATMENT. See Chapters 15 and 20.

INFECTIONS OF THE ORAL MUCOSA

Acute Necrotizing Ulcerative Gingivitis (ANUG), (Vincent's Infection; Trench Mouth; Vincent's Stomatitis)

Clinically, the infection produces painful, bleeding gums which result in bad taste and a distinctive halitosis. Gingivitis which may be mild or severe can either be localized around one or more teeth or one quadrant or generalized throughout the entire mouth. A distinct clinical finding of diagnostic value is the presence of a variable number of blunted papillae whose surfaces are partially or totally covered with a grayish, loosely adherent, necrotic slough.[16]

Most cases occur in young adults between the ages of fifteen and twenty-five years with the incidence decreasing thereafter and becoming exceedingly rare after fifty years of age. In a recent study, the highest incidence was found in females between sixteen and seventeen and in males between seventeen and twenty-two years of age. The case rate of this high incidence group was 8.3 per 10,000 inhabitants, which dropped to 4.8 between twenty and twenty-four years and became further reduced to 2.1 between twenty-five and twenty-nine years. Three seasonal peaks were noted, one in September and October, the other in December and January and the third in June. Also, the disease was frequently associated with the common cold.[79] Stress is thought by some authorities to be a significant predisposing factor as most patients are students, young nurses and young executives—persons who are likely to be under unusual physical or mental stress. The disease is one of closed communities such as barracks and dormitories and is associated with lowered resistance. Unless treated satisfactorily it has a tendency to recur.

ETIOLOGY. No reasons have been forthcoming to explain why certain apparently benign organisms begin to preferentially multiply under conditions of stress and produce together this infection. Therefore, the role which the "Vincent organisms" *Borrelia vincenti* and fusiform bacteria play in this infection remains obscure.

LABORATORY DIAGNOSIS. Exudates from ANUG characteristically reveal a mixed flora of various microorganisms, including *B. vincentii, Bacteroides fusiformis,* and *Treponema microdentium.* For diagnosis, smears of exudates may be best visualized by dark-field or phase microscopy.

TREATMENT. Penicillin V 250 mg q.i.d. orally for three days will relieve the acute symptoms. In patients who are allergic to penicillin Flagyl® 250 mg t.i.d. orally for three days may be administered. It is essential to scale the teeth, restore carious teeth, extract any roots and excise any periodontal pockets to prevent recurrence. The patient should be instructed in correct oral hygiene.

Syphilis

Primarily a venereal disease, syphilis can also be transmitted orally, placentally and presumably through contaminated instruments. The organism enters a break in the mucosa and the characteristically indurated chancre develops after a period of two to six weeks. It lasts for two to six weeks, is highly infectious and may appear on the lips, tongue, tonsils and less frequently on the gingiva, face or eyes. About six weeks after its appearance the secondary phase develops. This is characterized by a rash consisting of macules, papules and pustules and within the oral cavity, mucous patches. The mucous patch, appearing in about 40 percent of cases, is a grayish and slightly raised area teeming with spirochetes and highly infectious. After another undetermined period of quiescence, approximately two-thirds of those infected develop the tertiary stage. This phase is characterized by destructive lesions which are hypergic, chronic, proliferative and inflammatory involving the visceral, skeletal and cardiovascular system. Gummas may involve the hard and soft palate and the tongue.

The acquisition of syphilis by the fetus occurs through placental circulation after the fourth month of pregnancy. Infection at this time results in death or in an infant who presents symptoms of secondary syphilis soon after birth. Some patients do not manifest symptoms until later in life. Late congenital syphilis may affect growth and development, especially of the teeth and oral tissues. Interstitial keratitis produces a ground glass appearance of the cornea. Lack of development of nasal bones results in "saddle-nose"; scars or crease-lines radiating from the corner of the mouth are referred to as "rhagades." Delays in the formation and eruption of the teeth also occur, and in addition, alteration of tooth morphology produces Hutchinson's incisors with their characteristic incisal notch and screwdriver-shaped crowns and mulberry molars with their unusual formation of the crown surface.[6,21,64,65]

The occupational hazard of acquiring syphilis from an active case during oral examination or treatment warrants particular attention and surgical gloves and glasses should be used by the practitioner whenever the disease is suspected.

LABORATORY DIAGNOSIS. Presumptive diagnosis may now be easily carried out in the dentist's office by utilizing finger-prick blood in the RPR test*.[63] To avoid false positives due to such diseases as malaria or infectious mononucleosis, definitive diagnosis using the TPI (*Treponema pallidum* immobilization test), among others, can only be carried out in a diagnostic laboratory.

PREVENTION AND CONTROL. In the United States and most other countries, epidemiological control necessitates the reporting of all cases to the local health authority.[6,21,93] In some patients who have received early adequate antibiotic treatment the serologic test may remain positive. These patients are called seroresistant or Wassermann-fast.

TREATMENT. Penicillin is the antibiotic of choice. If the patient is allergic to penicillin, erythromycin or tetracyclines are used.

Gonorrhea

In adults, venereal infection with *Neisseria gonorrhea* can result, after an incubation period of three to nine days, in urethritis, cervicitis and salpingitis. Gonococcal proctitis occurs in homosexuals and orogenital contact may result in an oral infection closely resembling acute necrotizing gingivitis. Infants acquiring the infection at birth can develop *Ophthalmia neonatorum* and contact of exudates can also result in vulvovaginitis of children or conjunctivitis of adults.

In the oral cavity, the gingiva, tongue and soft palate are most frequently affected with lesions varying in appearance from white or yellow patches to gray adherent membranes covering large areas of the oral mucosa. When these membranes eventually slough off, an inflamed surface with numerous bleeding points remains. This is particularly painful on the gingiva and is associated with considerable inflammation and swelling. Scarring can result if infections are prolonged.[6,7,65]

LABORATORY DIAGNOSIS. Presumptive diagnosis may be carried out on clinical grounds although culture of the organism or specific fluorescent antibody staining of exudate smears confirms diagnosis. Serological tests are not used although concurrent infection with syphilis should be ruled out.

TREATMENT. Penicillin and tetracycline are the drugs of choice.

Tuberculosis

Tuberculosis is a chronic, granulomatous disease caused by *Mycobacterium tuberculosis* and less frequently by *M. kansasii, M. intracellulare* and with bone tuberculosis, *M. bovis*. The disease is transmitted through inhalation of droplet nuclei from sputum or in the case of *M. bovis,* through contaminated milk.[93]

Oral lesions develop in about 1 to 3 percent of patients with postprimary systemic infection but can also occur rarely without associated systemic infection.[6,65]

PREVENTION AND CONTROL. Recognition of suspect cases should be promptly referred to a physician for treatment. To control the disease, the local health authorities must be notified and they will check all the patient's intimate contacts for infection. As risk of infection is presently low among most populations in North America, testing for an individual's conversion to tuberculin positive by the Tine skin test is currently replacing the use of chest x-ray screening. Although BCG vaccination is available and confers good immunity, it does convert a tuberculin Tine test. Therefore, to check for active disease, submission to periodic x-ray examination is necessary

---

* Hynson, Westcott & Dunning, Inc. Charles and Chase St., Baltimore, Maryland.

among tuberculin positive individuals who have acquired tuberculin sensitivity through inapparent infection, previous infection or BCG vaccination. Periodic screening is especially important to those in the high-risk profession of dentistry. Although oral manifestations of tuberculosis are rare indeed, inapparent infection, especially among low socioeconomic populations where the disease may be endemic, warrants particular attention.[14] Instruments should always be handled with tuberculosis in mind. Transmission of tuberculosis from one patient to another by contaminated instruments is very possible, especially when inadequate sterilization procedures are employed.[25] The best means of ensuring complete sterilization is by autoclaving; the use of cold sterilizing solutions is only of limited value and quaternary ammonium compounds are useless. In treatment of patients with active disease, gowning, gloving and masking should always be part of the operating regimen.[6,25,93]

TREATMENT. The antituberculous drugs streptomycin, isoniazid and para-aminosalicylic acid (PAS) are employed.

FUNGAL INFECTIONS

Candidiasis (Moniliasis, Thrush, Candidosis)

Generally of endogenous origin, the yeastlike *C. albicans* and occasionally other species of *Candida* may be found on most moist and warm tissue surfaces of the body including the oral cavity. The disease is more frequently found in infants and elderly individuals and in those suffering from malnutrition, hypovitaminosis, alcoholism, uncontrolled diabetes and debilitating diseases such as chronic anemia, leukemia, pemphigus and terminal malignant disease. Oral moniliasis may also be triggered by prolonged topical applications of corticosteroids, or antibiotics, and after intense radiation therapy to the face, mouth and jaws. The disease is characterized by pseudomembranes on mucosal surfaces, eczematoid skin lesions and less frequently, granulomata in various tissues.[16]

Oral moniliasis must be distinguished from lesions of herpetic stomatitis, primary and secondary syphilis, erythema multiforme, lichen planus and keratosis.[65]

It is convenient to divide oral candidiasis into acute and chronic forms. Acute infection of the oral mucosa resulting in *thrush* occurs in both infants and adults and is characterized by white, flaky pseudomembranes covering part or all of the tongue, lips, gums or buccal mucosa. If the membrane is removed a bleeding surface is left. Following administration of antibiotics the normal oral flora is altered and the growth of *Candida* is encouraged. The so-called penicillin sore tongue is a form of acute candidiasis and is characterized by a red, painful tongue.[72]

Denture sore mouth and chronic angular cheilitis are forms of chronic candidiasis. The former condition presents as redness of the palatal mucosa under a denture. Angular cheilitis which has been present for longer than a month is nearly always caused by *Candida*. Candidal leukoplakia is discussed in Chapter 5.

LABORATORY DIAGNOSIS. The organism can easily be cultured and species differentiated on Pagano Levine Media or serum tube culture.[56]

TREATMENT. Mycostatin® oral tablets (500,000 units) are sucked q.i.d. for a few days in the treatment of acute candidiasis.

In the case of chronic candidiasis treatment may extend over four to six weeks or longer.

Actinomycosis

An infection of endogenous origin related to trauma is caused in many by *A. israelii, A. naeslundii* and *A. propionica,* and in cattle by *A. bovis.* These organisms have been found associated both with carious lesions and periodontal disease and are also considered normal inhabitants of the mouth. The disease is characterized by a chronic, suppurative or granulomatous infection frequently localized to the cervicofacial region, thorax and abdomen. The lesions develop as firm granulomata which spread slowly to contiguous tissues and break down focally to form multiple draining sinuses, penetrating to the surface and discharging distinctive colonies of the agent referred to as "sulfur granules." They appear as purplish nodules without fistulas in the tissues of the cheek and face as diffuse and firm swellings of the lower face and upper neck. Lymphadenitis is frequent in secondary bacterial infections. In uncomplicated actinomycosis the draining lymph nodes may remain unaffected, a characteristic which differentiates actinomycosis from other infections.

LABORATORY DIAGNOSIS. The demonstration of sulfur granules in tissues and exudates and the culture of the organism confirms clinical diagnosis.[6,65]

TREATMENT. Penicillin is the drug of choice. Tetracyclines can be used in penicillin-sensitive individuals.

HERPESVIRUS INFECTIONS

Four human herpesviruses are now recognized: herpes simplex, varicella-zoster, cytomegalovirus and the Epstein-Barr virus.[82]

Herpes Simplex

This viral infection is characterized by latency and repeated localized lesions. The primary infection, usually appearing in childhood, may be asymptomatic or include a variety of symptoms with fever, gingivostomatitis accompanied by vesicular lesions in the oropharynx, or a severe keratoconjunctivitis, a vulvovaginitis, a generalized cutaneous eruption as a complication of chronic eczema (Kaposi's varicelliform eruption), a meningoencephalitis, or a fatal panvisceral infection as seen in newborn infants, and as traumatic infection of the fingers, herpetic whitlow. The latter is occasionally seen in dentists.[29,66]

There are two types of herpes simplex virus which can be distinguished serologically. The oral strain or type I has been isolated from gingivostomatitis, herpes labialis, pharyngeal lesions, meningoencephalitis, eczema herpeticum and skin lesions (with the exception of those seen on the thigh and buttocks), and its presence in the saliva of asymptomatic carriers may account for its wide dissemination among the population.[24] Infection with the genital strain (type II) may be acquired venereally and systemic infection of the newborn may occur. The location of the lesion is often indicative of the serotype isolated. In this respect, skin lesions in the area of the thighs and buttocks generally are the result of type II infection, whereas those on the face and lips, are the result of type I infection. Also meningoencephalitis has been associated with type I virus and lower spinal cord involvement with type II.

ACUTE HERPETIC GINGIVOSTOMATITIS. The primary disease is self-limiting with symptoms of moderate to severe intensity characteristic within the fifth to eighth day after onset. Severe burning and paresthesia precede the appearance of the vesicular eruptions which may be scattered throughout the mouth and oropharynx. In acute primary gingivostomatitis, the fever, sore mouth and malaise disappear at the eighth to tenth day, concurrent with the appearance of neutralizing antibodies with complete recovery occurring before the twenty-first day. The virus may be isolated from saliva up to three weeks after recovery and may be found at all times in individuals with frequent recurrent episodes. Fatalities are rare and are generally associated with the more severe types of infections involving the central nervous system.[84]

LABORATORY DIAGNOSIS. The diagnosis of primary herpes infection may be corroborated by the demonstration of a rise in either complement-fixing or neutralizing antibody titre in preconvalescent sera collected at least seven to fourteen days after onset of symptoms. Tissue culture may be used for isolation and neutralizing tests and the virus produces characteristic cytopathogenic effects (CPE) in primary cells cultures such as kidney of monkey, human or rabbit origin, human amnion and chick fibroblast or in continuous cell cultures such as HeLa, Wi 38, Rep-2, MA 184 or L cells and pox lesions on the surface of the chorioallantoic membrane of the fertile hen's egg.[87]

Both herpes simplex virus and varicella-zoster virus, the causative agent of chickenpox and herpes zoster, produce typical ballooning degeneration, multinucleate giant cells and scattered intranuclear inclusion bodies (Lipschütz bodies). These changes can be easily seen on exfoliative cytologic smears from lesions up to forty-eight hours old, however, inclusion bodies are uncommon in oral smears. As oral ulceration, fever and malaise may also occur in acute leukemia and infectious mononucleosis, it is necessary to carry out white blood cell counts and heterophil antibody agglutination tests, particularly in the prepubertal and adolescent age groups, to exclude these diseases.[27,37,42,60,65,69]

TREATMENT. Specific treatment remains experimental. Antibiotics may be administered to control secondary infection. A vaccine may be used in severe recurrent cases.

Varicella-Zoster Virus

Oral and facial lesions may occur in both varicella (chickenpox) and herpes zoster. In the oral cavity the characteristic lesion is a vesicle surrounded by an erythematous margin; the buccal mucosa, tongue and palate are sites of predilection. Of the two diseases the most common is varicella which frequently develops in childhood as a systemic viral exanthem. Herpes zoster, the least common form generally seen in adults, is characterized by severe neuralgia in the distribution of the affected cutaneous or cranial nerve which precedes the appearance of the typical vesicular eruption on the skin or mucous membrane.

LABORATORY DIAGNOSIS. The virus may be isolated by the inoculation of appropriate cell cultures with fluid from newly appearing vesicles. The demonstration of a rising titre of complement-fixing antibodies is also helpful.

TREATMENT. There is no specific treatment. Analgesics are used to control the pain. Antibiotic creams may be used to prevent secondary infection of skin lesions.

Infectious Mononucleosis

Infectious mononucleosis is thought to be associated with infection of the Epstein-Barr virus (EBV). This virus has also been implicated in Burkitts Lymphoma and cancer of the postnasal space, as has the picornavirus Reo 3.[41,82]

Infectious mononucleosis develops after a two to six week incubation period and is a systemic infection characterized by fever and posterior cervical lymphadenopathy. In addition, splenomegaly occurs in about 50 percent of patients and more infrequently hepatitis, jaundice and muculopapular eruptions. When present the oral lesions are characteristic petechiae or purpuric spots appearing usually in the posterior palatal tissues. Bleeding, stomatitis affecting the buccal mucosa, acute gingivitis or small ulcers resembling those of recurrent aphthae are present not infrequently with pharyngitis, edema of the soft palate and uvula and tonsilitis.

Symptoms may be absent or mild in children and are more frequently seen within young adults. Oral manifestations usually occur five days before the onset of the systemic disease which persists for two to four weeks. In rare instances, neurologic involvement may also occur.[6,84]

LABORATORY DIAGNOSIS. A positive heterophil antibody titre (Paul-Bunnel, Heterol) within the first week of illness is diagnostic. Fluorescent antibodies to EBV develop and are retained thereafter. White cell counts reveal 50 to 70 percent lymphocytosis with characteristic abnormal "butterfly" lymphocytes.

TREATMENT. This is entirely symptomatic.

RECURRENT APHTHOUS ULCERS (APHTHOUS STOMATITIS, APHTHAE, CANKER SORES)

Although the clinical severity of recurrent aphthous ulcers (RAU) may vary, two distinct forms of the disease are recognized; one is mild and the other is severe and scarring. The mild form does not develop into the more severe form but rather both are characterized by their persistent chronicity with only rare instances of spontaneous, but temporary, remission. In the mild or minor form patients may either have one or two lesions a month or be persistently afflicted with twenty or thirty small lesions in various stages of development. The same pattern may also be seen in the severe or major form although the entire disease is greatly exaggerated, with large lesions developing which remain for weeks and months, resulting in scarring.[28,34,72]

In the *mild or minor* form a prodromal symptom of pain and burning with some localized swelling and inflammation may persist for one to two days before a white spot or raised bump in the mucosa slowly expands to 1 to 10 mm by two to three days. The round or oval lesion has a grayish or grayish-yellow covering of necrotic slough or serofibrinous exudate. On occasion the base of the ulcers may be composed of intensely raw, red tissue. The borders are distinct, rolled and indurated and surrounded by a narrow zone of inflammation rarely extending over 1 to 2 mm wide. They are associated with pain, tenderness and discomfort of variable intensity. Often functions such as eating, talking and swallowing are impeded and certain foods and beverages which are either salty, spicy, acidic or alcoholic can elicit acute and intense pain. In ten to fourteen days, healing occurs spontaneously without scarring. None of these exacerbations are preceded with an elevated temperature, regional node involvement or secondary infection.

In the *severe* or *major* form (periadenitis mucosa necrotica recurrens), the prodromal symptoms of pain and burning are much more intense and unlike the mild form much deeper tissues are involved and a slight fever is sometimes present. A white plaque or swelling of 1 to 5 mm develops, expands and ulcerates rapidly to a diameter of 10 to 30 mm which after several weeks or months heals with a scar. During this period the patient is in considerable discomfort from the tissue destruction and induration and frequently associated submandibular lymphadenopathy. Much of the oral tissue can become severely scarred after several years of these recurrent attacks.[39]

In both types, the ulcers may be found anywhere in the mouth, but they most commonly occur on the buccal and labial mucosa, tongue and lips and in the severe form can extend to the pharynx and palate and less frequently on the heavily keratinized tissue. The incidence of lesions occurring at any one time is also apparently closely related to the degree of keratinization occurring within the mouth. A significant increase in the number of lesions has been noted among susceptible individuals prior to menstruation when low estrogen levels result in a reduction in the cornification of the oral mucosa. Conversely, both a decrease of frequency and severity of these lesions has been found when keratinization of oral tissues has occurred as a result of smoking—an effect which is reversed once smoking ceases.

A genetic basis for predisposition has been suggested by several investigators who have found its incidence to be higher among certain family groups within the populations studied. Although the exact mechanism has yet to be determined, this predisposition may be related to certain inherent immunological defects. Not only is this type of lesion more frequently associated with atopic individuals but also occurs in significant numbers among persons having the likely autoimmune disorders ulcerative colitis and rheumatoid arthritis.[51]

The precipitating factor in each individual case may vary but trauma in one form or another is a predominant feature. Although the operational mechanism remains obscure, various foods, chemical irritants and physical and emotional stress have all been implicated. On the other hand, there is little significant relationship to seasonal incidence or drug allergies. It is not possible to predict from a patient's past experience either the number or severity of the lesions expected in the next episode, but rather statistical studies have indicated that the occurrence of lesions is quite random in nature.

The disease characteristically begins in childhood with the great majority of patients becoming afflicted by forty years. The milder form may affect as many as 20 to 50 percent of a population whereas the severe form is found rarely. The age of onset varies somewhat according to the type and sex. Males may acquire the severe form anytime within the first ten years, whereas its onset in females coincides a decade later, with the appearance of the milder form in both sexes. There appears to be a slightly higher incidence of mild aphthous ulceration among females and of the severe type among males.

ETIOLOGY. Cultures and histopathological examination of biopsy material has led several investigators to implicate the alpha hemolytic *S. sanguis* and its L-form. It was postulated that the L-form which does not possess a cell wall can remain within the tissue cells during periods of quiescence and is, during periods of stress, stimulated or encouraged by some unknown mechanism to convert to its bacterial form. Both transitional and bacterial forms are readily isolated from the lesion during periods of

TABLE 9-1
OTHER MICROBIAL DISEASES WITH ORAL MANIFESTATIONS

Disease	Causative Agent	Oral Manifestation
Burkitt's lymphoma	Herpesvirus: Epstein-Barr virus	Loosening of teeth, jaw tumors, orbital swelling; associated abdominal tumors.
Cancer of postnasal space	Herpesvirus: Epstein-Barr virus	Cancer of postnasal space.
Foot and mouth disease	Enterovirus: foot and mouth virus	Vesicles on mucous membranes of mouth, pharynx, lips.
Herpangina	Enterovirus: coxsackievirus A, serotypes 2,3,4,5,6,8	Severe pharyngitis, typical vesiculation on soft palate and anterior pillar of fauces.
Hand, foot and mouth disease	Enterovirus: coxsackievirus A16	Similar to herpangina lesions but more diffuse, occurring on buccal surface of cheek and gums, also on hands, feet and buttocks.
Acute nodular pharyngitis	Enterovirus: coxsackievirus A10	Firm, nodular lesions on uvula, and posterior pharynx.
Vesicular stomatitis	Rhabdovirus: vesicular stomatitis virus	Similar to herpangina or influenza-like disease.
Rabies	Rhabdovirus: rabies virus	Spasms of muscle deglutition leads to fear of swallowing.
Measles	Paramyxovirus: measles virus	Mild coryza, Koplik's spots.
Rubella	Alphavirus: rubella virus	Cervical lymphadenopathy, teratogenic effect.
Influenza	Orthomyxovirus: influenza virus, serotypes A,B,C	Sore throat, coryza.
Common cold	Enterovirus: echovirus; Rhinovirus; Paramyxovirus; Adenovirus types	Sore throat, pharyngitis, coryza.
Mumps	Paramyxovirus: mumps virus	Infectious parotitis, swelling of one or both parotid glands and sometimes, submaxillary and sublingual salivary glands.
Plague	*Yersina pestis*	Primary septicemic plague: pharyngeal and tonsillar infections.
Glanders	*Mallomyces mallei*	Acute form: primary ulceration of mucosae, particularly nasopharynx-leads to systemic disease.
Diphtheria	*Corynebacterium diphtheriae*	Infection of the tonsils, pharynx larynx and nose characterized by white spots which coalesce to form a pseudomembrane similar to ANUG and gonorrhea.
Leprosy	*Mycobacterium leprae*	Lepromatous form: ulceration and scarring of mucous membranes and leproma formation.
Sporotrichosis	*Sporothrix schenkii*	Nodular lesions in skin, lymph nodes and subcutaneous tissues—mucosal lesions are erythematous, ulcerative, suppurative, vegetative or papillomatous, easily confused with those produced by other oral infections.
Histoplasmosis	*Histoplasma capsulatum*	Chronic disseminated form: mucosal lesions which are nodular or vegetative appear on tongue, lips, buccal mucosa, hard and soft palate, larynx and vocal chords.
South American blastomycosis	*Paracoccidiodies brasiliensis*	Ulcerative lesions of oral mucosa.
Coccidioidomycosis	*Coccidioides immitis*	Rare: in both disseminated and cutaneous forms as ulcerations and punched out areas in the palate.
Mucocutaneous leishmaniasis	*Leishmania tropica*	Espundia type: ulcerative or indurated lesions on mucous membranes of buccal and nasopharynx.
Gonglyonema	*Gonglyonema pulchrum*	Inflammatory reaction during migration through mucosa and submucosa of oral cavity.
Trichinosis	*Trichinella spiralis*	Inflammatory tumors of mucobuccal folds of molar area due to encystment of parasite.

* References for this table include the following sources found on the reference list behind this chapter: 6, 21, 41, 84, 92, 93.

exacerbation and as they are released also free sequestered cell antigens which can incite an autoimmune response. During the active stages of either forms of this disease, increases of IgA and IgG can be detected in patients' sera and may represent antibodies against both oral mucosa and *S. sanguis*. In addition, IgG and IgM immunoglobulins can be found bound specifically to the cells of the spinous layer of the oral epithelium.[7,8,80]

The severity of the lesion is doubtless related to the degree of delayed hypersensitivity mediated by autoimmunity. The predominance of mononuclear leukocytes within the lesions, an increase in mast cells and the ability of oral mucosal antigen to transform patients' lymphoblasts, points to this conclusion.[50]

The type of lesion is a direct result of the inherent ability of leukocytes followed by plasma cells to infiltrate the oral mucosa. In the milder form only the corium and epithelium are involved, whereas in the severe form infiltration also occurs into the submucosal layers. The production of immunoglobulins, especially those involved in autoimmunity, may occur *in situ* by the plasma cells. Tissue destruction and inflammation are then a direct result of the interaction of this tissue fixed antibody with such host factors as complement.[64]

TREATMENT. Kenalog® in Orabase® can be applied to small lesions t.i.d.; it should not be rubbed on as this prevents its adherence, rather it should be dabbed on the lesion. In severe cases systemic corticosteroids may be required.

Other Oral Infections

Although it is not possible to discuss in detail all the infections which produce oral manifestations, Table 9-1 should serve as a quick reference. A more detailed analysis can be obtained from any current medical microbiology text or the recent, excellent review of communicable diseases edited by Benenson.[6]

It should be remembered that although the dentist may not be directly responsible for the treatment of these diseases, they may prove both infectious to him and, if adequate precautions are not taken, a source of infection to other patients. In this respect sterilization of instruments and the use of disposable needles should be a part of the normal operating regimen, especially to avoid transmission of both serum and infectious hepatitis. Whenever consultation requires the examination of patients with tuberculosis, syphilis, gonorrhea, tularemia, plague, rabies, glanders, leprosy and sporotrichosis, the additional precaution of masking, gloving and gowning should be carried out. In addition, the acquisition of diphtheria and mumps can be avoided by active immunization. Knowledge of the epidemiology of other infections may also aid in differential diagnosis.

REFERENCES

1. Alban, A.: An improved Snyder's test. *J Dent Res*, 49(3):641, 1970.
2. Adler, P.: Correlation between dental caries prevalences at different ages. *Caries Res*, 2:79–86, 1968.
3. Alexander, A. G.: The effect of lack of function of teeth on gingival health, plaque and calculus accumulation. *J Periodontol*, 41(8):438–441, 1970.
4. Allström, R.: Presence of leukocytes in crevices of healthy and chronically inflamed gingivae. *J Periodont Res*, 5:42–47, 1970.
5. Baboolal, R., Powell, R. N., and Prophet, A. S.: Hydrolytic enzymes in developing gingival plaque. *J Periodontol*, 41(2):87–92, 1970.
6. Benenson, A. S. (Ed.): *Control of Communicable Diseases in Man*, 11th ed. New York, The American Public Health Association, 1970.

7. Barile, M. F., and Graykowski, E. A.: Primary herpes, recurrent labial herpes, recurrent aphthae and periadentis aphthae: a review with some new observations. *J Dist Columbia Dent Soc*, 38:7–15, 1963.
8. Barile et al.: L-form of bacteria isolated from recurrent aphthous stomatitis. *Oral Surg*, 16(11):1395–1400, 1963.
9. Berglund, S. E.: Introduction to conference. *J Periodontol*, 41(4):195–196, 1970.
10. Berkenbilt, D. A., and Bahn, A. N.: Development of antibodies to cariogenic streptococci in children. *JADA*, 83:332–337, 1971.
11. Bickley, H. C.: A concept of allergy with reference to oral disease. *J Periodontol*, 41(6):2/302–12/312, 1970.
12. Brewer, H. E., Stookey, G. K., and Muhler, J. C.: A clinical study concerning the anticariogenic effects of NaH_2PO_4-enriched breakfast cereals in institutionalized subjects: results after two years. *JADA*, 80:121–124, 1970.
13. Brown, E. M.: Personal Communication. Sr. Dental Surgeon, Ridge Hospital, Accra, Ghana.
14. Brown, L. R., Merrill, S. S., and Lambson, G. O.: Microbiologic aspects of papillary hyperplasia. *Oral Surg*, 28:545–551, 1969.
15. Burnett, G. W., and Gilmore, E.: Incidence and distribution of oral pleuropneumonia-like L organisms. *J Dent Res* Research annotations), 38(3):632, 1959.
16. Burnett, G. W., and Scherp, H. W.: *Oral Microbiology and Infectious Disease*. A Textbook for Students and Practitioners of Dentistry, 3rd ed. Baltimore, Williams & Wilkins, 1968.
17. Candell, A., Scavizzi, F., and Marci, F.: The relationship between fluoride concentration and the caries frequency of different tooth surfaces in a high fluoride area. *Caries Res*, 4:69–77, 1970.
18. Critchley, P.: Metabolic activity of plaque as it relates to the gingival-dental structures. *Int Conf Dent Plaque*, 38–42, 1970.
19. Curzon, M. E. J., and Bibby, B. G.: Effect of heavy metals on dental caries and tooth eruption. *J Dent for Child*, 37(6):463–465, 1970.
20. Davies, R. M., Jensen, S. B., Schiott, C. R., and Loe, H.: The effect of topical application of chlorhexidine on the bacterial colonization of the teeth and gingiva. *J Periodont Res*, 5:96–101, 1970.
21. Davis, B. D., Dulbecco, R., Eisen, H. N., Ginsberg, H. S., and Woods, W. B. (Eds.): *Microbiology*. Hoeber Medical Division. New York, Harper & Row, 1968.
22. de Stoppelaar, J. D., van Houte, J., and Dirks, O. B.: The effect of carbohydrate restriction on the presence of *Streptococcus mutans*, *Streptococcus sanguis* and iodophilic polysaccharide-producing bacteria in human dental plaque. *Caries Res*, 4:114–123, 1970.
23. Dick, H. M., and Trott, J. R.: Immunity and inflammation as synergistic mechanisms in the pathogenesis of periodontal disease. *J Periodont Res*, 4:127–140, 1969.
24. Dowdle, W. R., Nahmias, A. J., Harwell, R., and Pauls, F.: Association of antigenic type of *Herpesvirus hominis* with site of viral recovery. *J Immunol*, 99:974–980, 1967.
25. Duell, R. C., and Madden, R. M.: Droplet nuclei produced during dental treatment of tubercular patients. *Oral Surg*, 30(5): 711–716, 1970.
26. Engel, L., and Kenny, G. E.: *Mycoplasma salivarium* in human gingival sulci. *J Periodont Res*, 5:163–171, 1970.
27. Fenner, F., and White, D. O.: *Medical Virology*. New York, Academic Press, 1970.
28. Francis, T. C.: Recurrent aphthous stomatitis and Behcet's disease. *Oral Surg*, 30(4): 476–487, 1970.
29. Frankel, M. A.: Tetracycline antibiotics and tooth discoloration. *J Dent for Child*, 27(2):117–143, 1970.
30. Frostell, G.: Proteolytic activity of plaque and its relation to soft tissue pathology. *Int Conf Dent Plaque*, 45–48, 1970.
31. Gelb, A. F., and Seligman, S. J.: *Bacteroidaceae* bacteremia, effect of age and focus of infection upon clinical course. *JAMA*, 212(6):1038–1041, 1970.
32. Genco, R. J.: Immunoglobulins and periodontal disease. *J Periodontol*, 41(4):196–202, 1970.
33. General discussion. *J Periodontol*, 41(4):232–239, 1970.
34. Gibbons, R. J.: Bacteriology of periodontal

disease. *Am Inst Oral Biol Ann Meet*, 49–56, 1969.
35. Gibbons, R. J.: Bacterial plaque as a common denominator in dental caries and periodontal disease. *Am Inst Oral Biol Ann Meet*, 39–46, 1969.
36. Gjermo, P., Baastad, K. L., and Rölla, B.: The plaque-inhibiting capacity of 11 antibacterial compounds. *J Periodont Res*, 5:102–109, 1970.
37. Gorlin, R. J., and Goldman, H. M.: *Thoma's Oral Pathology*, St. Louis, C. V. Mosby Co., 1970, vols. 1 and 2.
38. Graf, H.: Glycolytic activity of plaque and its relation to hard tissue pathology. *Int Conf Dent Plaque*, 42–45, 1970.
39. Graykowski, E. A., Barile, M. F., Lee, W. B., and Stanley, Jr., H. R.: Recurrent aphthous stomatitis, clinical, therapeutic, histopathologic, and hypersensitivity aspects. *JAMA*, 196(7):637–644, 1966.
40. Hennon, D. K., Stookey, G. K., and Muhler, J. C.: Prevalence and distribution of dental caries in preschool children. *JADA*, 79:1405–1414, 1969.
41. Henle, W., and Henle, G.: The relationship between the Epstein-Barr virus and infectious mononucleosus, Burkitt's lymphoma and cancer of the post nasal space. *East Afr Med J*, 46:1–5, 1969.
42. Horsfall, F. L., and Tamm, I. (Eds.): *Viral and Rickettsial Infection of Man*, 4th ed. Philadelphia, J. B. Lippincott Co.
43. Ingraham, R. Q., and Williams, J. E.: An evaluation of the utility of application and cariostasis effectiveness of phosphate-fluorides in solution and gel states. *J Tenn S Dent Assoc*, 50(1):5–12, 1970.
44. *International Conference on Dental Plaque*. American Dental Association and Warner-Lambert Pharmaceutical Co., 1970.
45. Jenkins, G. N.: The mode of formation of dental plaque. *Caries Res*, 2:130–138, 1968.
46. Kay, L. W.: Control of infections in dental practice. *J Dent Assoc S Africa*, 25:251–262, 1970.
47. Keyes, P. H.: Present and future measures for dental caries control. *JADA*, 79:1395–1404, 1969.
48. Lang, L. A., Thomas, H. G., Taylor, J. A., and Rothaar, R. E.: Efficacy of a self-applied stannous fluoride prophylactic paste. *J Dent for Child*, 37(3):27/211–32/216, 1970.
49. Leach, S. A., and Hayes, M. L.: A possible correlation between specific bacterial enzyme activities, plaque formation and cariogenicity. *Caries Res*, 2:38–46, 1968.
50. Lehner, T.: Autoimmunity in oral diseases, with special reference to recurrent oral ulceration. *Proc R Soc Med (Section on Odontology)*, 61:515–524, 1968.
51. Lehner, T.: Autoimmunity and management of recurrent aphthous ulceration. *Brit Dent J*, 122:15–20, 1967.
52. Lehner, T.: Autoimmunological investigation of recurrent aphthous ulceration. *J Dent Res* (Nov.–Dec. Suppl.):1164, 1965.
53. Loe, H.: Present day status and direction for future research on the etiology and prevention of periodontal disease. *J Periodontol*, 40(12):678–682, 1969.
54. Loe, H., and Schiott, C. R.: The effect of mouthrinses and topical application of chlorhexidine on the development of dental plaque and gingivitis in man. *J Periodont Res*, 5:79–83, 1970.
55. Losee, F. L., and Bibby, B. G.: Caries inhibition by trace elements other than fluorine. *NY Dent J*, 36:15–19, 1970.
56. MacKenzie, W. R.: Serum tube identification of *Candida albicans*. *J Clin Path*, 15:563–565, 1962.
57. Mergenhagen, S. E.: Complement as a mediator of inflammation: Formation of biologically-active products after interaction of serum complement with endotoxins and antigen-antibody complexes. *J Periodontol*, 41(4):202–205, 1970.
58. Mergenhagen, S. E. *et al.*: Significance of complement of the mechanism of action of endotoxin. *Curr Top Microbiol Immunol*, 50: 37–77, 1969.
59. Mergenhagen, S. E. *et al.*: Reactions and periodontal inflammation. *J Dent Res*, 49(2)(Part 1):256–261, 1970.
60. Mitchell, D. F., and Standish, S.: *Oral Diagnosis/Oral Medicine*. 2nd ed. Philadelphia, Lea & Febiger, 1971.
61. Muhler, J. C.: A clinical comparison of fluoride and antienzyme dentifrices. *J Dent Child*, 37(6):501–514, 1970.
62. Nisengard, R. J., and Beutner, E. J.: Relation of immediate hypersensitivity to perio-

dontitis in animals and man. *J Periodontol,* 41(4):223–228, 1970.
63. Nolte, W. A. (Ed.): *Oral Microbiology.* St Louis, C. V. Mosby Co., 1968.
64. Oppenheim, J. J., and Francis, T. C.: The role of delayed hypersensitivity in immunological processes and its relationship to aphthous stomatitis. *J Periodontol,* 41(4):205–210, 1970.
65. *Oral Manifestations of Bacterial, Viral and Mycotic Infections.* Council on Dental Therapeutics, American Dental Association, Chicago, 1968.
66. Platt, D., Crosby, R. G., and Dlabow, N. H.: Evidence for the presence of immunoglobulins and antibodies in inflamed periodontal tissues. *J Periodontol* 41(4):215–223, 1970.
67. Riethe, P., and Weinmann, K.: Caries inhibition with fluoride gel and fluoride varnish in rats. *Caries Res,* 4:62–68, 1970.
68. Rizzo, A. A.: Histologic and immunologic evaluation of antigen penetration into oral tissues after topical application. *J Periodontol* 41(4):210–213, 1970.
69. Robbins, S. L.: *Pathology.* Philadelphia, W. B. Saunders, 1967.
70. Schiott, C. R., Loe, H., Jensen, S. B., Kilian, M., Davies, R. M., and Glavind, K.: The effect of chlorhexidine mouthrinses on the human oral flora. *J Periodont Res,* 5:84–89, 1970.
71. Selvig, K. A.: Attachment of plaque and calculus to tooth surfaces. *J Periodont Res,* 5:8–18, 1970.
72. Shafer, W. G., Hine, M. K., and Levy, B. M.: Philadelphia, W. B. Saunders Co., 1967.
73. Sheft, D. J., and Shrago, G.: Esophageal moniliasis: the spectrum of the disease. *JAMA,* 213(11):1859–1862, 1970.
74. Silness, J.: Periodontal conditions in patients treated with dental bridges. *J Periodont Res,* 5:60–68, 1970.
75. Simon, B. I., Goldman, H. M., Ruben, M. P., and Baker, E.: The role of endotoxin in periodontal disease. I. A reproducible, quantitative method for determining the amount of endotoxin in human gingival exudate. *J Periodontol,* 40(12):695–701, 1969.
76. Simon *et al.*: The role of endotoxin in periodontal disease. III. Correlation of the quantity of endotoxin in human gingival exudate with the clinical degree of inflammation. *J Periodontol,* 41(2):81–86, 1970.
77. Sims, W.: The interpretation and use of Snyder tests and *Lactobacillus* counts. *JADA,* 80:1315–1319, 1970.
78. Sims, W.: The concept of immunity in dental caries. 1. General consideration. *Oral Surg,* 30(5):670–677, 1970.
79. Skach, M., Sabrodsky, S., and Mrklas, L.: A study of the effect of age and season on the incidence of ulcerative gingivitis. *J Periodont Res,* 5:187–190, 1970.
80. Stanley, H. R., Graykowski, E. A., and Barile, M. F.: The occurrence of microorganisms in microscopic sections of aphthous and nonaphthous lesions and other oral tissues. *O.S., O.M., & O.P.* 18(3):335–341, 1964.
81. Steinberg, A. I.: Evidence for the presence of circulating antibodies to an oral spirochete in the sera of clinic patients. *J Periodontol* 41(4):213–215, 1970.
82. Stewart, S.: Studies on the herpes-type virus recovered from Burkitt's tumor and other human lymphomas. *Adv Virus Res,* 15:291–305, 1969.
83. Sundstrom, F., and Ericsson, Y.: Oral carbohydrate clearance: Testing methods and clinical significance. *Caries Res,* 2:214–228, 1968.
84. Swain, R. H. A., and Dodds, T. C.: *Clinical Virology,* Baltimore, Williams & Wilkins Co., 1967.
85. Taichman, N. S.: Mediation of inflammation by the polymorphonuclear leukocyte as a sequela of immune reactions. *J Periodontol,* 41(4):228–232, 1970.
86. Tempel, T. R., Snyderman, R., Jordan, H. V., and Mergenhagen, S. E.: Factors from saliva and oral bacteria, chemotactic for polymorphonuclear leukocytes: their possible role in gingival inflammation. *J Periodontol,* 41(2):71–80, 1970.
87. *Viruses and the Cell Systems Useful in Their Cultivation. (A Provisional Chart).* Bethesda (Md.), Microbiological Associates, Inc., April 1969.
88. Volpe, A. R., Schulman, S. M., Goldman, H. M., King, W. J., and Kupczak, L. J.: The long term effect of antimicrobial formulation on dental calculus formation. *J Periodontol,* 41(No. 8):463–467, 1970.
89. Von Der Fehr, F. R.: The caries inhibiting

effect of topically applied hexafluorostannate on dentine and enamel. *Caries Res,* 4:269–282, 1970.
90. Von Der Fehr, F. R., Loe, H., and Theilade, E.: Experimental caries in man. *Caries Res,* 4:131–148, 1970.
91. Winer, R. A., O'Donnell, L. J., Chauncey, H. H., and McNamana, T. F.: Enzyme activity in periodontal disease. *J Periodontol,* 41(8):449–456, 1970.
92. Zegarelli, E. V. Kutscher, A. H., and Hyman, G. A. (Eds.): *Diagnosis of Diseases of the Mouth and Jaws.* Philadelphia, Lea & Febiger, 1969.
93. Zinsser, H.: *Microbiology,* 14th ed. New York, Appleton-Century-Crofts, Division of Meredith Corp., 1968.
94. Zipkin, I., Baer, P. N., Hawkins, G. R., Zucas, S. M., and Mantel, N.: The effect of fluoride and dietary protein levels on calculus formation, alveolar bone loss, selected salivary constituents and fluoride deposition in the bones and teeth. *J Periodontol,* 41(4):320–437, 1970.

Chapter 10
The Role of Laboratory Tests in Oral Diagnosis
LAWRENCE COHEN

THE PRACTISING DENTIST is frequently asked to provide dental treatment for patients with medical problems. On occasions he may see a patient whom he suspects has a systemic disease. There is no reason why a dentist with his training should not order laboratory tests to confirm his suspicions. If the dentist establishes that the patient has a medical problem, the correct procedure is for him to refer the patient to his physician for treatment.

The purpose of this chapter is to help the dentist to choose the correct clinical test for a patient and to interpret the results. Because a patient may consult his dentist before his physician, the dentist can play an important role in the early detection of systemic disease.

PLASMA PROTEINS

The plasma proteins include fibrinogen, albumin and globulin and constitute 6 to 8 gm/100 ml of the plasma. With the exception of γ-globulins, the plasma proteins are formed in the liver. Fibrinogen is important in the clotting mechanism. The globulin fraction comprises alpha-1, alpha-2, beta and gamma components. Electrophoretic analysis enables the approximate concentrations of these components in human plasma to be determined.

CONDITIONS AFFECTING THE RED BLOOD CELLS

"Anemia" is a decrease in the level of hemoglobin below the normal level. An increase above normal in the erythrocyte count, the hemoglobin level and hematocrit is termed "polycythemia." (Table 10-1)

Anemia

If the patient is pale and admits to breathlessness on exertion, lassitude, headaches and palpitations, he should be investigated for anemia. It should be remembered that a severely anemic patient will not tolerate an acute blood loss, and for this reason tooth extraction or an oral surgical procedure should not be carried out until the hemoglobin level is restored to the normal range, by transfusion if necessary. As a general rule a hemoglobin level of at least 10gm/100 ml and a hematocrit of at least 28, and preferably over 30, should be regarded as the lowest limits for surgery.

Tests Employed in the Diagnosis of Anemia

Although the red blood cell count (RBC) is frequently employed it is inaccurate, even machine counting techniques giving an error of 2 to 4 per cent. The hemoglobin level and hematocrit are the two most satis-

TABLE 10-1
NORMAL RANGE OF BLOOD CELL VALUES

	Men	Women	Children—Both Sexes (3 mo.–13 yr.)
Erythrocytes (millions/cu mm)	4.6–6.2	4.2–5.4	3.8–5.2
Hemoglobin (gm/100 ml)	14–18	12–16	10–14.5
Hematocrit	42–52	37–47	31–43

Note: This table is reprinted by kind permission of the publishers from Cohen, L.: *A Synopsis Of Medicine In Dentistry.* Philadelphia, Lea & Febiger, 1972.

factory tests in the diagnosis of anemia. When investigating a patient with anemia the red cell count, white cell count, differential white cell count, the hemoglobin and hematocrit levels are performed routinely.

Examination of a Stained Peripheral Blood Smear

This procedure allows observation of alterations in the size, shape and structure of individual red cells or white cells. In addition a reasonable estimate of the platelet count can be made in most cases from the peripheral smear alone.

Classification of Anemia

An erythrocyte may be of normal size (normocytic), smaller than normal (microcytic) or larger than normal (macrocytic). A red cell may contain a normal concentration of hemoglobin (normochromic) or less hemoglobin than normal (hypochromic). The term "hyperchromic" does not exist, as a mammalian erythrocyte cannot become supersaturated with hemoglobin. Anemias are classified as normocytic-normochromic, microcytic-hypochromic and macrocytic-normochromic (megaloblastic anemias).

NORMOCYTIC-NORMOCHROMIC ANEMIAS. This group of anemias is caused by acute blood loss, by hemolysis or by decreased blood formation in the bone marrow. The red cells are normal in volume and in hemoglobin concentration. Sickle cell trait and sickle cell anemia, which occur in the American Negro, are the most important forms of hemolytic anemia occurring in the United States of America. Sickling of the red cells is observed when the blood is sealed under a cover slip at a low oxygen tention. The Sickledex* test is a simple test which is available for diagnosing sickle cell anemia.

MICROCYTIC-HYPOCHROMIC ANEMIA. This type of anemia is caused by excessive loss of iron as a result of chronic hemorrhage from hemorrhoids, peptic ulcer or heavy menstrual flow or from deficient intake of iron in the diet. It may also be idiopathic.

MEGALOBLASTIC ANEMIAS. This group includes pernicious anemia and some anemias due to defective absorption of vitamin B_{12} and folic acid from the small intestine. Pernicious anemia is due to absence or deficiency of intrinsic factor which results in a deficient supply of vitamin B_{12} to the bone marrow. Tropical sprue and celiac disease which are folic acid deficiency anemias are characterized by diarrhea associated with sore tongue.

The Schilling Test

This test, which is a urinary excretion technique, is used to measure the absorption of radioactive vitamin B_{12}. Normal patients will excrete in the urine for twenty-four hours after an oral dose of radioactive vitamin B_{12} more than 15 percent of the administered radioactivity. Individuals with impaired absorption of vitamin B_{12}

* Ortho Diagnostics, Raritan, New Jersey.

excrete less than 5 percent (most patients with pernicious anemia excrete less than 2 percent).

Polycythemia

Patients with this disease have a bluish-red color of the skin and mucous membranes. They may bleed excessively following tooth extraction. The red cell count varies from 6 to 10 millions per cubic millimeter. The white cell and platelet counts are also raised.

CONDITIONS AFFECTING THE WHITE BLOOD CELLS

The normal white cell count in the adult varies between 4,000 and 10,000 per cubic millimeter. In the first two or three years of life lymphocytes make up 60 percent or more of the circulating leukocytes, but by the age of fourteen or fifteen the normal adult distribution is reached. (Table 10-2)

A circulating white cell count in excess of 10,000 per cubic millimeter is termed "leukocytosis" and occurs in a number of infections: a count below 4000 per cubic millimeter is known as leukopenia.

Leukemia

Leukemia is the malignant proliferation of the precursors of white cell in the bone marrow, resulting in large numbers of white cells in the peripheral blood, many of which are immature. The dentist should consider a diagnosis of leukemia when a patient feels unwell and is pale and there is spontaneous hemorrhage from the gingivae. The latter are swollen, bluish-red and tender, and often there may be an associated Vincent's infection due to the lowered resistance. In the lymphocytic and monocytic forms, gingival hypertrophy is often found. The white cell count and differential white cell count are employed in confirming the diagnosis.

Agranulocytosis

Agranulocytosis should be suspected when a patient develops severe ulceration of the mouth and fauces with little inflammatory reaction around the ulcers. The white cell count shows a severe form of leukopenia. The condition may occur following the administration of drugs such as aminopyrine, sulfonamides, gold or chloramphenicol.

In any unusual form of oral ulceration a complete blood count (CBC) is indicated.

TABLE 10-2
NORMAL RANGE OF WHITE CELL VALUES

Cell Type	Range of Normal Values %	Per cu mm
Neutrophils	40–70	1600–7000
Lymphocytes	20–45	800–4500
Monocytes	2–8	80–800
Eosinophils	0–5	0–500
Basophils	0–1	0–100

Note: This table is reprinted by kind permission of the publishers from Cohen, L.: *A Synopsis Of Medicine In Dentistry*. Philadelphia, Lea & Febiger, 1972.

CONDITIONS AFFECTING THE PLATELETS

The platelets may be reduced in number, *thrombocytopenia,* or they may be defective in function, *thrombasthenia.* Spontaneous bleeding from the gingivae may occur in *thrombocytopenic purpura.* The normal platelet count is 150,000 to 450,000 per cubic millimeter and thrombocytopenia is said to occur when the count is below 100,000 per cubic millimeter. Thrombocytopenia may be induced by sensitivity to drugs such as quinidine and Sedormid® or by an infection. When no cause can be found the condition is known as idiopathic thrombocytopenic purpura. In thrombocytopenic purpura due to any cause the bleeding time is prolonged (see below).

PURPURA. Purpura is defined as hemorrhages into the skin and joints and from mucous membranes. As stated above, it may result from a decrease in the number of platelets. In some conditions, the platelets are normal but hemorrhages result from capillary fragility, vascular purpura (*see* tests of platelet function).

CLINICAL TESTS EMPLOYED IN THE INVESTIGATIONS OF DISEASES OF THE BLOOD

The whole blood clotting time, partial thromboplastin and one-stage prothrombin time are tests of plasma clotting activity in common use. The bleeding time, platelet count, tourniquet test and clot retraction test are believed to measure platelet function. (Tables 10-3 and 10-4)

Tests of Clotting Function

Whole Blood Clotting Time

Venous blood is usually employed. A prolonged clotting time indicates that a problem exists which should be further investigated.

Partial Thromboplastin Time (PTT)

This is a one-stage test for stage I defects and is the usual test employed in the diagnosis of hemophilia (factor VIII deficiency) and Christmas disease (factor IX deficiency). If one of these factors is lacking, the time will be prolonged.

One-Stage Prothrombin Time

This is a test for stage II defects. The prothrombin time may be prolonged in patients with liver disease; it is prolonged in patients receiving anticoagulant drugs which inhibit the utilization of vitamin K by the liver and therefore decrease prothrombin synthesis. The time taken for the clot to form is recorded and compared with a normal control plasma.

Tests of Platelet Function

Bleeding Time

This test measures the time necessary for active bleeding to cease from a clean superficial wound. The two tests in general use are the Duke and Ivy methods. In hemophilia the bleeding time is normal.

Platelet Count

The normal platelet count is 150,000 to 450,000 per cubic millimeter. As stated above the count is reduced in thrombocytopenic purpura.

Tourniquet Test

This test, which is nonspecific, is an index of capillary fragility and platelet function. A blood pressure cuff is placed on the upper arm and inflated to the midpoint between systolic and diastolic pressure. It is left for five minutes, after which the forearm is examined for petechiae. Normal individuals have 0 to 10 petechiae; between 10 and 20 is equivocal; more than 20 indicates abnormal hemostatic function.

Clot Retraction Test

This test is used to measure platelet function. A test tube of blood, without anti-

TABLE 10-3
THE PHYSIOLOGY OF BLOOD COAGULATION
List Of Clotting Factors

Factor I—Fibrinogen
Factor II—Prothrombin
Factor III—Tissue Thromboplastin
Factor IV—Calcium
Factor V—Proaccelerin, labile factor
Factor VII—Proconvertin, serum prothrombin conversion accelerator (SPCA), stable factor
Factor VIII—Antihemophilic globulin (AHG)
Factor IX—Plasma thromboplastin component (PTC), Christmas factor
Factor X—Stuart Prower factor, Stuart factor
Factor XI—Plasma thromboplastin antecedent (PTA)
Factor XII—Hageman factor
Factor XIII—Fibrin stabilizing factor (FSF), fibrinase

Note: There is no Factor VI.

TABLE 10-4
DIAGRAM OF THE CLOTTING MECHANISM

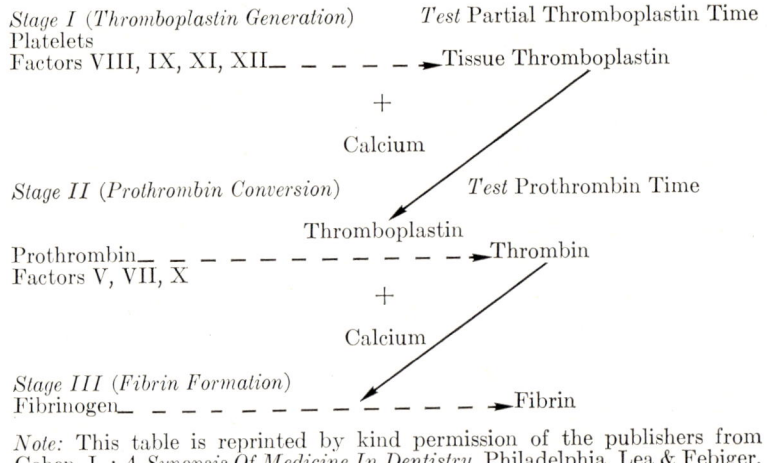

Note: This table is reprinted by kind permission of the publishers from Cohen, L.: *A Synopsis Of Medicine In Dentistry*. Philadelphia, Lea & Febiger, 1972.

coagulant, is placed in the incubator at 37 C. The clot should begin to retract in thirty minutes and should be retracted completely in twelve hours. The clot fails to retract when the platelets are reduced or there is a failure of the platelets to break up and initiate the clotting process.

Investigation of Anemia

For tests employed in the diagnosis of anemia see page 110.

BLOOD CHEMISTRY

Blood Urea Nitrogen

The normal range of blood urea nitrogen (BUN) is 5 to 25 mg/100 ml. In patients with renal failure levels in excess of 100 mg of BUN per 100 ml of blood are common.

Creatinine

The normal concentration of blood creatinine is 0.8 to 1.4 mg/100 ml and figures in excess of 1.5 mg/100 ml are regarded as significant. Diet has little effect on the blood creatinine, which is almost entirely endogenous, being produced from the breakdown of the body tissues. In advanced renal failure the concentration of plasma creatinine is significantly raised.

Uric Acid

The concentration of uric acid in the blood plasma normally varies from 2.5 to 7 mg/100 ml. It is the chief purine end-product of nucleoprotein metabolism in man and in the absence of renal insufficiency its level is not significantly affected by the ingestion of a diet rich in purine. The level of uric acid is raised in acute gout.

Blood Cholesterol

The blood cholesterol level is 150 to 250 mg/100 ml. Elevated values are found in hypothyroidism, nephrotic syndrome, idiopathic hypercholesterolemia, biliary cirrhosis and often diabetes.

Blood Glucose

The Dextrostix* test can be used in the dental office for estimating the level of blood glucose. The patient's finger is cleaned with an alcohol swab, dried and then pricked with a sterile needle. A large drop of blood is then placed on the treated paper and left in contact for exactly sixty seconds, when it is washed off with a stream of water. The color is then compared with the manufacturer's color standards and the blood glucose level is read.

If the fasting venous blood sugar is greater than 110 mg/100 ml or the blood sugar two hours after a meal is greater than 120 mg/100 ml, diabetes mellitus is the presumptive diagnosis. To confirm the diagnosis a glucose tolerance test is required.

URINALYSIS

The standard urinalysis includes the appearance of the specimen, pH, specific gravity, presence or absence of protein, presence or absence of glucose and ketones and microscopic examination of the centrifuged urinary sediment. For the microscopic examination of urine clean-voided specimens are needed which in the female require special preparation to prevent vaginal contamination. With the exception of microscopic examination and the specific gravity examination, it is possible for the dentist or his assistant to test a sample of urine in his own office by means of the Labstix* test.

1. *Appearance.* Occasionally the urine may be red due to the presence of blood or porphyrins.

2. *pH.* Normal urine is usually acid but on standing at room temperature will slowly become alkaline due to bacterial growth.

3. *Specific gravity.* If, on a random urine specimen, the specific gravity is 1.022 or greater and there is no significant glycosuria or marked proteinuria, then it is reasonable to conclude that the overall renal function is adequate.

4. *Protein.* Protein is normally absent from the urine. Its presence usually indicates some systemic disease or renal pathology. In some patients, however, protein appears in the urine when they are in the upright position but not when they are lying down. This condition of orthostatic proteinuria is diagnosed by testing the early morning urine produced during sleep and comparing it with one taken later in the day.

5. *Glucose.* Diabetes mellitus is the most

---

* Ames Company, Division Miles Laboratories, Inc., Elkhart, Indiana.

important cause of glucosuria. The normal renal threshold is about 180 mg/100 ml blood glucose level. Some patients have a low renal threshold and may spill sugar into the urine at levels below 180 mg/100 ml (renal glucosuria).

If a patient presents with a recent history of increased thirst and polyuria and examination of the urine shows the presence of glucose, a glucose tolerance test is required to confirm the diagnosis of diabetes mellitus. It should be remembered that a diabetic is prone to develop severe periodontal disease and apical infections and that dryness of the mouth is an early manifestation of diabetes mellitus. In addition, patients with recurrent boils and long-standing angular cheilitis associated with *C albicans* should always be suspected of being diabetic until proved otherwise.

6. *Ketone bodies (acetone and diacetic acid).* These are classic findings of diabetic acidosis. However, acetonuria may also occur in starvation and in children who have difficulty in eating because of acute herpetic stomatitis. In the latter, the administration of a glucose solution by mouth will soon remove the ketone bodies. In diabetes, the presence of large amounts of ketones is one of the major indications of diabetic acidosis or impending acidosis.

BLOOD ENZYMES

The dentist should be aware of the fact that in certain diseases there is an alteration in the level of specific enzymes in the blood which are of value in establishing or confirming a diagnosis.

Alkaline Phosphatase

This is an enzyme produced mainly in the liver and bone. In obstructive jaundice the alkaline phosphatase level is raised.

The osteoblasts in bone produce large amounts of alkaline phosphatase. Paget's disease, hyperparathyroidism, rickets and osteomalacia, and osteoblastic metastatic carcinoma to bone all give consistently elevated values. Although carcinoma of the prostate gives rise to osteoblastic metastases (see below) there is in addition a specific rise in the serum acid phosphatase level (*see* below).

Acid Phosphatase

This enzyme is produced in the prostate. Carcinoma of the prostate frequently metastasizes to bone and most of the metastases are osteoblastic in nature, appearing as radiopaque lesions on the radiograph. On occasion the jaws may be involved, in which case the serum acid phosphatase is raised.

Serum Transaminases

The enzymes serum glutamic-oxaloacetic and glutamic pyruvic transaminase (GOT and GPT) are found in many tissues, but the highest concentrations are found in the liver and myocardium. Normally, less than 40 Karmen units are found in the serum. Tissue injury as found in disorders of the liver and in myocardial infarction will increase the level of GOT and GPT in the serum.

DISEASES OF BONE

There are a number of diseases of bone in which the serum calcium, phosphate* and alkaline phosphatase levels are altered. For convenience it is proposed to consider the laboratory findings in deficiency states and general diseases of bone.

Deficiency States

Rickets

The serum calcium level is generally normal or at the lower limit of normal. Serum phosphate values are reduced from the normal childhood level of 5 to 6 mg/100 ml to 2 to 4 mg/100 ml. The alkaline phosphatase level is generally elevated.

Osteomalacia

The serum calcium values are normal or at the lower limit of normal and the serum phosphate concentrations are reduced from the normal adult levels of 3 to 4 mg/100 ml. Alkaline phosphatase activity is increased.

Scurvy

In the infant there are subperiosteal and cutaneous hemorrhages and bleeding occurs around erupted teeth. In the adult cutaneous hemorrhages occur and when teeth are present there is bleeding from the gingivae.

When an adequate amount of vitamin C is being absorbed, it is excreted in the urine. If after 200 mg of vitamin C, none is excreted, this indicates that the body stores are depleted and that the patient is vitamin C deficient.

General Diseases of Bone

Osteitis Deformans (Paget's Disease)

The serum calcium and phosphate are normal but the serum alkaline phosphatase is markedly raised (*see* Ch. 7).

Fibrous Dysplasia of Bone

The serum calcium and phosphate are normal but the serum alkaline phosphatase may be raised. It should be noted that the latter level is never as high as in Paget's disease (*see* Ch. 7).

Hyperparathyroidism

The serum calcium is usually greater than 11 mg/100 ml and the serum phosphate is low. Serum alkaline phosphatase may be increased especially in the presence of significant bone disease (*see* Ch. 7).

ENDOCRINE DISORDERS

Some of the endocrine glands are dependent on and controlled by a specific hormone produced by the anterior pituitary. The pituitary gland itself is controlled by the hypothalamus.

The secretion of parathyroid hormone is dependent on a low blood calcium level.

When the blood calcium rises, the hormone secretion is suppressed. The laboratory findings in hyperparathyroidism have been previously discussed (*see* Ch. 7).

The dentist may encounter patients whose periodontal status has worsened over a relatively short time and who present with a periodontal infection. He should always suspect diabetes and carry out the necessary tests (*see* Ch. 3). It should be emphasized that dryness of the mouth is

---

* The terms 'serum phosphorus' and 'serum phosphate' are used synonymously. Serum inorganic phosphorus levels are measured in terms of the phosphate ions, for ionized free phosphorus does not circulate.

an early manifestation of this disease.

The thin patient with exophthalmos, a rapid pulse, moist sweating palms and tremor of the outstretched fingers is an obvious case of hyperthyroidism. Myxedema (hypothyroidism) is the obvious diagnosis in a patient with loss of the outer third of the eyebrows and puffiness around the eyes particularly when the speech is slow and deep toned.

Two tests which the dentist can order in suspected thyroid disease are the protein-bound iodine and butanol-extractable iodine. In hyperthyroidism both are raised and in hypothyroidism both are lowered.

The tests involved in the diagnosis of adrenal disorders are outside the scope of the dentist.

REFERENCES

1. Goodale, R. H., and Widman, F. K.: *Clinical Interpretation of Laboratory Tests*, 6th ed. Philadelphia, Davis, 1969.
2. Ravel, R.: *Clinical Laboratory Medicine*. Chicago, Year Book Medical Publishers, 1969.

Chapter 11

The Role of the Oral Pathologist in Oral Diagnosis

HERMAN MEDAK

A VARIETY of diseases of local and systemic origins can be found in the oral mucosa. Some of these are of infectious nature, some are neoplastic and some of unknown etiology. A unique feature of the oral cavity is that the oral flora has the potential of destroying hard tissue, such as teeth and bone.

The dental clinician is primarily concerned with the commonly painful, disfiguring and disabling diseases that attack the teeth and supporting structures, necessitating repair and reconstruction. The clinician also has a responsibility of identifying and initiating treatment of the diseases of the soft tissue, whether benign or malignant, hopefully in their early stages when a cure is frequently possible.

In all forms of cancer, early detection and early therapeutic intervention is critical. Because the oral cavity is so frequently inspected by clinicians, most oral cancers should be detected in relatively early stages. Yet, even clearly diagnostic symptoms are frequently overlooked or disregarded in dental practice.

In 1971, 24,300 new cases of oral cancer were expected in the United States and 11,000 deaths due to oral cancer.[1] Tragically, many of these cases are identified too late for effective therapy, and only one patient out of three survives five years. Despite the fact that oral cancer is more accessible than cancer in any other part of the body, it has a rate of cure lower than cancer of any other part of the body with the exceptions of cancer of the lung and stomach.

Other diseases of the oral mucosa also can cause widespread damage if not identified and treated promptly. The dental clinician, therefore, has a responsibility to his patients to identify and follow the progress of every lesion or abnormality discovered in or around the oral cavity.

It is the role and function of the oral pathologist to make a definitive diagnosis of abnormalities in the oral cavity, since the structural changes in oral diseases are relatively specific. It is essential that the practicing dental clinician utilize the oral pathologist's laboratory to assist in diagnoses.

In general, the rules for the clinician to follow are these:

1. Relatively inexpensive and painless cytological examination by smears should be conducted whenever an abnormality is discovered.

2. A biopsy should be ordered whenever a lesion is suspected of being malignant, a cytological examination is suspicious or positive, whenever soft tissue is removed by surgery or whenever an abnormal condition persists for any length of time despite treatment.

THE ORAL PATHOLOGIST

The American Academy of Oral Pathology is the organization dedicated to the advancement of the science of oral pathology. Fellowship in the Academy is granted to a graduate dentist who passes the appropriate examination in oral pathology, clinical oral pathology and general pathology. His knowledge of general pathology will make it possible for him to relate the local disease to the overall systemic picture.

The specialist in oral pathology is, therefore, a dental clinician as well. He may be affiliated with a dental school, a laboratory or a hospital.

The oral pathologist is aware of the specific and unique cellular structure of the oral mucosa. Contrary to most other anatomical areas, the epithelium of the normal oral mucosa varies in different sites in accordance with variation in function and mechanical influences. The interpretation of cytological material demands a knowledge of the specific location from which a sample is taken, because cellular characteristics that would be pathological in one area are perfectly normal if found elsewhere.

It is the function of the oral pathologist to provide a tentative diagnosis of disease on the basis of smears and a definitive diagnosis on biopsies. Smears or biopsies taken by the clinician or specialist are submitted for laboratory analysis. It is essential that oral smears be sent to a laboratory experienced in oral cytology due to the peculiarities of oral mucosa.

ORAL CYTOLOGY

Oral cytology does not provide as definitive a diagnosis as a biopsy, but it is recommended for any area in the oral cavity which exhibits abnormal change, such as ulceration, a red area, a white patch on an inflammatory base or a fissure. It is indicated in cases where a lesion is small and cancer is not suspected. If cancer is suspected, a biopsy is indicated immediately, but a smear may be taken for rapid preliminary evaluation.

The cytologic smear is relatively inexpensive and painless, compared to the biopsy. It is indicated in patients who object to a biopsy as a follow-up after surgery and during radiation therapy. If a large lesion is seen which is usually benign but may become malignant like erosive lichen planus, where multiple biopsies would have to be done repeatedly, it is simpler to take repeated multiple smears to detect possible malignant changes.

A commercially available Cyto-Kit is recommended for taking a scraping. It consists of one spatula, two glass slides, a bottle of fixer, a history sheet and mailing container and canvas bag.

In using the Cyto-Kit, the clinician should fill out all blanks on the history sheet and mark the area of the lesion on the chart on the reverse side of the history sheet.

The patient's full name is placed on the ground glass portion on both of the slides.

In taking a smear, the area should be isolated. If dry, it should be slightly moistened with a drop of saline solution or with the patient's saliva. Excess saliva should be removed. The lesion should then be scraped with the spatula several times, avoiding severe bleeding when possible, but being sure to obtain cells from the affected area. The scraped material is smeared on the glass slide, and enough fixing solution to cover the smear is immediately poured over the glass. A second smear is obtained in the same manner. After fifteen minutes, the fixing solution is poured off, and the slides are allowed to dry. They are then placed in a plastic container and mailed to the oral pathologist.

If a commercial kit is not available, glass slides can be obtained from the drugstore. Any flat spatula in the dental cabinet or a wooden tongue depressor can be used for scraping and the smear can be fixed, if necessary, in rubbing alcohol. The patient's name, age, sex and address, the doctor's name, address and phone number, the location and description of the lesion should be written on a sheet of paper and mailed to a pathologist or cytology laboratory, qualified for oral cytology.

In reporting results to the clinician, five classes of cytological findings are specified:

Class I. Only normal cells observed.

Class II. Minor abnormalities observed, but are within benign limits.

Class III. Atypical cells suggestive of cancer observed. A biopsy is mandatory.

Class IV. Findings strongly suggestive of cancer. A biopsy is mandatory.

Class V. Positive of cancer. A biopsy is mandatory.

Though numerical classifications are simple and demand little interpretation by the clinician, the tendency among pathologists is to rely more on descriptive interpretations of the material. In our opinion, the descriptive interpretation is of greater value to the pathologist for follow-up and recommendation to the clinician. However, the numerical classification still has value for the clinician.

False negatives are more frequent than false positives, depending on the technique of taking a smear and the condition in each laboratory. However, positive reports require confirmation by biopsy before treatment. A negative interpretation (class I or II) may indicate a benign lesion or may represent the absence of abnormal cells from the smear or inadequate technique of obtaining material.

If a lesion persists, even if the original cytological examination was negative, it is essential that further smears or biopsies be taken. The dentist is not relieved of responsibility by one negative cytological report, particularly if a lesion or clinical abnormality persists.

It must be emphasized that oral cytology, although quite accurate when properly used, is only an adjunct and not a substitute for a biopsy when cancer is suspected.

Although the primary purpose of a cytological test is to detect early and unsuspected cancer, it may also be used in the differential diagnosis of viral and dermatologic lesions and other benign conditions.

It is difficult to overestimate the importance of the oral cytologic examination to the dentist in general practice. It is perhaps indicative that in one study,[2] 20 percent of all oral cancers under treatment were completely unsuspected by the patient or the dentist but were discovered by routine cytological smears of presumably benign lesions. Early manifestations of oral cancer simply cannot be distinguished from benign abnormalities on the basis of clinical observation.

In Sandler's study[3] it may be presumed that two out of three of the patients in whom oral cancer was discovered through cytologic examination would have died within five years. It may also be presumed that early detection made it possible to save their lives through prompt treatment. For this reason, cytological smears are strongly indicated whenever clinical abnormalities are observed by the general dental practitioner, regardless of how harmless or benign they may seem.

BIOPSY

The term "biopsy" is usually used when tissue or material is removed from a living subject for examination. The purpose of a biopsy is to determine the nature of a lesion and to establish a definitive diagnosis and give some indication for treatment and prognosis. No radiation therapy or surgery will ordinarily be started without a positive tissue biopsy.

Though the dentist is well qualified to remove tissue from the oral cavity, it is usually desirable for the clinician performing a biopsy to be well acquainted with the technique or to refer the patient to a specialist. In cases of suspected malignancy, it is advantageous to request the clinician who will perform the surgery in addition to take the biopsy.

A biopsy is mandatory whenever the results of a cytologic examination is in class III, IV or V or if the lesion is suspicious of malignancy. Furthermore, any tissue or growth removed surgically from the oral cavity should be submitted for pathologic examination.

It is advisable not to biopsy indiscriminately, since there is a small possibility of spread of the original tumor. This is more pronounced in connective tissue tumors. Also, the emotional trauma to the patient may deter him at a later time from returning to the dentist or physician.

There are four different types of biopsies: incision biopsy, excision biopsy, aspiration biopsy and punch biopsy.

Incision and Excision Biopsy

In general, in any form of biopsy, it is essential that an adequate amount of material is removed. Also, the biopsy should be taken from a significant area, including the border of normal and abnormal tissue, if possible. In deep-seated lesions, especially in lesions beneath the intact mucous membrane, it is very important to remove deep tissue in order to avoid missing the actual tumor. Pinching of the material with a forceps should be avoided.

In the case of a small lesion, a complete excision is advisable (excision biopsy) together with primary closure of the defect. In larger lesions, where only a portion is excised, great care has to be taken in the selection of the location. Necrotic tissue from the center of a lesion should be avoided. If the tumor or lesion is large, multiple biopsies may be advisable. Primary closure of the wound should be accomplished to avoid hemorrhage. The only danger associated with an excision or incision biopsy may be in the presence of a vascular tumor, where a severe hemorrhage may result.

The tissue biopsy should be immediately placed into the fixative, commonly 10% neutral formalin, and sent to a competent pathologist for processing and diagnosis.

A positive biopsy is usually the final conclusion of the diagnostic procedure, while a negative biopsy is not always conclusive and may have to be repeated.

Aspiration Biopsy

This procedure is used in cases when the lesion is too deep or not easily accessible. A large diameter needle on an empty syringe is inserted into a solid or cystic area, and tissue fragments or fluid are aspirated. The tissue fragments are fixed in 10% neutral formalin, centrifuged, and the pellet is treated like an ordinary biopsy. Aspirated fluid can be smeared, stained and examined or concentrated by centrifuging and sectioned like a tissue specimen.

This type of biopsy requires more experience than the incision or excision biopsy.

Punch Biopsy

The punch biopsy requires a special instrument and has limited use in the oral cavity.

SUMMARY

In summary, the oral pathologist should act as a consultant to the clinician and assist in the interpretation of the laboratory test. He establishes the definitive diagnosis from the biopsy and can be of assistance in planning therapy.

REFERENCES

1. *Cancer Statistics, 1971.* New York, American Cancer Society, p. 7.
2. Hutter, R. V. P. and Gerrold, F. P.: Cytodiagnosis of clinically inapparent oral cancer in patients considered to be high risks. *Am J. Surg, 112*:541, 1966.
3. Sandler, H. C.: A retrospective study of a head and neck cancer control program. *Cancer, 25*:1158, 1970.

Chapter 12

Occlusion and Its Relation to Oral Diagnosis and Treatment Planning

VINCENT E. URBANEK

ONLY within the past decade has it become fashionable for most clinicians and dental educators to openly proclaim that an evaluation of a patient's dental occlusion should serve as the foundation or starting point for oral diagnosis and treatment planning. Yet, judging from the controversy that surrounds the science of occlusion, it has obviously developed into one of the major enigmas of contemporary dentistry.

During the past eighty years it was not uncommon for various clinical specialties to formulate occlusal dogmas, most of which competed with one another and were primarily based on mechanical devices rather than biological principles. Confusion and frustration were further compounded when theorists finally accepted what had always been clearly self-evident, that occlusions occur and exist in innumerable combinations. They are as unique as individuals and snowflakes. The imposition of a stereotyped occlusal scheme as the panacea for all occlusal problems has about as much rationale as the mandatory extraction of teeth in all cases of arthritis.

While there is almost unanimous agreement as to the overall importance of occlusion, there exists likewise much disagreement as to which occlusal concept or method will best meet the needs of the patient—especially in those cases requiring comprehensive treatment. Paradoxically, while the various concepts of occlusal adjustment and reconstruction vary in their approach and method many have survived the test of time. As an example consider the following clinically proven but diametrical techniques:

1. Gnathological instrumentation versus functionally generated registrations.
2. Completely adjustable articulators versus semiadjustable articulators.
3. Check-bite techniques versus pantographic tracings.
4. Cusp-fossa occlusion versus cusp-embrasure occlusion.
5. Cuspid protection versus group function.

Essentially, the preceding methods demonstrate a variation in "mechanics." Clinical success with any of these methods should continue to accrue as long as the mechanics are structured within the anatomic and physiologic framework of the patients' stomatognathic systems.

THE STOMATOGNATHIC SYSTEM

The masticatory or stomatognathic system, like other bodily systems, consists of various tissue components which are functionally related and proprioceptively coordinated. It consists of the craniomandibular joint, jaws, teeth with their occlusal surfaces and contiguous-supporting structures and the neuromuscular complex. In any final functional analysis of this system it is important to consider the component structures, not only individually but in their relationship to each other. In spite of extractions, meniscectomies, condylectomies and even hemimandibulectomies the system can continue to function physiologically but in an impaired manner. Without coordinate neuromuscular function, however, mandibular movements of a purposeful nature are no longer feasible and the masticatory complex ceases to function as an integrated biological system. It is the neuromuscular complex that is inherently responsible for the forces that are generated during occlusal contacts between opposing teeth. It is somewhat ironic that the neuromuscular component which activates a contiguous assortment of structures into a physiological functional unit could also have the capacity to effect a pathological breakdown.

Parafunctional Mandibular Movements

If mandibular movements were limited to the primary physiologic functions such as mastication, swallowing and speech, occlusion per se would occupy a less important position. Unfortunately, we are also confronted with a variety of nonphysiologic mandibular functions that are categorized as parafunctional or pernicious depending upon their magnitude. These are characterized clinically by bruxism and/or clenching and various other interocclusal habits such as pencil and pipe-stem chewing. In most instances parafunctional masticatory muscle activity is the result of various combinations of stimuli from voluntary or involuntary tension-relieving habits and proprioceptive impulses from occlusal interferences. While the question as to which of these two contributing factors occurred first is the source of some controversy they are notwithstanding always present. When a patient with bruxism has pronounced occlusal interferences psychological counseling will be of little or no value. If the same occlusal interferences are first modified or removed so that occlusal compatibility is reestablished, then psychological counseling is normally not necessary. Conversely, when a patient with overt bruxism has minor occlusal interferences combined with severe psychic tension then psychotherapy is usually necessary.

The occlusal forces that are generated during physiologic mandibular functions are short term and of low magnitude. Furthermore, these forces are developed by isotonic muscle contractions which in themselves facilitate an adequate blood supply to and from the involved muscles. The significance of this becomes readily apparent when one recalls that muscle tissue has one of the highest metabolic requirements of any tissue. Conversely, parafunctional mandibular movements are developed primarily by isometric muscle contractions and are characterized by occlusal forces that are relatively long term and of a much greater magnitude.

Pernicious mandibular movements occur when the muscles of mastication through sustained or habitual bruxing and/or clenching override the normal protective (proprioceptive) feedback mechanism. As a result, injurious occlusal forces are produced and dissipated through the teeth and their supporting apparatus and through the tissues of the temporomandibular joints. Normally the dental components break down before the tissues of the joints. Sometimes the adaptive capacity of either of these tissues to occlusal forces is so great that the muscles become fatigued, to the point that a transient myospasm is developed thereby initiating the masticatory pain-dysfunction syndrome.

The ultimate clinical effect of occlusal stress depends on the adaptive tissue capacity of the masticatory components. This is why younger or healthy persons normally tolerate occlusal prematurities more effectively than persons who are debilitated or older.

Bruxism

Parafunctional muscle activity of the masticatory muscles can be transient or become a long-term, habitual response. Concomitant with masticatory parafunctional muscle activity, there is a nonfunctional grinding and clenching of the teeth that is referred to as bruxism. The following are clinical signs of bruxism:

1. Nonfunctional wear facets, incisal and occlusal.
2. Breakdown of restorations.
3. Pulpal hyperemia.
4. Pulpal necrosis.
5. Increased tooth mobility.
6. Gingival recession.
7. Periodontal pathosis.
8. Hypertrophy of masticatory muscles, especially the masseter muscles.
9. Increased muscle tenderness to palpation.
10. Myalgia.
11. Masticatory pain dysfunction syndrome due to masticatory myospasm.
12. Chronic occipital or temporal headaches.

Many patients are unaware of grinding and clenching their teeth. Frequently a parent, spouse or roommate may be the first to bring attention to the audible and somewhat annoying sounds of nocturnal bruxing habits. The most severe forms of bruxism usually occur during sleep when psychic factors are symbolically depicted in dreams and the patient lacks conscious awareness and control.

MASTICATORY PAIN-DYSFUNCTION SYNDROME

Within the past two decades it has finally become apparent that the mechanism which causes the masticatory pain-dysfunction syndrome (MPD syndrome) is an asynchrony of the masticatory muscles. Parafunctional muscle activity is brought on by chronic oral habits and is sequentially manifested as muscle fatigue, muscle tenderness and ultimately as muscle spasm (myospasm). Previously, it was assumed that mandibular dysfunction was the result of pathology or derangement of the tissues of the temporomandibular joint, and hence the term "temporomandibular joint pain-dysfunction syndrome." Instead of joint dysfunction we are usually confronted with muscle dysfunction, thereby contraindicating in nearly all cases surgical and sclerosing procedures of the temporomandibular joints as a mode of treatment. It is important to bear in mind that psychic tension increases muscle tension, and in the case of the stomatognathic system, occlusal disharmonies function as predisposing factors or "occlusal triggers" (Fig. 12-1).

To understand fully the MPD syndrome, it is necessary to consider in some detail the occlusal and psychogenic factors.

Occlusal Factors

The *Glossary of Prosthodontic Terms* defines occlusal disharmony as that condition occurring when the contacts of opposing occlusal surfaces of teeth are not in harmony with other tooth contacts and with

Occlusion and Its Relation to Oral Diagnosis and Treatment Planning

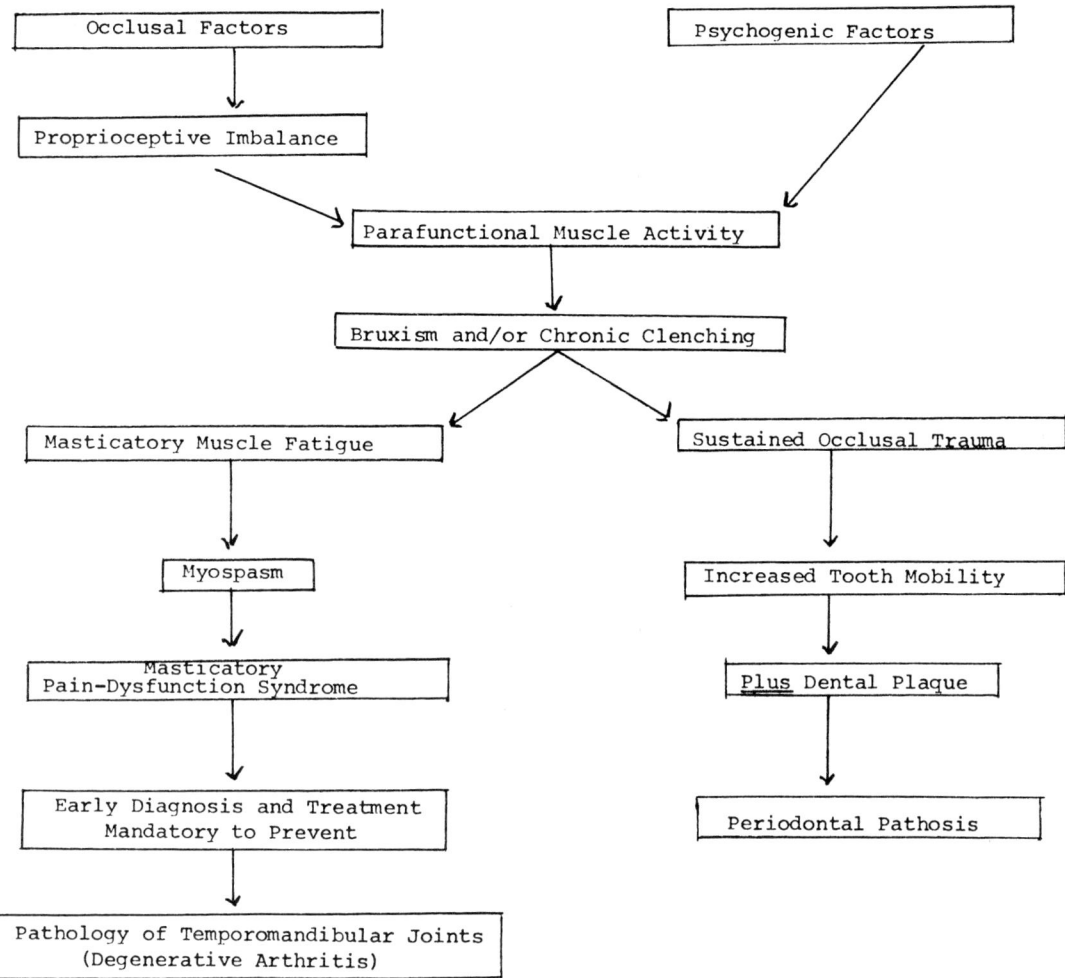

Figure 12-1. Schema depicting the dual etiology of the masticatory pain dysfunction syndrome and the possible pathological sequelae.

the anatomic and physiologic control of the mandible. It may result from a number of causes:
1. Premature contacts occurring in the following mandibular positions:
   a. Centric relation.
   b. Centric occlusion.
   c. Working side.
   d. Balancing side.
   e. Lateral protrusive.
   f. Protrusive.
2. Iatrogenic (dentist-produced) causes.
   a. Restorations.
   b. Orthodontic therapy.
   c. Occlusal equilibration.
   d. Extractions: (1) mesial and distal drift and (2) extrusion.
3. Developmental disturbances:
   a. Incongruous arch forms.
   b. Incongruous tooth forms.
   c. Anodontia.
   d. Supernumerary teeth.
   e. Malpositions of individual teeth: (1) mesioversion, (2) distoversion,

(3) labioversion or buccoversion, (4) linguoversion, (5) supraversion, (6) infraversion, (7) transversion, (8) axiversion and (9) torsiversion.

Psychogenic Factors

Psychogenic factors are those attitudinal factors which influence the psyche or mind and include the various manifestations of anxiety, worry, emotional tension, repressed aggression, and so forth. These factors are not associated with structural brain lesions or any clearly defined physical cause. Psychogenic factors of a prolonged or unresolved nature have been implicated in a variety of somatic disturbances. Some examples are diabetes mellitus, high blood pressure, tension and migraine headaches, myocardial infarction, bronchial spasm, myospasm affecting various functional muscle units, ulcers, etcetera.

Parafunctional Muscle Activity

Psychogenic conditions frequently induce increased tonus in various muscle groups. The following functional muscle units are frequently involved:

MUSCLES OF THE LOWER BACK. The patient complains of lower back pain.

MUSCLES OF THE UPPER BACK AND POSTERIOR CERVICAL AREA. The patient complains of shoulder and neck pain and occipital headache.

MUSCLES OF MASTICATION. The patient complains of muscle tenderness and limited mandibular movements. Hypertonicity of these muscles may be of a short duration, from a few hours to a few days, followed by a gradual return to normal tonicity. While occlusal factors may not by themselves precipitate increased muscle tonus, they apparently play a predisposing role when the patient is under stress. This would tend to account for the observation that most persons have some degree of occlusal disharmony and yet do not present with any of the clinical symptoms of bruxism, periodontal pathosis or mandibular dysfunction.

Clinical Features of the Masticatory Pain Dysfunction Syndrome

The syndrome consists of the following symptoms:

1. Unilateral myogenic pain that is centered in the auricular and temporomandibular joint areas with possible extension to the temporal area, zygomatic area, angle of the mandible or the lateral cervical area.

2. Tenderness of one or more of the masticatory muscles which can be best established by digital palpation.

3. Limitation and midsagittal deviation of mandibular movements (Fig. 12-2, A and B).

4. Clicking sounds during condylar excursions which appear to be the result of muscle incoordination rather than the cause.

5. A transient malocclusion in acute cases of myospasm of the lateral pterygoid muscle (Fig. 12-3, A and B).

As seen from the schematic outline depicting the etiology of the MPD syndrome (Fig. 12-1), pathological involvement of the temporomandibular joints per se can occur, but if so, only in the late and final stages. Therefore, in order to rule out possible joint pathology, a radiographic survey is necessary. A simple, but unfortunately not infallible method is to palpate the external auditory meatus and note the presence or absence of tenderness. If tenderness to digital palpation is noted, it is highly probable that tissue-joint pathology is present. The cause-and-effect relationship between these symptoms and fatigue,

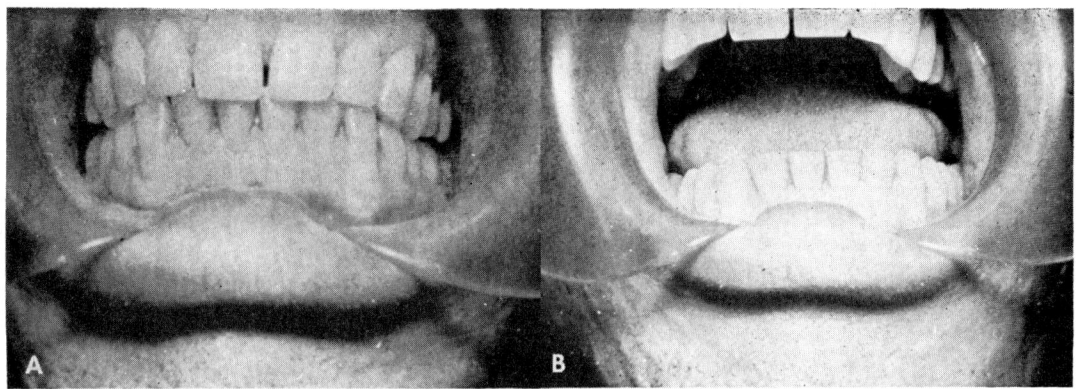

Figure 12-2. (A) Patient with masticatory muscle dysfunction with teeth in centric occlusion. Note relative relationship between the maxillary and mandibular incisor midlines. (B) Patient was instructed to "open his jaw" in the midsagittal plane. Note deviation of the lower incisor midline to the patients left side. The right lateral pterygoid muscle was very sensitive to intraoral digital palpation.

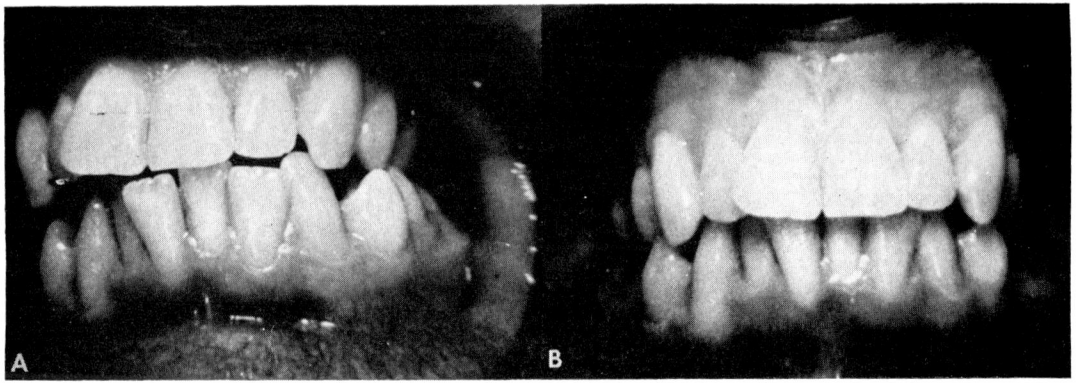

Figure 12-3. (A) Patient with a transient maloccusion and trismus due to acute myospasm of the right lateral pterygoid muscle. Patient was a second-year medical student and developed the above condition during examination week (psychogenic stress). The posterior teeth on the right side were completely out of occlusal contact. (B) Same patient 24 hours later. The myospasm had been reduced by a provisional unilateral occlusal splint made of autopolymer resin. Construction was carried out directly in the patient's mouth and placed on the symptomatic side. Patient had numerous occlusal disharmonies.

spasm and asynchrony of the masticatory muscles becomes readily apparent as one reviews the anatomical makeup and the physiological functions of the masticatory system. In addition, a small percentage of these patients (less than 2 percent) will present with otalgia, vertigo and tinnitus without discernible organic involvement of the ear structures, eustachian tubes or semicircular canals. Needless to say, whenever any of the three latter symptoms are present, consultation with an otologist is mandatory to rule out such otological disorders as external otitis, otitis media, mastoiditis and Meniere's disease. It is axiomatic that a thorough differential diagnosis is always indicated and one should consider and rule out the following: (a) diseases of the teeth, periodontium, jaws, oral mucosa, salivary glands, paranasal sinuses; (b) typical and atypical neuralgias; and (c) any systemic disease.

It has been clinically substantiated that the two common denominators in the majority of patients with MPD syndrome are occlusal deficiencies coupled with psychogenic problems. These two factors reinforce one another and their summation is manifested in the form of masticatory parafunctional muscle activity; that is, such chronic oral habits as bruxism, clenching, etcetera. Since problems of a psychogenic nature are occasional to most individuals, it is grossly unfair to indiscriminately categorize all such patients as ambulatory neurotics or psychotics. Less than 6 percent of these cases require psychotherapy, and with early diagnosis and treatment, this figure could be reduced to one-half. Most patients who experience "lockjaw" as a result of masticatory myospasm are baffled and frightened and understandably so. The latter response, through the mechanism of feedback input, ultimately induces additional muscle dysfunction and myogenic pain. The overall result is a self-sustaining cycle (Fig. 12-4) which in many of these patients becomes an established episodic response. The longer that this response is condoned the more difficult it becomes to eradicate. Hence, the need for early diagnosis and treatment.

Unfortunately, delay on the part of the patient in seeking treatment is fairly common. When the patient finally presents for treatment professional procrastination is also not uncommon. Once a tentative diagnosis is made of the MPD syndrome, the very first step in treatment should be to help the patient comprehend the nature and interrelationships of the etiological mechanisms. Empathy and reassurance will alleviate much of the psychic tension resulting from the symptoms of the MPD syndrome and in a small percentage of patients will provide complete resolution.

As a general rule any occlusal changes by grinding should not be performed at the

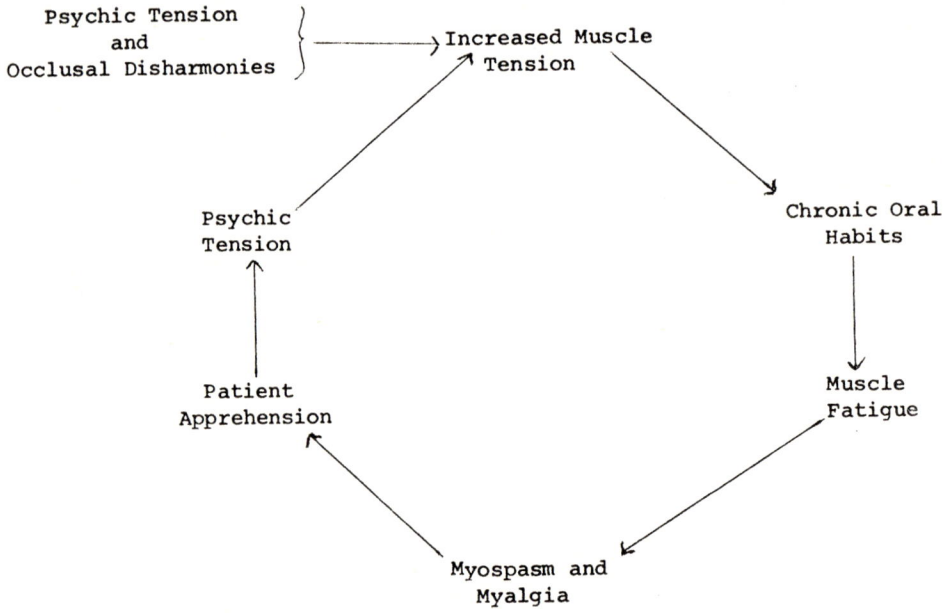

Figure 12-4. "Feedback input" of patient apprehension.

first visit since the result of such procedures are irreversible and may result in permanent damage. It is important to keep in mind that the contacts between occlusal and incisal surfaces are mechanical in nature and the manifestation of neuromuscular activity. Also in the presence of neuromuscular dysfunction the existing occlusal and incisal relationships are frequently of a transient and misleading nature (Fig. 12-3, A and B).

Treatment

A rational approach to successful treatment demands cognizance of the etiologic factors. Since we are primarily confronted with increased muscle tension, fatigue or spasm of one or more of the main muscles of mastication and a concurrent degree of occlusal incompatibility, the treatment plan should be directed towards their resolution. Muscle imbalance or asynchrony prevents physiologic placement of the mandible in the functional border positions, especially in centric relation. For this reason, occlusal modification should be delayed until all traces of myospasm and pain have been eliminated. Until then a functional occlusal analysis is impractical. When the external (lateral) pterygoid muscle is involved it usually pulls the affected side partially or completely out of occlusion thereby effecting a transient type of malocclusion (Fig. 12-3, A). Equilibration at this time would result in irreparable destruction of the occlusal morphology. It can also provoke an exacerbation of the original symptoms. About the only exceptions to this principle, however, are recent dental restorations or individual teeth that obviously are responsible for the proprioceptive imbalance. Not infrequently, the offending tooth will be an unopposed, extruded maxillary or mandibular third molar whose mesial aspect at the time of complete mandibular closure is contiguous with the distal aspect of the opposing second molar (Fig. 12-5). Such a relationship frequently results in a traumatic protrusive or retrusive displacement of the mandible with eventual degenerative changes in the temporomandibular joints or the periodontal structures. To prevent these sequelae an early diagnosis is essential and in such circumstances equilibration or even extraction of the offending third molar will produce dramatic results.

Interocclusal "Bite Opening" Appliances

Over the years it has been demonstrated by clinical trial and error that neuromuscular asynchrony of the masticatory system can be eliminated or attenuated through the use of removable, interocclusal "bite plates" or splints. They are effective in the majority (70 to 80 percent) of such cases. Of the various modes of treatment for masticatory muscle dysfunction these appliances are by far the safest since they are of a provisional nature. With proper follow-up any changes in tooth and occlusal relationships are normally of a transient and reversible nature. While the exact

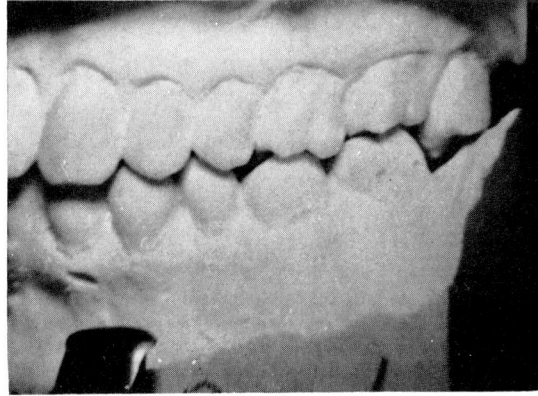

Figure 12-5. Unopposed, extruded maxillary third molar. During centric relation closure the mandible was deflected in an anterior-medial direction. The temporomandibular joint on the contralateral side was sensitive to palpation.

mechanism by which they alleviate hypertonicity is somewhat speculative it is difficult to dispute success. The following explanations for the effectiveness of interocclusal "bite opening" appliances have been generally accepted:

1. They negate cuspal inclines that function as occlusal triggers.

2. They provide a greater degree of mandibular stability at the horizontal and vertical levels of occlusal closure.

3. They provisionally provide for modified occlusal and incisal contacts which in turn effect a compensatory change in mandibular movements.

All of the above rationales imply a change in the occlusal scheme. By temporarily modifying the nature and force of occlusal contacts among opposing teeth there are concomitant changes in the neural feedback signals from the proprioceptors situated in the periodontal ligaments. Since the afferent impulses of proprioception, which are transmitted through the mesencephalic root of the trigeminal nerve to the brain, are now different the resultant motor impulses to the muscles which control the movements of the mandible are likewise altered. The desired end result is a diminution of muscle tension and such parafunctional habits as bruxism and chronic clenching. Again, it is important to emphasize that early diagnosis and treatment is mandatory. Otherwise, if episodic masticatory muscle dysfunction has been present and allowed to persist for a period longer than six months, the condition has *ipso facto* become established and the prognosis is guarded.

A cardinal rule of thumb is to limit the increase in vertical opening between the anterior incisors to a maximum of 2 mm. It has been noted in some myogenic dysfunction cases that an increase in the occlusal vertical dimension greater than 2 mm will precipitate an acute exacerbation of symptoms; namely, pain and mandibular dysfunction. Under these conditions the involved masticatory muscles are in a hypertonic state. As such their sensitivity is increased and they become extremely responsive to spatial changes in the vertical plane. It is possible that such changes induce contraction of the antigravity muscles through activation of the stretch reflex. Sustained encroachment on the interocclusal distance is usually indicated by increased muscle, tooth or temporomandibular joint tenderness. A physiologic resting range for muscle equilibrium between the opening and closing muscles must exist to permit optimal muscle synergy. The significance of the interocclusal rest space has been long noted by prosthodontists. In complete denture cases there is a tendency to increase the occlusal vertical dimension (or decrease the free way space) in order to facilitate the placement of artificial teeth and to enhance esthetics. Any infringement on the free way space results in irritation and trauma to the mucosal bearing surfaces while the long-term effect is irreversible resorption of the residual ridge.

Since the primary purpose of a bite opening appliance in the overall treatment plan is of an intermediate and provisional nature, the material of choice for construction is any of the plastic resins. Acrylic and thermoplastic vinyl splints can be easily constructed in the dental office and lend themselves readily to adjustment and modification at the chairside.

For purposes of discussion and clinical evaluation interocclusal bite opening appliances may be grouped into two major categories: palatal bite plates and occlusal splints.

Palatal bite plates are essentially modified Hawley-type appliances with a flat horizontal bite plane in the anterior region. During mandibular closure the six mandibular anterior teeth make premature incisal contact with even biting pressure on the bite plane (Fig. 12-6); as a result, the posterior teeth are unable to make occlusal contact. Since the main concern is a short-term treatment appliance the use of a labial arch wire is normally not necessary.

Occlusal splints are likewise designed to temporarily change occlusal proprioception by an increase of 1 to 2 mm in the occlusal vertical dimension. They differ from palatal bite plates in the following ways:

1. They may be fabricated for either the maxillary or mandibular dental arch.

2. During mandibular closure the posterior and usually the anterior teeth are in contact with the splint interposed between the occlusal and incisal surfaces.

3. They help to stabilize the remaining teeth of one dental arch through a mechanical locking and bracing effect at the occlusal and incisal surfaces.

The latter is accomplished by first surveying the teeth on the diagnostic cast. The splint is constructed so that the terminal occlusal edges on the buccal and lingual surfaces end slightly in the undercut areas (Fig. 12-7, A and B). The resiliency of the acrylic and vinyl resins permit insertion, passive mechanical retention and removal.

The type of appliance most commonly used is the palatal bite plate probably because it is easier to construct and adjust. However, it should not be worn for longer than a period of several weeks without close supervision. Extrusion of the posterior teeth and intrusion of the mandibular anterior teeth are common sequelae. During longer periods of treatment a labial divergence of the maxillary anterior teeth may occur. Occasionally, during treatment of acute cases of the MPD syndrome with a palatal bite plate, an exacerbation of the presenting symptoms will occur. Close examination will usually reveal one or both of the following conditions: the occlusal vertical dimension has been increased greater than 2 mm and/or the external auditory meatus on the symptomatic side is sensitive to digital palpation. The latter condition is suggestive of tissue pathology or possible trauma within the confines of the temporomandibular joint. Many of these patients present with class II type malocclusions characterized by a pronounced vertical overlap of the anterior teeth (deep overbite) and comparatively steep condylar pathways. In these cases an occlusal splint is the appliance of choice since it tends to reduce rather than increase joint pressure during mandibular closure by providing posterior interocclusal support.

In order to satisfy individual clinical needs many variations of both basic types of splints are possible. For example when the mandibular anterior teeth are periodontally involved a palatal bite plate is contraindicated for obvious reasons. In such cases a complete occlusal splint is in-

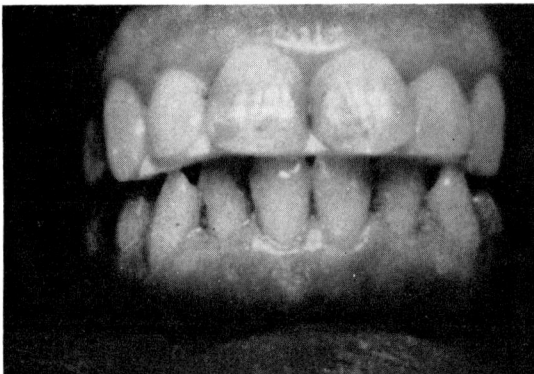

Figure 12-6. Palatal bite plate in equalized contact with the mandibular anterior teeth. The posterior teeth are not in physical occlusal contact.

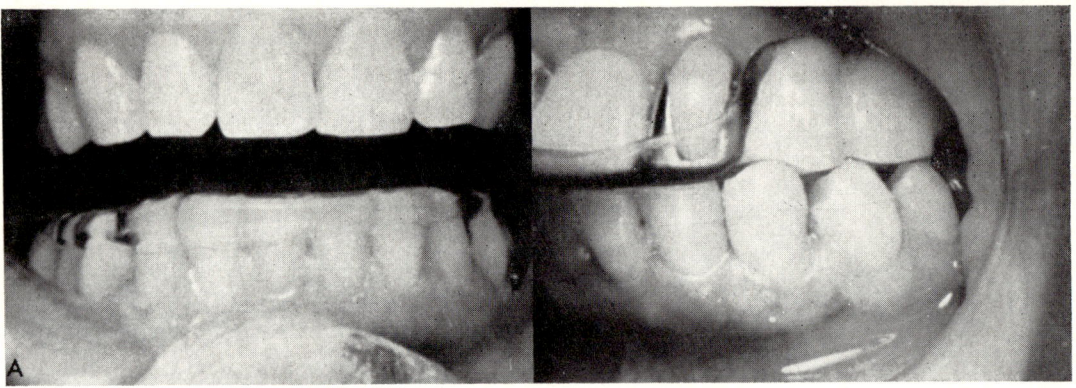

Figure 12-7. (A) An occlusal splint at insertion. At this time the occlusal resinous surfaces should be equilibrated as well as at subsequent follow-up visits. (B) Maxillary occlusal splint with added acrylic denture teeth to replace both maxillary premolars.

dicated because of its built-in stabilization feature. If the periodontal pathology has not progressed to the stage of moderate alveolar bone loss and the teeth manifest minimal clinical mobility (class I) then a simpler, modified form of the complete occlusal splint can be utilized. This particular type is the posterior, unilateral occlusal splint in which the interocclusal segment is placed on the affected or symptomatic side. The unilateral occlusal splint is simple to construct and with proper precautions can be fabricated directly in the patient's mouth with any of the autopolymer resins. During polymerization of the resin the splint should be removed and replaced several times to permit partial disengagement of the undercut areas. The simplest forms of posterior unilateral occlusal splints are ordinary cotton rolls, sections of wood tongue blades and strips of gutta percha.

FUNCTIONAL OCCLUSAL ANALYSIS

All existing deflective occlusal contacts (occlusal interferences or prematurities) are potential causes of abnormal tooth mobility or masticatory muscle dysfunction. Whether this actually occurs depends on the magnitude and frequency of the generated physical forces, the adaptive capacity of the periodontal supporting structures and the extent of the psychogenic component. The basic purpose of a functional occlusal analysis is to locate these "occlusal triggers" and eliminate them by means of selective grinding without initiating future occlusal dysfunction.

The method by which occlusal interferences are identified is most important since some type of a reproducible reference position must be established. With this need in mind we invariably note the presence of two temporomandibular joints. The latter are an inherent and vital component of the stomatognathic system since they provide a moveable connecting link between the cranium and the mandible. Articulation occurs between the mandibular condyle and the articular eminence of the temporal bone. The two bones are separated by a pliable fibrous meniscus which conforms to the contours of the articular surfaces and subdivides each temporomandibular joint into two distinct synovial compartments forming, from a functional point of view, a double joint. Condylar movement below the meniscus (lower compartment) occurs as a rotational or hingelike movement. Movement above the meniscus (upper compartment) occurs along the articulating surface of the articular fossa and eminence as a translatory or sliding movement since the meniscus is attached to the medial and lateral poles of the condyle. As both mandibular condyles are situated at opposite ends of the same bone, movement on one side effects a simultaneous compensatory movement on the other side. Furthermore, since movements of the condyles normally involve both compartments of both joints simultaneously it becomes readily apparent that condylar positions and movements can be extremely variable and therefore difficult to register and reproduce—as long as the opposing teeth are not in occlusal contact.

After some reflection it becomes evident that the only feasible reproducible mandibular position occurs when translation is completely blocked and condylar rotation is permitted in the most retruded or the so-called terminal hinge position. In this position both condyles are in their most posterior and cranial positions and are stabilized by the ligaments and structures of the temporomandibular joints. It is important to envision this positional relationship as bone-to-bone (mandible to maxillae) which, by convention, is intentionally independent of the guiding influence of the occlusal surfaces; this is *centric relation*. Since this position requires that the masticatory musculature be free of any asynergy or hypertonicity, other than normal physiological tonus, it is sometimes referred to as a *ligamentous position*.

In the majority of people examined it is noted that as the mandible closes in the terminal hinge position a deflection, slide or shift of the mandible will occur as the teeth make their initial contact, which gives origin to the expression "deflective occlusal contact." The final placement of the mandible is determined by the maximum intercuspation of the teeth and is called *centric occlusion*. As such it should be envisioned as a tooth-to-tooth relationship. This relationship is at times referred to as a *muscle position*, as most persons are able to close from any open mandibular position directly into centric occlusion. This voluntary response is attributed to the proprioceptive signals that are generated during occlusal contacts and the ability of the neuromusculature to record, remember and repeat the necessary contraction pattern. This cause-and-effect response is commonly called "muscle memory" and has given rise to the expression that "the occlusion programs the neuromuscular response." As the overall occlusal scheme changes through normal attrition, physiological drift, new restorations, loss of teeth, extrusion and so forth, the resulting proprioceptive pattern brings about compensatory changes in the muscle synchrony patterns. Also, since compensatory programming incorporates any occlusal deficiencies that may be present in centric occlusion, the latter position cannot be relied upon as a reference position in the overall evaluation of maxillomandibular relationships.

Thus far we have established the existence of two basic jaw relationships—centric relation and centric occlusion—which may or may not coincide. In most patients a discrepancy, difference or range will exist between these two positions and a deflective occlusal contact can be demonstrated. Thus, when mandibular closure occurs with both condyles in the terminal hinge position (centric relation) the initial solitary physical contact between the guiding inclines of two opposing teeth may cause the mandible to be forcibly deflected. This is sometimes referred to as a "slide in centric." The physical forces that are generated by such initial contacts are usually resolved as horizontal vectors. Teeth and their supporting structures are best suited to withstand occlusal forces in a vertical or axial direction. When such horizontal forces suddenly become induced and sustained it is primarily through the mechanism of parafunctional masticatory muscle activity.

Ideally the *guiding principle of treatment* is to locate and negate those centric relation interferences that under optimal conditions serve as occlusal triggers. With regard to symptoms they are manifested in various forms such as muscle tenderness, muscle asynchrony, atypical occlusal wear, increased tooth mobility, alveolar bone sclerosis or resorption, root resorption and the MPD syndrome (Fig. 12-1). The nature of the pain may be extremely variable since its origin can be pulpal, periodontal, muscular or temporomandibular.

The most difficult part in doing a functional occlusal analysis is for the examiner to guide or direct the mandible into the terminal hinge position and effect a centric relation closure. Patients with any of the symptoms of the mandibular dysfunction syndrome usually present with some degree of active muscle resistance thereby making centric relation closure a dubious, difficult and sometimes painful procedure. While certain drugs such as meprobamate, Valium® and Robaxin® may allay psychogenic influences, they should not be expected to serve as panaceas. The safest way to alleviate neuromuscular imbalance and thereby facilitate centric relation closure is by means of a removable bite plate or splint. By preventing maximum intercuspation (centric occlusion—a muscle position) the occlusal proprioceptive pathways responsible for programming group muscle coordination (muscle memory) will no longer be operational. Thus, by provisionally modifying tooth-to-tooth contacts, closure in the most retruded jaw-to-jaw relationship can be facilitated. While construction of a bite plate or splint may appear to be an unnecessary time-consuming procedure, the best interests of the patient should be our primary concern since "fools rush in where angels fear to tread." Moreover, if patient education, empathy and reassurance have been genuinely implemented time is now on the side of the operator.

Centric relation prematurities can be identified by markings with articulating paper, ribbon or perforations with 30 gauge wax. Since by definition centric relation is a diagnostic border position and is therefore reproducible, all premature contacts should be verified by repeated registrations. Assuming the patient to be educable, he should ultimately be capable of performing centric relation closure without any external guidance and should be able to determine and stop at the first position of occlusal contact. The position is noted and then the patient is instructed to resume closure. The direction and length of mandibular deflection is noted and verified by repetition. Normally if the deflection or shift is in an anterior direction and less than 1 mm grinding is not indicated. In the main, those centric prematurities that cause lateral mandibular shifts are considered to be the most detrimental. Clinically and electromyographically it has been demonstrated that a lateral shift from centric relation to centric occlusion is more likely to initiate parafunctional muscle activity than an anterior shift. When the psychogenic climate is right, bruxism may become insidiously established as a behavioral response. Conversely, reduction of such prematurities can either resolve or lessen the extent of bruxism.

Interferences between centric relation and centric occlusion are usually removed by increasing the width and depth of the involved fossae. When the interference is formed by opposing cuspal inclines, it is reduced by following the rule of "MUDL" which pertains to the *mesial upper* incline of the buccal cusp and the *distal lower* incline of the lingual cusp. Cusp tips are necessary to maintain occlusal stability in the centric range and the functional eccentric range. Therefore, they should never be reduced unless they constitute an interfering contact in all maxillomandibular positions—which seldom is the case. Unfortunately, the guiding philosophy of some practitioners in regard to selective grinding is to "eliminate those damn cusps."

Tooth contacts of a functional and parafunctional nature also occur during eccentric mandibular excursions. As such, a functional occlusal analysis should also take into consideration the relationships of teeth during protrusive and lateral movements.

With the teeth in contact a protrusive movement of the mandible originating from centric occlusion should occur as a smooth, gliding movement with no "bumps" or interferences. Initially there may be interferences in the molar region but as the condyles move downward and forward the posterior teeth disengage. Even so, any posterior interferences should be noted—especially in cases of missing and malposed molars. Since the protrusive movement is not a "border movement," it is subject to variation and the examiner must rely on his clinical acumen. As the movement occurs, the mandibular incisors, cuspids and first premolars glide downward and forward along the palatal surfaces of the maxillary anterior segment until interincisal contact is established.

Displacement of individual teeth (fremitus) can be best determined by digital palpation. The ideal end position is one in which most or all of the incisors and cuspids occlude simultaneously and evenly; thereby, effecting a uniform distribution of the concomitant physical stresses. This unit relationship of the anterior teeth is referred to as anterior group function.

Protrusive interferences in the posterior area are selectively ground by following the rule of "BULL" which pertains to the *buccal upper* cusps (reduce the distolingual incline) and the *lower lingual* cusps (reduce the mesial buccal incline). The "BULL" cusps are horizontally adjacent to the centric holding cusps and therefore do not normally affect the occlusal vertical dimension. Next, the interferences in the anterior segment are corrected by reducing the lingual incisal surfaces of the involved maxillary teeth. The mandibular incisors being the most susceptible teeth to attrition are normally not subjected to selective grinding.

On the working (chewing) side, interferences are noted in the lateral glide from centric occlusion to the end-to-end contact position of the opposing buccal and lingual cusps. The buccal cusps of the lower teeth normally glide along the inner inclines of the opposing buccal cusps. As in the protrusive movement selective grinding of the working side is limited to the "BULL" cusps; namely, the lingual (inner) inclines of the *buccal upper* cusps and the buccal inclines of the *lingual lower* cusps. At times during working side excursions the opposing cuspids come into contact and cause the remaining posterior teeth to disengage. This effect is commonly referred to as a "cuspid rise." Some operators regard a cuspid rise as desirable since the cuspids absorb most of the lateral stresses. By virtue of their size, crown-root ratio and location, the cuspids are usually well adapted for this purpose. In the absence of cuspid mobility, periodontal pathology and bruxofacets a natural occurring cuspid rise should be maintained without modification. In contradistinction to the cuspid rise concept, others advocate that the cuspid, premolar and molar teeth should contact together in a simultaneous and uniform manner. Such a group relationship of the teeth on the working side is commonly referred to as "group function." Either of these two philosophies is acceptable and the guiding principle should be to avoid or minimize any selective grinding that will cause a decrease in the occlusal vertical dimension as this predisposes to "overclosure." If this occurs, cuspal interferences may be introduced on the balancing side and/or the anterior incisal segment. The possibility of overclosure becomes a critical consideration in patients with an extreme anterior vertical overlap. If such a patient presents with overt symptoms of mandibular dysfunction occlusal reconstruction of the posterior teeth within the physiological limits of the interocclusal distance (freeway space) is sometimes the only recourse available. While bite plates or splints are used primarily to alleviate masticatory neuromuscular asynchrony, they can also be used as trial appliances to determine the amount of vertical opening that a patient can physiologically accept.

The balancing (nonworking) side can be examined for interferences during the same lateral movement. Occlusal contacts occur between the opposing centric holding cusps; namely, the lingual (inner) incline of the lower buccal cusp and the buccal incline of the upper lingual cusp. The balancing condylar pathway is usually the most inclined of all condylar pathways. Balancing cuspal contacts usually occur on guiding inclines that have the greatest slope. This combination encourages a horizontal rather than a vertical or axial resolution of occlusal forces. Balancing contacts must be carefully evaluated as to whether they are functioning in a physiological capacity or as interferences. As a rule balancing side occlusal contacts are not necessary for optimal or normal masticatory function. Their only indication is in complete dentures where bilateral "balanced occlusion" helps to stabilize the denture bases. A missing mandibular first molar should alert the examiner as the second and third mandibular molars tend to tip forward, a relationship which frequently produces severe balancing interferences.

It is not uncommon for unilateral balancing interferences in the second and third molar areas to cause dysfunction in either the ipsilateral or contralateral jaw-joint and the associated lateral pterygoid muscle. The symptoms that are most frequently encountered are "clicking," muscle tenderness and midsagittal deviation of the mandible.

Occlusal contacts on the balancing side occur between the centric holding cusps which play a vital role in maintaining the occlusal vertical dimension. When a balancing interference is located and verified the examiner must decide which of the cusps, maxillary or mandibular, better maintains or "holds" the centric range (retrusive zone) after which the opposing cusp tip is reduced. The reduction of both cusp tips is seldom necessary and is normally contraindicated.

It is common knowledge that teeth can be expected to shift into a new occlusal relationship when they are taken out of occlusion. Therefore, the most difficult aspect of selective grinding is to end up with a stable occlusion. It is for this very reason that indiscriminate grinding cannot be justified. As a treatment procedure it is irreversible and is at times more destructive than the disease. A rule of thumb is to minimize all grinding procedures and when in doubt "don't." The operator must proceed cautiously and in most cases several visits are necessary and are to be encouraged, as time is on his side. Complete diagnostic casts mounted on an adjustable articulator with a centric relation registration and face-bow transfer provides the soundest and safest method. This becomes especially significant when one considers the myriad combinations of dental occlusions as they actually occur and exist. By cross-checking and verifying interferences between the mouth and the articulated diagnostic casts, and by equilibrating the diagnostic casts first, the operator is demonstrating a professional concern for the welfare of the patient. At the same time he is reducing the possibility of iatrogenically inducing another "occlusal neurotic."

A functional, compatible neuromuscular response can be effected by providing uniform occlusal contacts with axial loading in the following positions:

1. *The retrusive zone*—the area that lies between and includes centric relation and centric occlusion. Interferences in this zone are believed to be the most harmful and the most likely to initiate bruxism.

2. *Protrusive excursions*—removal of interferences necessary since "short" protrusive movements take place during mastication and frequently combine with the lateral component to form the lateral-protrusive movement.

3. *Lateral excursions*—freedom from interferences necessary to insure bilateral masticatory capability which is a mandatory "must" since sustained unilateral chewing promotes neuromuscular asynchrony.

   a. *Working side*—removal of interferences effects bilateral group function which enhances bilateral chewing.

   b. *Balancing side*—next to centric relation interferences balancing side interferences are the most destructive. When they are condoned they are frequently the cause of jaw-joint dysfunction.

SUMMARY

The purpose of selective occlusal grinding is to have as many teeth as possible occlude evenly in the basic maxillomandibular relationships. Thus, the main objective is to effect a uniform distribution of the physical stresses which are generated by the neuromusculature and dissipated through the teeth (in an axial direction) and their supporting structures. When these conditions are satisfied the ensuing compatible relationship will normally preclude the insidious inception of chronic parafunctional habits. Once established such habits have the potential to effect the breakdown of any of the vital tissue components of the stomatognathic system.

REFERENCES

1. Beyron, H.: Optimal occlusion. *Dent Clin N Am,* July 1969, p. 537.
2. Freese, A. S., and Scheman, P.: *Management of Temporomandibular Joint Problems.* St. Louis, C. V. Mosby Co., 1962.
3. Goldman, H. M., and Cohen, D. W.: *Periodontal Therapy,* 4th ed. St. Louis, C. V. Mosby Co., 1968.
4. Guichet, N. F.: *Occlusion—A Collection of Monographs.* Anaheim (Calif.), The Denar Corporation, 1970.
5. Posselt, U.: *Physiology of Occlusion and Rehabilitation,* 2nd ed. Oxford, Blackwell Scientific Publications, 1968.
6. Ramfjord, S. P., and Ash, M. M.: *Occlusion,*

2nd ed. Philadelphia, W. B. Saunders, 1971.
7. Sarnat, B. G. (Ed.): *The Temporomandibular Joint*, 2nd ed. Springfield, Charles C Thomas, 1964.
8. Schuyler, C.: Freedom in centric. *Dent Clin N Amer,* July 1969, p. 681.
9. Schuyler, C.: Fundamental principles in the correction of occlusal disharmonies, natural and artificial. *JADA,* 2:1193–1202, 1935.
10. Schwartz, L., and Chayes, C.: *Facial Pain and Mandibular Dysfunction.* Philadelphia, W. B. Saunders, 1968.
11. Schwartz, L. et al.: *Disorders of the Temporomandibular Joint.* Philadelphia, W. B. Saunders, 1959.
12. Shore, N. A.: *Occlusal Equilibration and Temporomandibular Joint Dysfunction.* Philadelphia, J. B. Lippincott Co., 1959.

Chapter 13
Oral Diagnosis and Treatment Planning in Periodontics

ZIGMUND C. PORTER

Correct diagnosis is essential for intelligent treatment. Because our interest is in the patient who has the disease and not simply the disease itself, diagnosis must include a general evaluation of the patient. The diagnosis must be systematic and organized. It is not enough to gather facts. The findings must be pieced together so that they provide a meaningful explanation of the patient's periodontal problem.

The secretary takes the name, address, phone number(s) of the patient and the name of the referring dentist.

When the patient calls the periodontist's office for a consultation, inquiry is also made as to whether the patient has had a recent full set of long-cone radiographs. Most dentists realize that periodontists prefer to have a long-cone set of radiographs and if they have not been taken will arrange for their office to take a set. When they are taken by the periodontist, duplicates should be taken and a set sent to the dentist before the initial consultation appointment.

THE HISTORY

The patient is sent a history form or given this form when the radiographs are taken. The history form consists of a medical questionnaire (see Ch. 3), a dental habit history and a dental history (Figs. 13-1 and 13-2). The advantages of the patient filling this form out at home are multiple. It is more complete and thorough than questioning the patient at the chairside, it gives the periodontist a legal document in the patient's own handwriting and it saves time. Only those questions which are answered "yes" does the patient have to explain more fully in the space provided. Time may be spent at the chairside detailing the "yes" answers more carefully.

The patient is also required to fill out a form in the waiting room asking for his birthdate, address and occupation. The periodontist should see the radiographs before the first appointment and confer with the referring dentist. The dentist is able to provide a general outline of the case history and other pertinent information which might prove invaluable.

THE CONSULTATION APPOINTMENT

The examination of the patient begins with the consultation appointment. Observations are made as to the weight-to-height relationship, obvious physical deformities and general hygiene and appearance of the patient. Before examining the mouth of the

Answer with a check or yes or no.

1. Do you have any particular mouth habits with which you are familiar? _____
2. Do you ordinarily place foreign objects between your teeth? _____
3. Do you bite your lip? _____ tongue? _____ cheek? _____
4. Do you clench or grind your teeth during the day? _____ night? _____
5. Do you awaken in the morning with the teeth together? _____ with aches in the jaw joint? _____ with aches in the face or temple? _____ Numb feeling in teeth? _____
6. Do you "doodle" or play with the teeth? _____ Is one tooth ever sore? _____ loose? _____
7. Do you feel your teeth come together evenly? _____ Does one tooth hit before the others? _____
8. Are you conscious of sore teeth? _____ loose teeth? _____ High or rough fillings? _____ Rough teeth? _____ Movement of teeth? _____
9. Are you conscious of any habit with your tongue (thrusting, etc.)? _____
10. Do you have difficulty opening or closing the mouth? _____ pain? _____ clicking? _____ popping? _____
11. When do you brush your teeth? _____ How often a day? _____ Direction of brushing? _____ Do you use floss? _____ toothpicks? _____ stimudents? _____

Figure 13-1. Habit history.

patient, it is important for the periodontist to talk with him. It is sometimes startling for a patient to be asked to give an opinion of his dental and oral condition before an examination has even been made. Further questioning often reveals that this is the first time a dentist has even bothered to ask the patient's opinion. Sometimes the patient does not know how to begin to answer this question, and it is suggested that the next question should be: "What importance do you attach to your teeth?" With a conversational atmosphere and with guidance from the periodontist, after five or ten minutes the patient will have revealed some of the reasons for wanting to keep his teeth, how far he is willing to go in retaining his teeth, what his motivation might be and finally, his overall opinion as to what his oral health might be.

It cannot be stressed sufficiently that this initial period of discussion must take place. It is suggested that the periodontist should be seated facing the patient, either in the operatory, which is preferred, since an examination is to follow, rather than stand-

Reason for present visit:

1. Chief complaint _____

2. Duration of complaint _____
3. Last visit to dentist _____ What was done? _____
4. Date of last full dental x-rays? _____ Were models taken for diagonistic purposes? _____
5. In your opinion what is your general dental condition? _____
6. What would the loss of your teeth mean to you (dentures)? _____

7. Are your teeth painful to: Heat? _____ Cold? _____ Sweets? _____ Chewing? _____ Touch? _____
8. What side do you chew on? _____ Why? _____
9. Does food catch between teeth? _____ Where? _____ When? _____
10. Do your gums bleed? _____ Where? _____ When? _____
11. Do tartar and stain return quickly? _____ Do cavities develop quickly? _____
12. Are you conscious of bad taste? _____ Bad breath? _____
13. Do you have any sensation or feeling in your gums? _____ Pain? _____ Itching? _____
    Numbness? _____ Other? _____
14. Have you had difficulty following a dental extraction? _____
15. Have you had previous periodontal treatment? _____ Where, when, and by whom? _____

16. Orthodontic treatment? _____
17. Are you conscious of your teeth in any way? _____ Satisfied with the way they look? _____
18. Do you chew satisfactorily? _____
19. Missing teeth? _____ When lost? _____ Why? _____
20. Replacements? _____ Why not? _____
21. Patient evaluation of replacements _____

Figure 13-2. Dental history.

ing, because it changes the dialogue to one of question and answer. It also makes the patient feel that he is being considered as an individual with individual problems. From the periodontist's side, much valuable information is gathered about the total individual.

Three factors are necessary for successful treatment of a periodontal patient: the patient's motivation, the periodontal condition and its ability to be repaired by the periodontist, and the dentist's ability to do the necessary restorative work. Without sufficient motivation little or nothing can or should be done because the patient will be unwilling to undergo any periodontal or dental work and, more important, take care of it after the work is completed.

It has been asked whether one can determine motivation during such a short dialogue. Although this information may not always be forthcoming, those individuals who are motivated at the beginning soon become apparent after a short period of questioning. For those who cannot be discerned as being motivated at this time, the total therapy should not be detailed until the motivation can be established or, better still, developed, as will be outlined under initial therapy.

EXAMINATION OF THE PATIENT

The lips are examined for lip habits, such as a mentalis habit, lip biting or chewing, or mouth-breathing. Mouth-breathing will often be associated with gingivitis in those gingival tissues which are allowed to dehydrate. They will be clearly demarcated from the gingival tissues which are covered by the cheeks or lips. The appearance is one of localized enlargement with redness and a diffuse surface shininess. Attempts to reproduce these changes in experimental animals could not be achieved.[1] The cheeks, tongue, floor of the mouth and palate are examined by direct vision and with a mirror: the tongue is grasped with a gauze and pulled gently upward and out of the mouth. The visual examination enables one to observe changes in color and texture from the normal appearance, the presence of swelling and other abnormalities. A digital examination with the forefinger is made, checking for enlargements, swelling or sore areas which might be present. The submental, submandibular and cervical lymph nodes are also palpated and any tender or enlarged nodes are noted.

The Gingiva

Color Changes

The gingival color is usually the first thing that is observed. Changes in the gingival color may vary from the normal of coral pink to that of dark red, reflecting the degree of inflammation present. Usually the more acute the inflammation, the more red the gingiva becomes. In long-standing, chronic, periodontal disease, fibrosis may occur, giving a color which does not reflect the degree of involvement. Color is only one of a series of criteria for diagnosis. Color changes should be noted as to the location, whether they are in the papillae, along the marginal or attached gingiva, and whether the affected part or parts is confined to a specific area or generalized throughout the mouth. A significant find, though rare, is the absence of a mucogingival line which is often found in leukemia. Pigmentation of the gingiva is a common finding in many dark-skinned individuals.[2] According to Dummet, 60 percent of the gingiva and 61 percent of the hard palate in Negroes are pigmented.[3]

Enlargement of the Gingiva

Gingiva enlarges by *hyperplasia* which is an increase in the number of cells in normal arrangement in the tissue. The clinical size of the gingiva corresponds to the total of the cellular and intercellular elements present and their vascular supply. The alteration in the size of the gingiva is another of the most common findings of gingival disease. This enlargement must not be confused with that of bony enlargement; the differential diagnosis can easily be made by observation, probing and palpation. Most gingival enlargement is due to inflammation but other common causes, which may also have inflammation present, are the hormonal changes of pregnancy and puberty and Dilantin sodium (Fig. 13-3). The initial enlargement of gingival disease is usually seen at the gingival margin or in the papillae.

Normal gingiva is stippled, from the light stippling seen when the tissues are dried, to that of a noticeable orange peel effect (Fig. 13-4). The presence of inflammation causes the stippling to disappear.

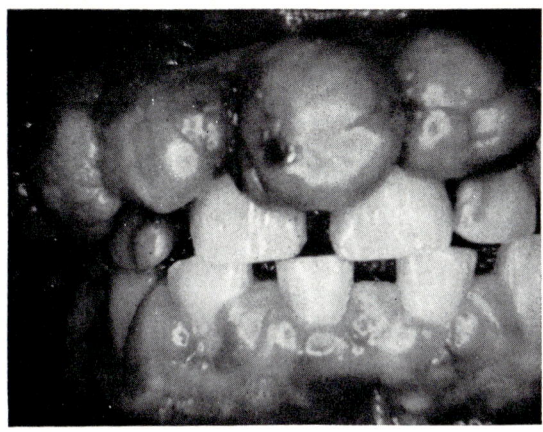

Figure 13-3. Dilantin hyperplasia. Note the greater enlargement of the maxillary labial gingivae due to the drying effect of mouth breathing.

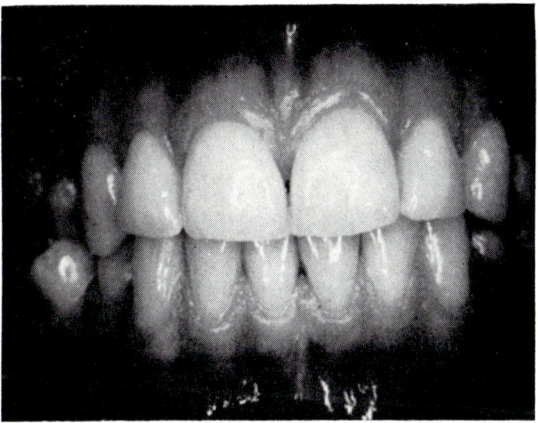

Figure 13-4. Normal gingivae. Note the sharp free gingival margin, a tight adaptation to the teeth and the stippled "orange peel" effect.

Thus the presence of inflammation is inversely proportional to the presence of stippling because of the presence of edema.[4] However, in longstanding, chronic inflammatory disease where fibrosis has occured, stippling might return. The presence of pockets in this instance will give a positive diagnosis of disease.

Frena

Frena are noted, especially in the presence of marked recession. Formerly it was thought that the pull of the frena alone causes gingival recession. This is only partially true, for in addition to the pull of the muscles, a malposed tooth with little or no bone on the facial aspect is also necessary; thus the pull of the muscles is directly onto the fibrous tissue labial to the tooth and unsupported by bone. High or wide frena also mean a reduction or absence of the attached gingiva at that point.

Charting the Mouth

Using a chart, the missing teeth are recorded with appropriate lines. The gingival margin is drawn with a line that is in direct relationship to the cemento-enamel junction of the teeth which are drawn on the chart. Cases of delayed or altered passive eruption, where the gingival margin does not recede from the enamel of the tooth by the age of twenty-three,[5] are detected easily in this manner, when pockets extending to or just beyond the cemento-enamel junction are also present.

Areas of recession and frena are noted on this chart. Before pocket measurements are taken, the mucogingival line is also drawn on the chart by its relationship to the gingival margin. There is no mucogingival line on the palate as it is entirely keratinized. Bowers[6] has shown that as little as ½ mm of attached gingiva is sufficient for normal function. The functional adequacy of the attached gingiva can be predicted by a simple tension test.[7] By pulling on the lips or cheeks, lateral tension is created. If this causes the gingival margin to pull away from the teeth surfaces, it is not adequate (Fig. 13-5). The buccal aspect of the lower first bicuspids has the least amount of attached gingiva in the mouth, usually because of the high and wide muscle attachments (Fig. 13-6).[6]

The sulci and pockets are probed for depth and contents. A thin calibrated periodontal probe is used, directed parallel to

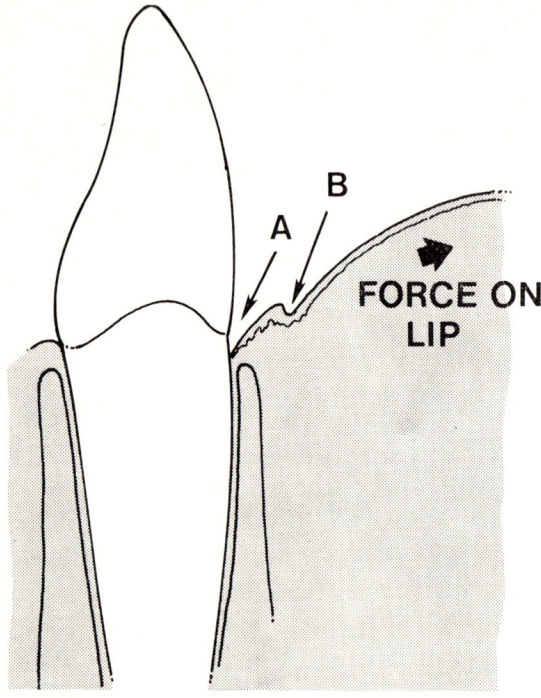

Figure 13-5. The labial frenum causes pocket formation by pulling the attached gingiva away from the tooth and allowing food impaction (A). The vestibular fornix is shallow because of the presence of the frenum (B).

the long axis of the tooth. Angulation of the probe will lead to errors in measurements. Six measurements are taken on each tooth: facially and lingually at the mesial, radicular and distal. The probe is inserted until resistance is felt and then moved slightly laterally to see if the bottom of the pocket has been reached. Sometimes scaling must be done to allow the probe to reach the bottom of the pocket. A curved explorer or curette is used to probe the furcations. These pockets are marked on the chart by points. The chart has millimeter lines drawn across, starting at the cementoenamel junction and extending past the apices of the teeth that are drawn on the chart. By extending the points with a line and lightly shading the portion between the gingival margin and the line representing the base of the pocket, a "gingival profile" will be obtained which will graphically depict the depths of the pockets and their relationship to the mucogingival line.

Probing can cause hemorrhage if the lining of the pocket is ulcerated. Suppuration

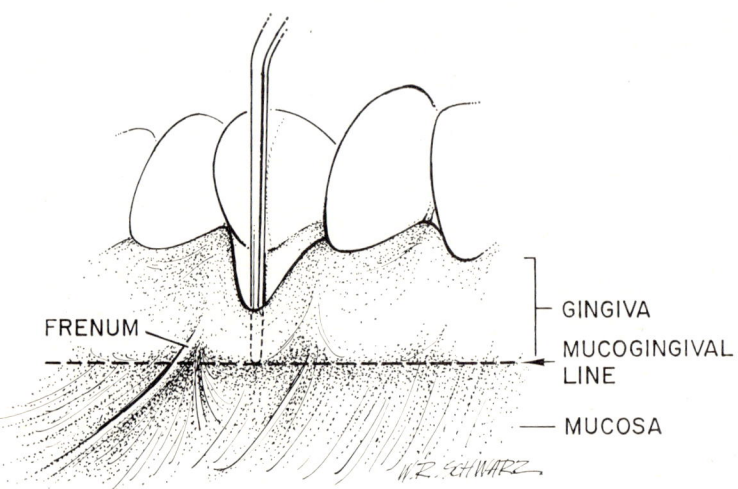

Figure 13-6. The pocket indicated by the probe and the recession around the first bicuspid are due to several factors: the pull of the frenum on the attached gingiva, the positioning of the bicuspid in a buccal position causing this portion of the tooth to be outside the alveolar bone housing. Thus, the gingiva attaches directly to a greater portion of root without the intercession of bone. The pull of the frenum together with the constant trauma of toothbrushing, etcetera, give rise to recession and pocket formation.

depends upon the condition of the epithelial lining rather than the depth of the pocket. The presence of bleeding or suppuration, or both, is noted.

Tooth Mobility

The mobility of the teeth is checked using the forefinger and the handle of an instrument, such as a mirror. Usually the mobility is graded using a system of one to three, but many periodontists have differently calibrated systems. What is important is that the system be consistent from tooth to tooth in the same individual and from individual to individual and that the periodontist be able to explain the divisions in his system. The mobility is recorded on the chart. The degree of mobility is too often equated with the loss of teeth. The prognosis for teeth with extreme mobility depends upon the cause of mobility: crown-root ratio, the amount and morphology of the remaining bone and the traumatic forces placed on the tooth. According to Pritchard,[8] the prognosis is not always hopeless, even when a tooth can be elevated and depressed in its socket. *Mobility is not proportional to the amount of bone loss.*

To complete the chart, malposed and rotated teeth are noted. Poor margins and open contacts are checked and other iatrogenic factors, such as the impingement of prosthetic replacements upon the gingival margin, are noted. The resulting chart will become one of the most important parts of the case record and is vital for diagnosis, prognosis, planning other treatment, for insurance claims and in the event of a misunderstanding with the patient.

Caries

Caries is noted as to the degree of active caries present and whether there is any endodontic involvement. Caries control will be spoken of during the optional phase of the treatment plan.

Angle's Classification and Arch Form

Angle's classification is noted, as is the arch form. Where the arch is wide and the tooth is invested in a thick width of bone, there is cancellous bone between the cortical plates. Cancellous bone is destroyed more rapidly by inflammation than is the cortical plate. If this resorption is unchecked, the interradicular bone may be destroyed without much loss of the cortical plates, leaving the tooth sitting in a defect with bone only at the apex.[9-11] Ramadan demonstrated that radiographically such a defect would not be noted.[12]

Tooth Position

A tooth that is prominent in the arch usually has thin bone and gingiva on the facial aspect. Teeth that are recessed have thick marginal bone on the facial aspect; on the lingual aspect, just the opposite is found. If the tooth is extremely prominent, a complete absence of bone is sometimes noted.[13] This is called a dehiscence (Fig. 13-7).[14] The result of a dehiscence with a frenum was previously noted. The areas

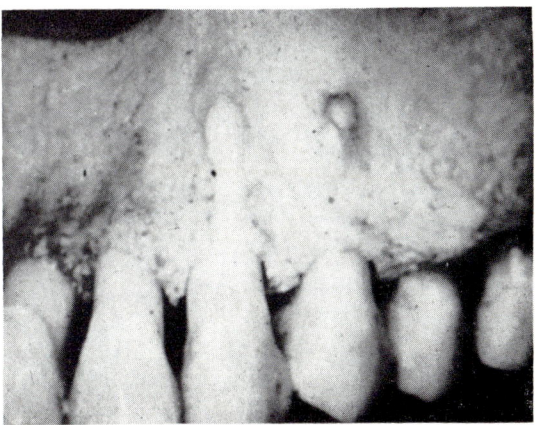

Figure 13-7. An area of dehiscence is present over the labial aspect of the cuspid. A fenestration is visible near the apex of the first bicuspid.

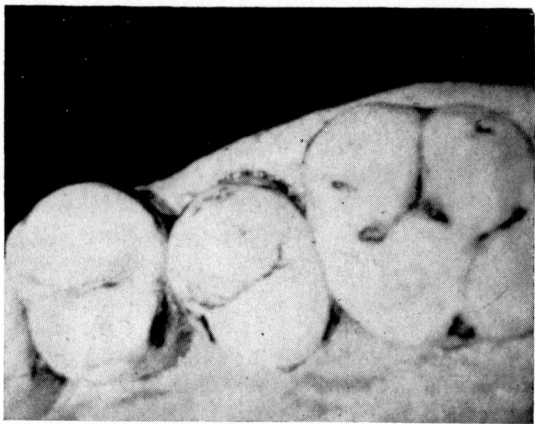

Figure 13-8. Occlusal view of the skull showing the rectangular shape of the first maxillary molar which together with its rotation result in prominence of the mesiobuccal root.

which most commonly have thin or absent bone over the root surfaces are the maxillary and mandibular molars, which are often slightly rotated toward the facial, making the mesial or mesiobuccal root prominent (Fig. 13-8).[14] Cuspids, particularly mandibular cuspids, are usually prominent. The plane of the mandibular cuspid in relation to the plane of the lateral incisor, in a square or ovoid arch form, leads to a broad, flat, bony septum. This anatomic deviation predisposes this area to bony deformities (Fig. 13-9).[15] This is also

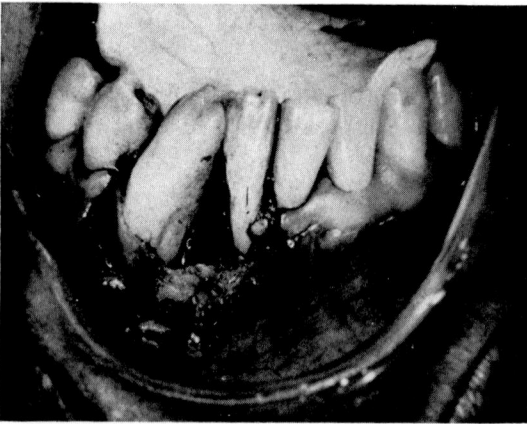

Figure 13-9. The mesial aspect of a mandibular cuspid showing a wide bony septum which predisposes this area to intraosseous defects.

true of the buccal of recessed teeth, the lingual of prominent teeth or the interproximal areas of the posterior teeth. A wide bony septum is vulnerable to crater formation or other bony defects because of the available cancellous bone and the centrally located blood vessels.

Oral Hygiene

Notation of the oral hygiene is made, such as the amount and type of calculus (supragingival or subgingival type), materia alba and food. It is suggested that staining for plaque not be done at this time, since a complete explanation should accompany the demonstration.

Occlusion

The occlusion is examined for wear and the presence of facets.[16,17] If wear facets which match are observed in teeth where the mandible must be moved beyond the envelope of mastication to or near the border movements of the mandible, these facets are indicative of bruxism.[18,19] Abnormal movement of the teeth other than that noted during the mobility examination will be noticed by placing the fingers on the buccal of the maxillary posterior teeth and asking the patient to move his jaw in right and left lateral excursion.

Most patients are unaware that they grind their teeth at night or even that they do it during the day. Usually, once it is pointed out to the patient, he will return at a later visit to comment that he has since noticed the habit.

Evidence from studies and agreement among periodontists is leading to the following conclusion: that bruxism is the chief cause of damaging occlusal forces.[20-22] Normal function—chewing, swallowing and talking—does not damage a healthy periodontium.[23] The frequency of contact of the natural teeth during mastication and swallowing indicates that it is occasional and fleeting and that the forces do not exceed eight to ten pounds.[24-26]

It has been stated that these forces are vertical in direction and conducive to periodontal health. Tension habits, such as bruxism, introduce horizontal components of force which are injurious to the supporting structures of the teeth, especially if the teeth do not wear. Forces of one hundred pounds or more have been found during clenching.[27] What is important about traumatic forces is *magnitude, distribution, direction* and *frequency* (Fig. 13-10). Traumatism is probably not caused by the type of occlusion or the articulation of the teeth. Occlusal traumatism does not affect the depth of the gingival sulcus, thus it has no primary effect upon the gingiva.[27] On the other hand, inflammation does deepen the sulcus and cause pockets. *Inflammation is the primary cause of pocket formation.* There is evidence to show that trauma from occlusion in the presence of inflammation will change the direction of the pathway of inflammation to cause angular bone loss (Figs. 13-11, 13-12).[28] Thus, *occlusal traumatism is not a primary cause of*

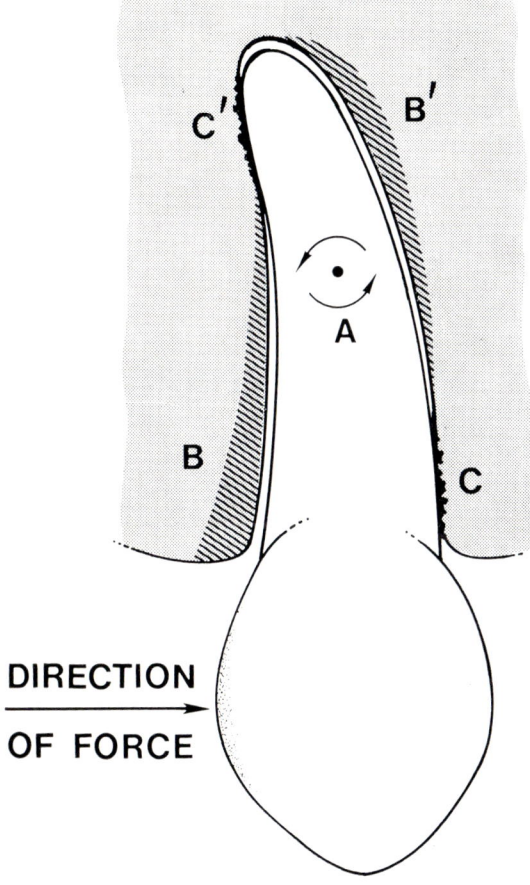

Figure 13-10. The effect of applying a mesial force to an upper cuspid as in occlusal trauma. A, a point situated at the junction of the middle and apical one-thirds of the root, indicates the center of rotation of a single-rooted tooth. B and B′ indicate areas of bone apposition: the areas of tension. C and C′ indicate areas of bone resorption: the areas of pressure.

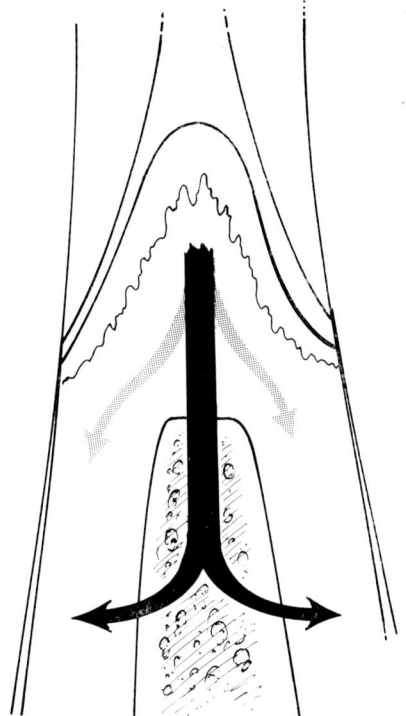

Figure 13-11. Pathways of inflammation occurring interdentally. The dark arrows indicate the direction of the spread of inflammation from a marginal lesion in the absence of occlusal trauma. The lighter arrows indicate the direction of the spread of inflammation associated with occlusal trauma.

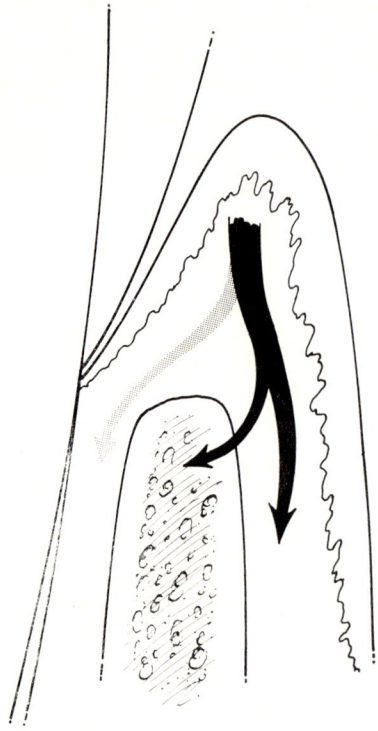

Figure 13-12. Pathways of inflammation. The dark arrows indicate the direction of the spread of inflammation from a marginal lesion in the absence of occlusal trauma. The lighter arrows indicate the direction of the spread of inflammation associated with occlusal trauma.

periodontal pocket formation but a secondary cause. This is not to be confused with secondary traumatic occlusion, where the ratio of the root in bone to that portion of the tooth above the bone is so unfavorable that torque and lateral forces may occur with normal function.

Statistically, the most common primary prematurity is the mesiolingual aspect of the lingual cusp of the maxillary first bicuspid (Fig. 13-13).[7] This is found when the patient has his head slightly tilted backward, the tip of his tongue placed dorsally and superiorly and the jaw guided into its most retruded position. The patient is then instructed to close until the teeth begin to contact: centric relation or the retruded cuspal position. The next most common prematurity is the same point of the second bicuspid. Once this point is found and the patient allowed to close his jaw further, the direction of closure from this point is noted and is called the slide or glide.

With the teeth in centric occlusion (habitual position or the intercuspal position), the first tooth to strike in a lateral excursion—either right or left—is noted and the patient is allowed to continue into this lateral excursion until cusp tip meets cusp tip. This will indicate either a cuspid rise or the degree of group function: that is, some or all of the teeth on the working side. Carbon paper or typewriter ribbon placed on both sides of the mouth will indicate the most prominent areas of occlusal interferences. On the side away from which the jaw is moving (the balancing side) any prematurities are noted (Fig. 13-14). These interferences are called balancing side interferences and are generally considered to be the most injurious to teeth other than nonfunctional movements such as bruxism.[29]

The problems in occlusion are vast. It is not known as yet if function occurs during

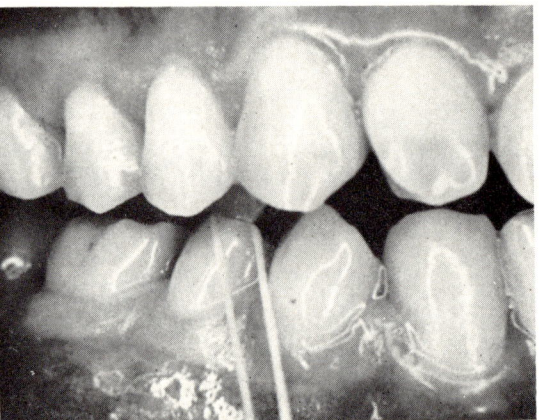

Figure 13-13. A balancing side interference demonstrated with dental floss which indicates contact between the opposing teeth.

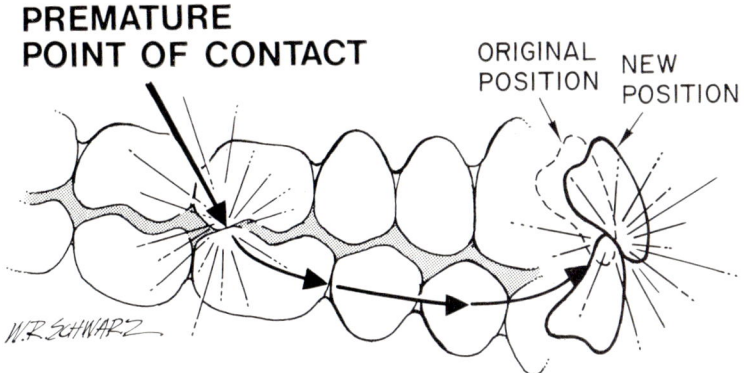

Figure 13-14. One of the major causes of pathologic migration of the anterior teeth is a premature point of contact on one of the posterior teeth driving the mandible anteriorly. This in turn causes the mandibular incisors to strike the lingual surfaces of the maxillary teeth. With loss of bone resulting from periodontal disease, the teeth migrate anteriorly.

lateral excursion or whether that position is used only during bruxism. The evidence, though scanty, points to the fact that lateral excursion is used mainly during parafunctional movements such as bruxism.[30] Parafunctional movements are bruxism, clenching, clamping or tapping the teeth; that is, those tooth contacts which are other than chewing, talking and swallowing. Most people rarely put their teeth together during the protrusive movement, except during parafunctional habits, but rather use a lateral protrusive movement and then grasp the food with the teeth apart and tear it with the hand. The teeth may come close together for shearing action but probably do not touch, except fleetingly, during this position.[31] It is important to note if the posterior teeth touch when the patient moves toward or is in the protrusive position. The "mutually protected" occlusion implies that the anterior and posterior groups of teeth function at different times to protect one another. A common cause of pathological migration of the anterior teeth is the presence of a posterior prematurity which forces the lower jaw anteriorly with the lower incisors striking the lingual of the maxillary incisors and driving them labially (Figs. 13-14 and 13-15).[7] The degree of overbite and overjet are thus important and should be observed.

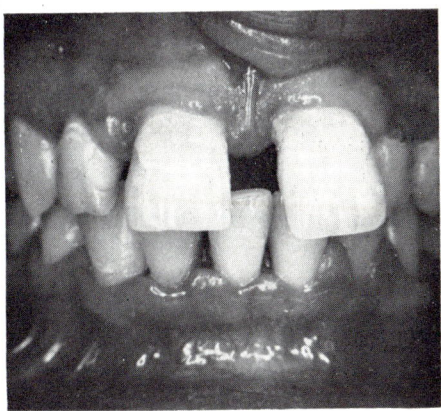

Figure 13-15. A clinical case illustrating pathological migration resulting from periodontitis and a posterior prematurity.

Habits

Tongue thrust habits are important and often overlooked. The obvious open bite anteriorly is easy to see and thus diagnose, but some pathological migration of anterior teeth can be initiated by the tongue. A syndrome [32] is seen which includes a palate hyposensitive to palpation with the finger, an enlarged tongue with crenulations on the borders, splayed anterior teeth and open bite. The movement of the tongue during swallowing is against the anterior teeth and this causes food to be pushed against the soft palate, reverse swallowing (Figs. 13-16, A, B and C).

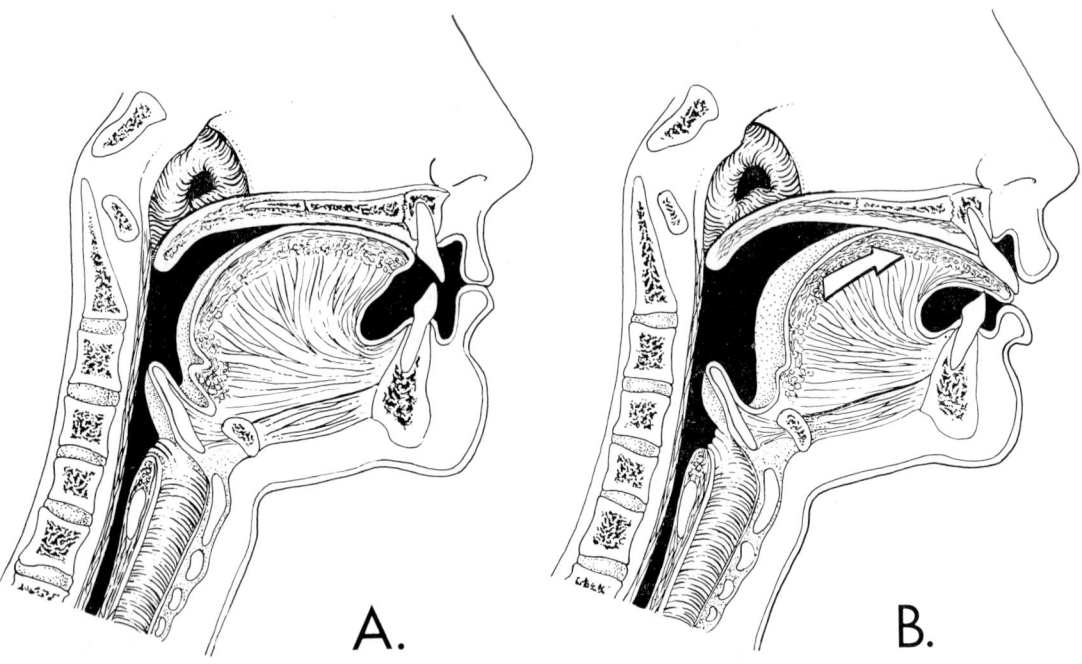

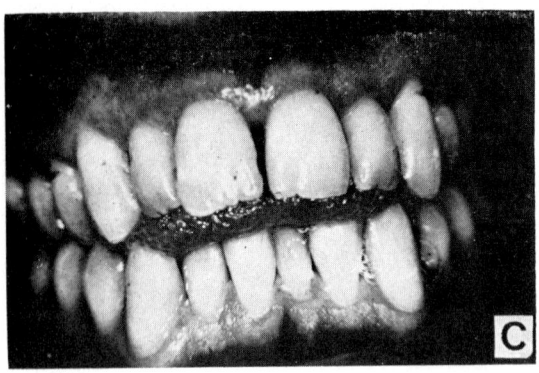

Figure 13-16. (A) The normal position of the tongue during swallowing. The dorsum of the tongue is against the hard palate with the tip of the tongue against the mucosa and gingivae and on occasions against the teeth, anteriorly. (B) The position of the tongue during "reverse swallowing" or "tongue thrusting": the tongue pushes anteriorly between the incisors causing flaring of these teeth and resulting in an "open bite." Flaring is associated with bone loss due to periodontal disease and is one of the causes of "pathologic migration." (C) Note the tongue position during reverse swallowing and the anterior open bite.

THE IMPORTANCE OF THE RADIOGRAPH IN DIAGNOSIS

The radiographs should have been consulted initially and throughout the clinical examination for correlation. They are now examined thoroughly to help tie the clinical findings together. A periodontal pocket cannot be seen on the radiograph, nor can the morphology of the bony deformities. However, the approximate gross amount of bone disruption can be seen, as can the most coronal position of the bone in septal regions. The position or condition of structures on the buccal or lingual aspects of the teeth cannot be seen, nor can the radiographs tell whether there is mobility or even the gingiva-to-bone relationships, since the gingiva may have receded with the bone and no pocket may be present. A radiograph gives invaluable information concerning the location of the maxillary sinus, crown-to-root ratio, endodontic pathology, the fit of various restorations on the proximal surfaces and other abnormalities which may be present (see Ch. 6) and most important, the condition of the alveolar bone and periodontal ligament on the mesial, distal and apical aspects of the root.

Ramfjord[33] has indicated that the direction of traumatic occlusion forces is perpendicular to the plane of the remaining proximal bony wall. Radiographic findings correlated with the clinical findings of mobility, pocket depths and prematurities are invaluable.

The radiograph is a valuable aid, a diagnostic tool, in the determination of periodontal disease, but the radiograph alone is not of great value unless correlated with clinical findings.

The distribution and type of bone loss is an important diagnostic sign. It points to the location and destructive local factors in different areas of the mouth and in different surfaces of the same tooth. In periodontal disease, the destructive pattern in the interdental septa is a critical index of the destructive effects of the various local factors. The interdental septa undergo changes that affect the lamina dura, density of bone at crest of the ridge (marginal radiodensity), size and shape of the medullary spaces, and the height and contour of the bone. Bone loss in the interdental septa, perpendicular to the long axis of the teeth or parallel to a line joining adjacent cemento-enamel junctions, is referred to as horizontal bone loss and is generally conceded to occur in inflammatory processes without occlusal trauma. Bone loss which is at an angle to a plane perpendicular to the long axis of the teeth is referred to as angular or vertical bone loss and may involve traumatic occlusion in addition to inflammation.[33] Fuzziness and a break in the lamina dura in the crest of the interdental septum are among the earliest radiographic signs of periodontal disease.

It cannot be stressed too strongly that poor radiographic technique produces distortions that limit the value of the radiograph. The exposure, development time, type of film and especially the angulation can modify the radiographic appearance. Standardized, reproducible techniques such as the long-cone technique are required to obtain reliable radiographs for pretreatment and posttreatment comparisons.

SYSTEMIC DISEASE AND THE PERIODONTIUM

Consultations may be requested with the physician if, for example, a long interval has expired since the last physical examination. The patient may be sent for laboratory tests to eliminate suspected systemic factors (see Ch. 10). The common systemic factors which have an influence on periodontal disease are *diabetes mellitus* and those of hormonal influence such as *pregnancy* (Fig. 13-17) and *puberty,* although many other diseases are possible. What is most important to remember is *most systemic diseases usually make a pre-existing periodontal condition worse rather than affecting the periodontium directly.*

DIAGNOSIS

A diagnosis of the periodontal disease present is a summation of the carefully collected findings. The most common periodontal disease is *periodontitis*. The most common gingival disease is *gingivitis*. One should familiarize oneself with the various periodontal diseases; a comparison with the findings of the clinical examination should, in most cases, give an accurate diagnosis. It cannot be emphasized sufficiently that all the clinical findings together are meaningless unless the signs and symptoms of each disease are known, as are their differential diagnosis.

PROGNOSIS

The prognosis of a case is the sum total of the following:

1. The extent, type and duration of the periodontal disease.
2. The motivation of the patient.
3. The number and distribution of the remaining teeth and their condition.
4. The ability of the periodontist to achieve a predictable and acceptable result.
5. The type of restorative work necessary and the ability of the dentist to perform this work correctly.
6. The age, health and financial resources of the patient.

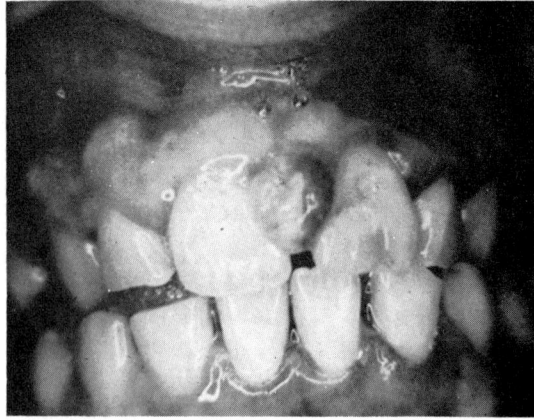

Figure 13-17. Pregnancy tumor. Note the obvious inflammation present in other areas of the mouth.

The question of prognosis arises in every case. Obviously, there is no problem in slightly or moderately involved teeth, especially if the dental work to be done afterward is minimal in amount and cost and the patient is motivated to practice good oral hygiene. The six points become important in the advanced and borderline cases which involve a great deal of time, periodontal and dental work, and make the motivation of the patient a key factor.

Any rules stating the amount of bone loss in relation to the extraction of a tooth have little value. Any tooth or teeth that are able to function in health are considered cured of disease. There is no point in retaining a tooth just for the sake of retaining it. On the contrary, we may encounter a line of seriously involved teeth. The question is whether to extract or to decide that together these teeth may function well. If the degree of involvement can be determined to have remained static for a number of years, it may be reasonable to assume that the tooth may do rather well after therapy. Acute problems respond well to therapy. If the rate of destruction is severe and is over a long period of time, then the prognosis is usually not favorable.

The next question is whether it is possible to change the local environment so that the destructive factors are no longer present or whether they can be reduced within the physiologic limits of the teeth. Can the patient keep the teeth clean? It has been said that elimination of pockets should be looked at from the point of view of treating the mouth so that the patient can keep it clean. This is the rationale for gingival surgery. There is no point at which the bone loss is so severe that a tooth has to be extracted;[34] for every example shown, someone can show a tooth that has been retained (Fig. 13-18). Basically, if the tooth and the surrounding tissues can be returned to health and the tooth can maintain itself in function, with or without the help of its neighbors, it should be retained, even if three-fourths of its bone is lost. We have all seen teeth with extensive bone loss that have surprising stability because of a good physiologic response by the remaining supporting structures. On the other hand, there are some teeth with one-half the bone missing that have a hopeless prognosis because they cannot be returned to health. An example of this is a maxillary cuspid-bicuspid area with roots so closely approximated that a pocket is formed because of the absence of bone. Thus, one of the teeth has a hopeless prognosis or both teeth will eventually be lost.

Root form, length and crown-ratio are critical for obvious reasons, especially if fixed or removable prosthetics are considered. Osseous defects are really not a factor, as with present knowledge most of them can be managed successfully.

The prognosis is better in older patients.[34] This is contrary to most theories of resistance and disease that the younger patient will recuperate faster and has better resistance. If the younger patient, who ordinarily is resistant to periodontal disease, succumbs so completely as to con-

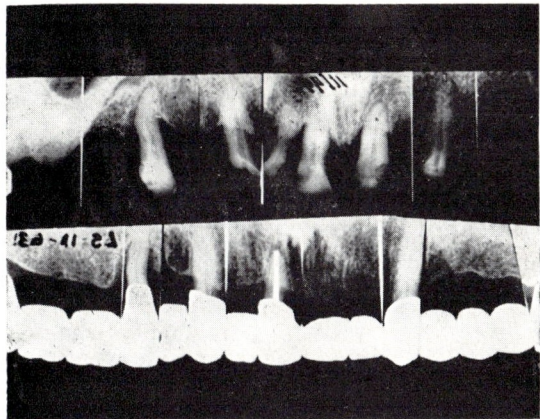

Figure 13-18. The upper radiographs show advanced periodontal disease which was treated and the missing teeth were restored. The lower set of radiographs, although still demonstrating osseous defects, were taken nineteen years later.

stitute a moderate or advanced case, he must seriously lack resistance or the factors promoting the disease are those of an overwhelming nature. The older patient has withstood the factors possibly for a longer time than the younger patient and it must be assumed that his resistance is better.

Some periodontists feel that the periodontal procedure should be predictable. The predictability is not in the procedure alone but also in the hands and experience of the operator. The procedure which fails at the hands of one operator may be consistently successful in the hands of another. The periodontist should be aware of his limitations.

It is stressed, however, that "heroic" procedures, which are done when the outcome is doubtful, should be used only as long as the effort that is expended to save a tooth would change the entire treatment plan of the mouth, such as from a partial denture to a fixed bridge. In addition, the patient should be fully aware of the consequences and the purposes of the procedure. To save teeth and then have a removable prosthesis placed is sometimes folly. Unfortunately, removable prostheses do not always live up to the claims made for them and compared to fixed prostheses they generally are more injurious to the periodontium.[35] On the other hand, if because of secondary traumatic occlusion, full-mouth reconstruction might be deemed necessary, one has to consider whether the dentist is prepared to carry through the proposed treatment plan. Is the cost of the treatment commensurate with the prognosis or will the patient lose the teeth anyway in a time span which is less than sufficient to warrant the cost? Is the patient sufficiently motivated to take care of the mouth? There is no formula which can be used, but all six points and their obvious ramifications should be considered separately and then together. This will help toward establishing a prognosis.

TREATMENT PLAN

It is preferable to carry out the treatment plan in a series of five steps.

Optional Phase

The first step of a treatment plan is the optional phase. This step refers to those procedures which may have to be performed by other specialists, the dentist or by the periodontist. It precedes what is considered the first step in most cases: initial therapy. During the optional phase all hopeless teeth are removed; extraction of these teeth undoubtedly will make the oral environment healthier, lessen the possibility of emergencies and make the access to the remaining teeth during the other procedures much easier. It will allow for healing of the extraction sites, so that upon completion of the periodontal therapy, these areas will be healed and ready for final prosthetic consideration. There are some instances where the extraction of a tooth with a doubtful prognosis in the midst of a line of periodontally involved teeth will allow, after healing, some bone fill. This is called a "strategic extraction." Extraction of any anterior teeth is done by the dentist, who has previously constructed a temporary partial denture for esthetics and phonetics. If long periodontal therapy or a long interval after therapy is contemplated before the patient returns to the dentist, a posterior temporary partial denture is constructed which will prevent migration and supereruption. If fixed bridgework is agreed upon and the prognosis is good for the remaining teeth, the dentist may elect to prepare the remaining teeth and place a temporary fixed bridge of acrylic. This is the most ideal solution, if it is made correctly. Emphasis is placed on contour, marginal fit and occlusion. It will help stabilize the teeth and is not as injurious as the removable appliance. Correctly made, it will give the patient an idea of the final appearance of the prosthetic work, help improve the occlusion and help to eliminate some of the local factors such as overhangs, caries and overcontoured restorations which may be present. In addition, it helps to open embrasures to allow for interproximal cleaning and helps to shunt the food away from the gingival margin by improved contours.

Endodontically Involved Teeth

Endodontic therapy should be instituted on all those teeth demonstrating endodontic signs and symptoms and all those teeth which might be possible future endodontic problems after the insertion of the prosthetic work (Figs. 13-19, 13-20, 13-21). If the periodontist contemplates removing the root of a molar and the prognosis for retaining the remainder of the tooth is favorable and there is no question as to which root is to be removed, endodontic therapy should be performed. A silver point is placed partially down the canal of the root to be removed. If the prognosis is questionable or there is some doubt as to which root is to be removed, the endodontic therapy should wait and

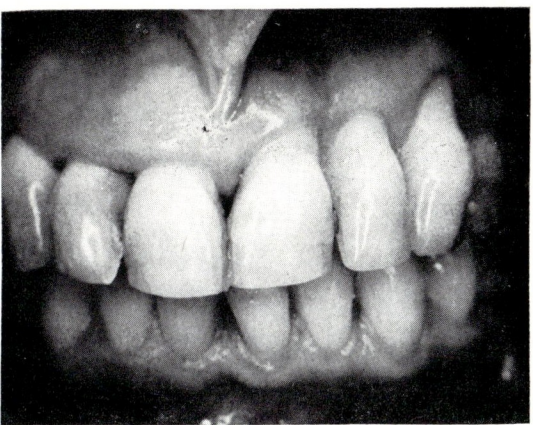

Figure 13-21. Same case as Figure 13-19, three months postoperatively. The splint has been removed.

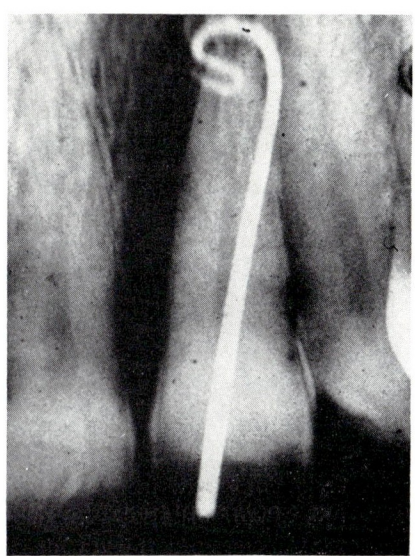

Figure 13-19. Radiograph of an endodontic-periodontic problem with gutta percha in place on the labial aspect of the tooth.

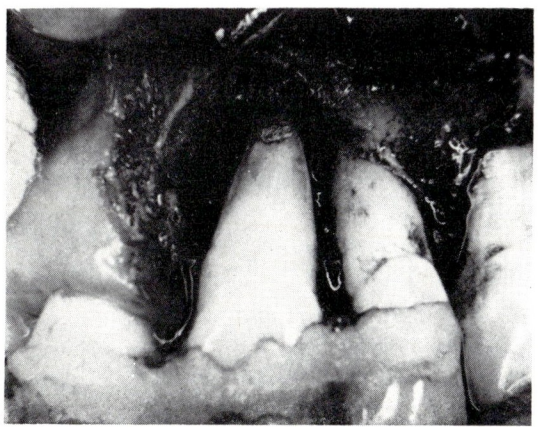

Figure 13-20. Same case as Figure 13-19 showing tooth splinted, gingival flap reflected, granulation tissue and calculus removed. The apex of the incisor has been beveled and filled with amalgam.

be done as soon as possible after the prognosis has improved. Morris[36] has stated that bone will not fill readily around an endodontically filled tooth. If the canal is filed and cleaned but not filled, the prognosis is as good for bone to fill as if there were no endodontic therapy needed. Therefore, on those teeth on which osseous procedures to graft bone are contemplated, endodontic therapy should either wait for the periodontal therapy or stop short of restoring the tooth.

Temporary Splinting

Temporary splinting or therapeutic immobilization is usually done in this phase (Figs. 13-22, A, and B). There are usually only two indications: (a) to help stabilize a tooth on which bone surgery is contemplated and (b) to splint teeth with secondary traumatic occlusion to its neighbors to see how these teeth will act if they are permanently splinted. Mobile teeth without secondary traumatic occlusion should never be splinted, but occlusal equilibration should be considered. If a mobile tooth is tied to a neighbor, especially if little or no care is taken to eliminate the traumatic forces which have most likely

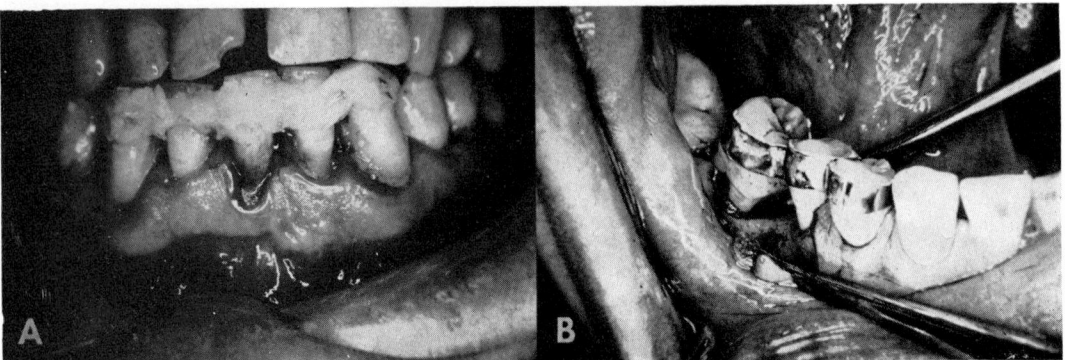

Figure 13-22. (A) A temporary wire and acrylic splint placed prior to surgery. (B) Orthodontic bands soldered together and placed prior to surgery as a splint.

caused the mobility, the tooth will not be able to avoid these traumatic forces and further damage will result (Fig. 13-23).[37] It is known that splinting a tooth to its neighbors will increase its mobility after a period of time because of the lessened amount of function. Furthermore, the temporary splints which are extracoronal, decrease the ability of the patient to cleanse the proximal areas of the teeth, especially with floss, and many themselves irritate the gingival margin.

Initial Therapy

Initial therapy is important for the overall success of the case. During this phase the patient is given a thorough explanation of the etiologic causes of their particular problem. They are instructed in how to clean their mouth, with particular emphasis on plaque control. They are given thorough scaling, curettage and root planing sessions and occlusal equilibrations.

The patient should be given repeated instructions on the intrasulcular brushing technique,[38] the use and abuse of dental floss and the interdental stimulator. The importance of plaque[39] is explained as to the importance of its concentration at the gingival margin. The patient is informed why it is important to break up this plaque in order to prevent further damage. The fact that it takes up to twenty-four hours for plaque to reform is stressed. Calculus is demonstrated in the patient's mouth. It is explained that the fastest calcification of plaque is two days[40] and thus calculus formation is relatively easy to prevent. If calculus does form, the outer surface of the calculus has plaque which can be removed and thus further calculus formation stopped. Plaque has the ability, especially in children, to take the refined sugars and convert them into acid thus initiating decay within minutes after eating.[41] Plaque is the cause of the release of toxins, which after eight days, can cause the destruction of the epithelial lining of the sulcus and give the clinical appearance of redness, swelling and hemorrhage.[42]

The explanations of what plaque can do, how one should clean one's mouth and the rationale behind these methods are constantly repeated, until the patient can demonstrate good plaque control. The need for a well-motivated patient in periodontal therapy is important. The patient should accept periodontal therapy and its benefits for his own reasons, which may not be identical to those of the periodontist. The patient should also accept the responsibility for keeping his mouth clean and free of plaque and for the health of his own mouth after completion of therapy.

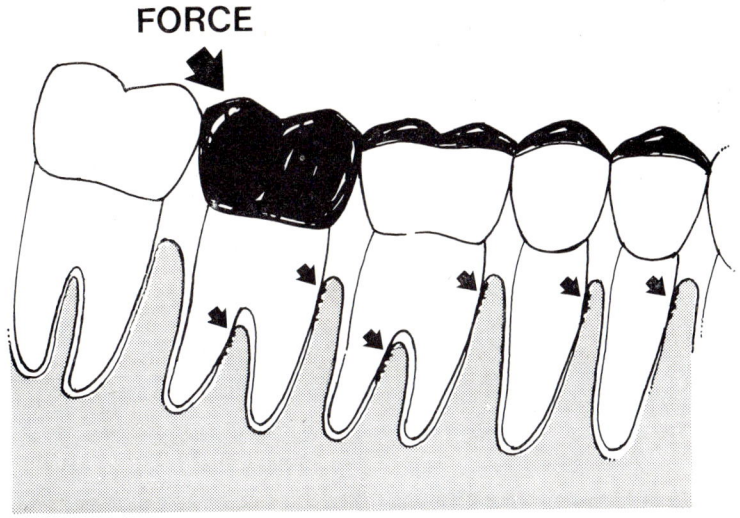

Figure 13-23. A premature contact on one tooth of a group of splinted teeth, the force being transmitted throughout the entire group. A tooth thus tied to its neighbors cannot avoid a traumatic force and thus a more grievous injury may occur.

Scaling and Curettage

Concurrently, scaling and curettage is done with root planing. It is suggested that the scaling be done under local anesthesia and that not more than a quadrant be done per sitting. The scaling should be checked with an explorer to help ensure the removal of all calcified debris and a smooth root. If the pockets are too deep and there is too much hemorrhage, the area should be scaled again. Curettage should be done to the pocket lining to ensure its complete removal for maximum shrinkage. Theoretically, the epithelial attachment should not be removed, but in practice this is hard to ensure. Thus, with the complete removal of plaque and calcified bacterial debris, the development of smooth roots along with continued plaque control by the patient, the pocket will shrink. How much it shrinks depends upon the amount of edema and cellular elements present. Those patients with a great amount of fibrosis will have the least amount of shrinkage. It is important to get maximum shrinkage and reduction of inflammation since it is not easy to raise a flap on soft, friable tissue. It is better to work in an area where the inflammation is reduced (Figs. 13-24 and 13-25). The patient is usually able to see the results of these procedures by the periodontist along with those home-care procedures which they have been shown. This procedure, in total, may reduce the pockets to such an extent that a different type of surgery may be contemplated; possibly elimination of some surgery altogether. Most important of all, it allows the periodontist to evaluate the patient's motivation. *If the individual is unwilling to take care of his mouth at this point, it is futile to contemplate any further periodontal or dental therapy.*

Occlusal Equilibration

The occlusal equilibration is performed in the initial therapy phase. Since there are more than forty recognized methods of adjusting the occlusion, it would be superfluous to describe a method at this point. The aims of occlusal equilibration are

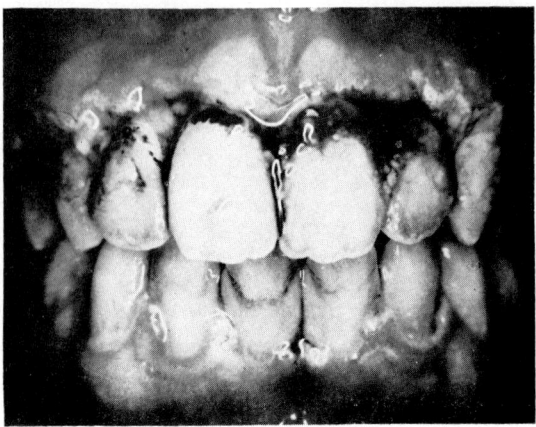

Figure 13-24. Acute necrotizing gingivitis. Note the bleeding and ulcerated areas in the maxillary incisor region.

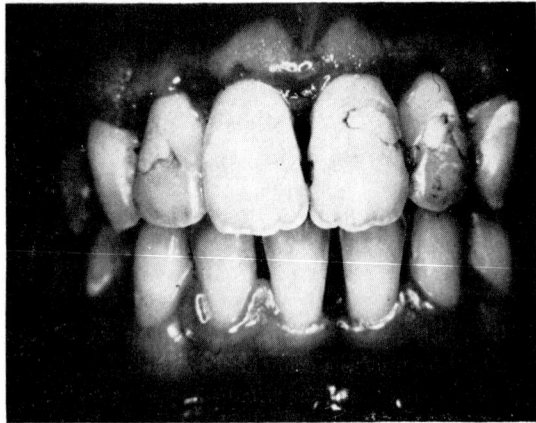

Figure 13-25. Same case as Figure 13-24, five days after scaling, curettage and home-care instructions.

nearly the same for most methods: (a) to eliminate the excessive lateral forces, (b) to achieve maximum intercuspation, (c) to eliminate slides and glides with the possible exception of a horizontal slide from the retruded cuspal position to the intercuspal position ("long centric") and (d) to direct the forces in the long axis of the tooth. In other words, an occlusal adjustment is performed to reduce forces applied to the teeth and direct these forces apically. If mobility continues and the patient demonstrates little or no lessening of the degree of mobility with repeated adjustments, it might be necessary to construct a night guard appliance to prevent damaging forces while the patient is grinding his teeth.

During the day it is suggested to those patients who grind or clench that they chew gum. The rationale is that masticatory forces are only fleeting and light and in the light of recent research, considered physiologic.[43] Certainly these forces are less damaging than that of the lateral forces seen during grinding.

Night Guards

The purpose of the various night guards is not to prevent the patient from bruxing; on the contrary, it allows him to brux but prevents him from doing any damage due to lateral stresses on the teeth by either keeping the teeth apart, as in the Hawley appliance, or allowing the teeth of one or both jaws to hit upon a smooth surface which is free of any interference.

At night the patient should wear one of three most common types of night guards:

1. *The Hawley type.* This is an acrylic and wire appliance constructed for the maxillary teeth which has a biting surface wide enough to accommodate all or most of the lower incisors and cuspids. This biting surface is located at a level behind the upper incisors which will allow the posterior teeth to avoid contact when the mandible goes into a lateral excursive movement. This is the smallest of the three types and the easiest to insert and adjust. It is contraindicated when the bony support of lower anterior teeth are very poor; there is also the possible eruption of the posterior teeth. Eruption of the posterior teeth is an uncommon finding because it is doubtful if the cellular change necessary for eruption will occur during an eight-hour sleep

period. There is a gross extrusion of the posterior teeth and for the first five to ten minutes in the morning the patient may not be able to feel a positive occlusal sense. Another use of the Hawley is to effect minor tooth movement of the upper anterior teeth.

2. *Full occlusal splint.* Acrylic is placed over the occlusal surfaces of the posterior teeth of a minimal thickness and extends 1 mm over the buccal and lingual surfaces for retention; a wire or wires may also be placed for retention. Usually, this type is constructed for the maxillary arch, except in cases where the mandibular anterior segment is at a level which is at least 3 to 5 mm higher than the plane of the posterior teeth. In this case, the splint is constructed for the mandibular posterior area with a major connector of wire and acrylic. This type of splint requires the models to be mounted on an articulator. Care must be taken to have most of the posterior teeth hitting the appliance at the same time. No interferences should be allowed during lateral excursion of the jaw; this is not easy to achieve with a flat plane appliance. It is suggested that small indentations be made that are no deeper than 1 mm to give the patient a "home base" when placing the opposing jaw against the appliance. The appliance loses its effectiveness if the cusps of the opposing teeth can catch upon its edge and receive torquing forces. No supereruption is seen.

3. *Double full occlusal splint.* This appliance is made of two full occlusal appliances. As in the second type, the casts must be mounted on an articulator. However, the adjustment of the appliances in the mouth is somewhat easier since a "home base" does not have to be provided and the problem of torque on the teeth on the opposing arch, when catching upon the edge of the appliance, is not present. The serious drawback is that two full occlusal splints are not the easiest appliances to wear during sleep.

Judging the Effects of Therapy

Although constant evaluation of each procedure during initial therapy is performed, a final step to evaluate and coordinate all of the procedures is done before the next phase: pocket elimination. The re-evaluation will provide information concerning the patient's motivation, oral hygiene effectiveness and healing capacity. The pockets should be reevaluated as to changes in depth, the gain or loss of attached gingiva and possible radiographic changes. These new pocket levels may be placed upon the original chart.

In essence, the initial therapy can provide the clinician with a logical sequence to a sometimes unpredictable and slow healing process. It can act as a protector to the patient in terms of time and money and to the clinician of time and effort. It can help assure a successful case.

The Surgical Phase

Having followed a careful plan of treatment during the initial therapy phase, the surgical phase becomes easier, for there will be less surgery to perform than when the patient was first seen. The type of surgery to be done in this phase depends upon the depth of the pockets, the relationship to the mucogingival line and the presence and type of osseous defects. Any pocket, whose base is above the mucogingival line, when there are no osseous defects present, lends itself to a gingivectomy (Fig. 13-26, A). A gingivoplasty is identical to a gingivectomy except that it is done to recontour soft tissue; the gingivectomy is done to remove tissue pockets. Some slight bone contouring in the interseptal areas can be done with a gingivectomy.

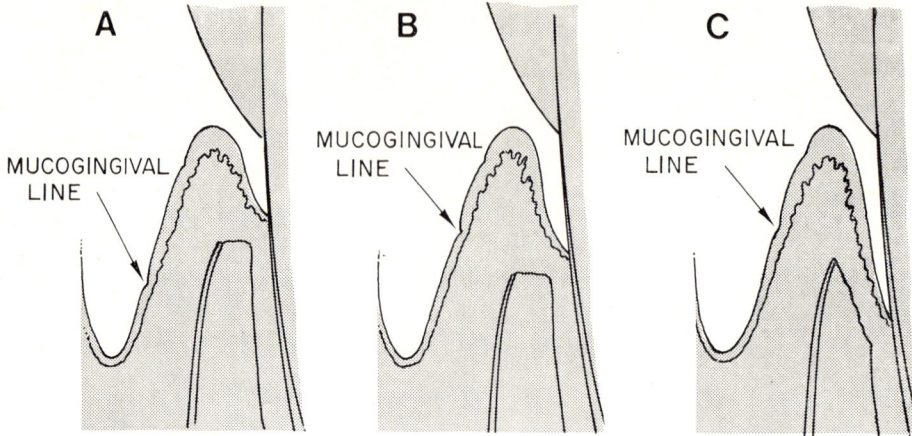

Figure 13-26. (A) A periodontal pocket with its most apical position above the mucogingival line. This is usually seen in gingivitis or early periodontitis. (B) A periodontal pocket with its most apical point below the mucogingival line. (C) A periodontal pocket with its most apical point below the crest of the alveolar bone. This lesion is now an "intraosseous" periodontal lesion and is usually seen in advanced periodontal disease.

For those pockets that extend to or beyond the mucogingival line, and where there is an insufficient width of attached gingiva (usually less than 1 to 2 mm), one of a number of mucogingival procedures should be considered (Fig. 13-26, B). Mucogingival procedures are usually mutilating, painful and heal by secondary intention so that the healing period is longer. The results are not always predictable. If possible, these procedures should be avoided.

If the pocket extends to or beyond the mucogingival line and there is more than 1 or 2 mm of attached gingiva present, with or without osseous lesions, repositioned flap techniques should be considered (Fig. 13-26, C). An example is the apically repositioned flap (Figs. 13-27, A, B and C). Although healing is not by primary intention, it approaches it to a greater degree that of the mucogingival procedures. These repositioned flaps will help to protect the bone, some will lower the vestibule and some will give a wider zone of attached gingiva. Most important of all, they can allow access to the bone for the various osseous procedures.

There are some osseous procedures, such as a transplant, which will not work unless completely covered with tissue. The gingivectomy and mucogingival procedures cannot do this.

There is not sufficient space nor is it the purpose of this chapter to discuss the types of periodontal surgery. It is important to remember that the initial therapy phase simplifies the surgical phase. The clinician is now able to determine the procedure which he must use and which will eliminate those pockets that remain, based upon their depth, relationship to the mucogingival line and the presence and type of osseous defects.

In planning a surgical procedure the clinician should only plan to do what he can within a given time interval, considering the patient's health and attitude. Surgery can vary from an area of one tooth to a sixth of the mouth, a quadrant, an arch, a half-mouth and, finally, to that of a full-mouth procedure. Some periodontists

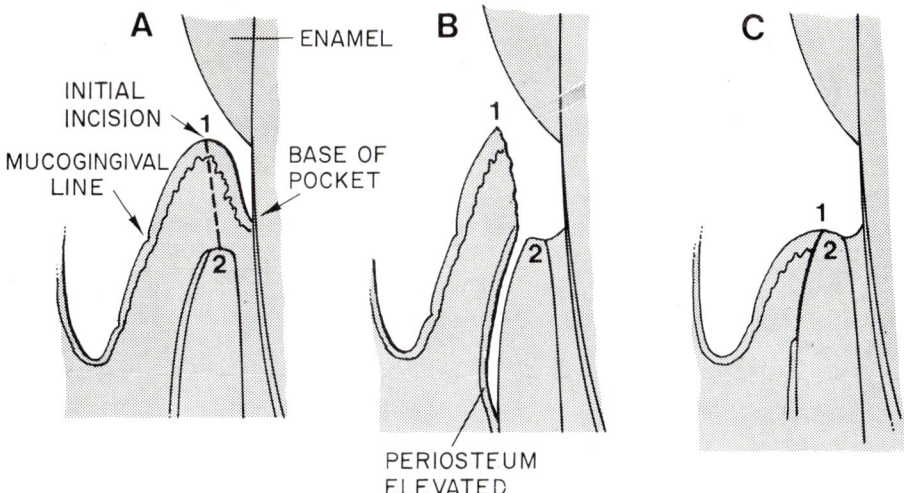

Figure 13-27. The apically repositioned flap. (A) The initial incision is made from the crest of the gingival margin (1) to the crest of the bone (2). (B) The flap is elevated away from the bone (mucoperiosteal flap) although the periosteum could be left with a sharp dissection (split thickness flap). The tissue lining the pocket is removed. (C) The flap is moved apically placing the crest of the marginal gingiva (1) at the crest of the bone (2). The gingiva can be placed either slightly apical to the crest of bone or slightly coronally on to the tooth root.

prefer to work in a hospital, some under local anesthesia with sedation, some under general anesthesia; some prefer to work only in the office. The choice of amount of surgery and place is left to the discretion of the clinician.

After healing, any remaining calculus is removed and the occlusion is refined. If mobility is still present six to eight weeks after surgery, further equilibration should be contemplated. Mobility, incidentally, is the only clinical criterion we have to test the effectiveness of our occlusal equilibrations. At this time, evaluation is made of those teeth with a doubtful prognosis; their prognosis depended upon the outcome of the surgical procedures. However, some osseous transplants may not give a final result for as long as six months to a year.

The restorative phase is now reviewed, and the original treatment plan is viewed in the light of what is now possible. The patient's ability to remove plaque is constantly rechecked. The surgical phase, theoretically, has made it easier for the patient to keep the mouth clean since there are no longer pockets present. However, in practice this is not always the case, since the gingival margin is now at a more apical level and the gingival recession has allowed larger food traps interproximally. Fluting or grooving of the posterior root surfaces which formerly were inaccessible to floss are now accessible and a method of hygiene should now be shown (Fig. 13-28). The interproximal brush seems to be more effective than floss for reaching these areas.

Should the patient change her mind about undergoing any restorative work or elect to wait for a period of time, little or no breakdown should occur except in those cases where there is secondary traumatic occlusion or a removable prosthetic appliance. The question then may arise, Why should prosthetics need be performed? The

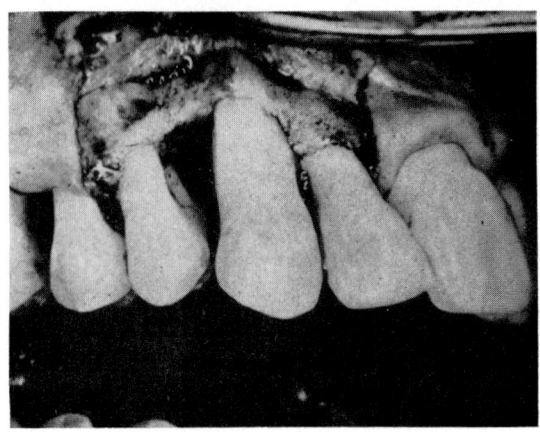

Figure 13-28. Note the "fluting" or grooving on the mesial aspect of the first bicuspid root.

answer is simply that prosthetics will be able to achieve a better occlusion than that of occlusal equilibration; it will provide the necessary contours that the present restorations cannot give, and it will help in closing open contacts, in splinting teeth with secondary traumatic occlusion and in providing better esthetics and phonetics.

Restorative Phase

The restorative phase is the fourth step (*see* Ch. 14).

Maintenance Phase

This is the fifth and final phase and is the one that insures the continued good oral health of the patient. With the philosophy which we have developed—the patient being responsible for the hygiene of his own mouth—the clinician is in the happy role of seeing his patients at intervals which are commensurate with the patient's ability to perform plaque control. The dentist is responsible for the dental care, which incidentally should be minimal from this point onward, since total mouth care was planned and performed. The periodontist is responsible for the care of the supporting structures of the teeth and overseeing the continued good hygiene of the patient.

Recall visits can easily be handled by the hygienist, since the primary concern here is usually some supragingival calculus, confined to a few teeth, and stain. The patient understands that "cleaning" is now a checkup to see if they have been doing their job. The periodontist should check the patient on each recall visit to ensure that there are no pockets which may have begun to appear; the occlusion is checked by the presence of increased mobility. Full-mouth, long-cone radiographs should be taken every two to three years to check the bony picture. Any slips in oral hygiene are thoroughly discussed and corrections are instituted.

Neither the periodontist, the dentist nor the patient can do it alone; together they can achieve a predictable result.

REFERENCES

1. Klingsberg, J., Cancellaro, L. A., and Butcher, E. O.: Effects of air drying on rodent oral mucous membrane: A histologic study of simulated mouth breathing. *J. Periodontol,* 32:38, 1961.
2. Dummett, C. O.: Clinical observations on pigmentation variations in healthy oral tissues of the Negro. *J Dent Res,* 24:7, 1945.
3. Dummett, C. O.: Physiologic pigmentation of the oral and cutaneous tissues in the Negro. *J Dent Res,* 25:422, 1946.
4. Greene, R.: A study of the characteristics of stippling and relation to gingival health. *J. Periodontol,* 33:176, 1962.
5. Gottlieb, B., and Orban, B.: Active and passive eruption of the teeth. *J Dent Res,* 13:214, 1933.
6. Bowers, G.: A study of the width of attached gingiva. *J Periodontol,* 34:201, 1963.

7. Glickman, I.: Clinical periodontology. Philadelphia, W. B. Saunders Co., 1964, p. 608, 723, 419.
8. Pritchard, J. F.: *Advanced Periodontol Disease: Surgical and Prosthetic Management.* Philadelphia, W. B. Saunders, 1965, pp. 146–147.
9. Weinmann, J. P.: Progress of gingival inflammation into the supporting structures of the teeth, *J Periodontol 12:*71, 1941.
10. Ochsenbein, C.: Rationale for periodontal osseous surgery. *Dent Clin North Am,* March, 1960, p. 27.
11. Pritchard, J.: A technique for treating intrabony pockets based on alveolar process morphology. *Dent Clin North Am,* March, 1960, p. 85.
12. Ramadan, A. B. E., and Mitchell, D. F.: A roentgenographic study of experimental bone destruction. *Oral Surg,* 15:930, 1962.
13. Cogswell, W. W.: *Dental Oral Surgery.* Colorado Springs, Out West Printing Co., 1932.
14. Nabers, C. L., Spear, G. R., and Beckham, L. C.: Alveolar dehiscence. *Tex Dent J,* 78:4, 1960.
15. Sibley, L., and Pritchard, J.: Etiologic factors contributing to bony deformities in the mandibular cuspid-lateral incisor area. *J Periodontol,* 34:101, 1963.
16. Beyron, H. L.: Occlusal changes in the adult occlusion. *JADA,* 48:674, 1954.
17. Weinberg, L. A.: Diagnosis of facets in occlusal equilibration. *JADA,* 52:26, 1956.
18. Ramfjord, S.: Bruxism, a clinical and electromyographic study. *JADA,* 62:21, 1961.
19. Thaller, J. L.: Bruxism, a factor in periodontal disease. New York Dental Journal *31:* 17, 1965.
20. Bruxism. Report of 14th Congress of A.R.P.A. Internationale, Venice, Italy. *Acad Rev,* 4:9, 1956.
21. Lipke, D., and Posselt, U.: Parafunctions of the masticatory system (bruxism): Report of panel discussion. *J West Soc Periodontol,* 8:133, 1960.
22. Nadler, S. C.: Bruxism, a classification: Critical review. *JADA,* 54:65, 1967.
23. Anderson, D. J.: A method of recording masticatory loads. *J Dent Res,* 32:785, 1953.
24. Jankelson, B., Hoffman, G. M., and Hendron, J. A.: The physiology of the stomatognathic system. *JADA,* 46:375, 1953.
25. Muhlemann, H. P., Herzog, H., and Vogel, A.: Occlusal trauma and tooth mobility. *Schweiz Monatsschr Zahnheilkd,* 66:527–44, 1956.
26. Yurhstas, A., and Manly, R. S.: Measurements of occlusal contact area effective in mastication. *Am J Orthod,* 35:185, 1949.
27. Macapanpan, I. C., and Weinmann, J. P.: The influence of injury to the periodontal membrane in the spread of inflammation. *J Dent Res,* 33:263, 1954.
28. Glickman, I., and Smulow, J. B.: Alterations in the pathway of gingival inflammation into the underlying tissues induced by excessive occlusal forces. *J Periodontol,* 33: 7, 1962.
29. Schuyler, C. H.: Factors contributing to traumatic occlusion. *J Prosthet Dent,* 11:708, 1961.
30. Graf, H., and Zander, H. A.: Tooth contact patterns in mastication. *J Prosthet Dent,* 13:1055–56, 1963.
31. Muhlemann, H.: Tooth mobility, a review of clinical aspects and research findings. *J Periodontol* 38:686, 1967.
32. Ray, H. G., and Santos, H. A.: Consideration of tongue thrusting as a factor in periodontal disease. *J Periodontol,* 25: 250, 1954.
33. Ramfjord, S.: Periodontal reaction to functional occlusal stress. *J. Periodontol* 30: 95, 1959.
34. Goldman, H. M., and Cohen, D. W.: *Periodontal Therapy.* St. Louis, C. V. Mosby, 1968, p. 354, 356.
35. Krogh-Paulsen, W.: Partial denture design in relation to occlusal trauma and periodontal breakdown. *Int Dent J,* 4:847, 1954.
36. Morris, M. L.: Healing of human periodontal tissues following surgical detachment from non-vital teeth. *J Periodontol* 28: 222, 1957.
37. Weinberg, L. A.: Force distribution in splinted anterior teeth. *Oral Surg,* 10:484, 1957.
38. Bass, C. C.: An effective method of personal oral hygiene. *J La State Med Soc, 106:* 100, 1954.
39. Arnim, S. S.: Microcosms of the human mouth. *J Tenn Dent Assoc,* 39:3, 1959.
40. Turetsky, S., Renstrup, G., and Glickman, I.:

Histologic and histochemical observations regarding early calculus formation in children and adults. *J Periodontol, 32:*7, 1961.
41. Massler, M.: Personal communication.
42. Ash, M. M., Gitlin, B. N., and Smith, W. A.: Correlation between plaque and gingivitis. *J Periodontol, 35:*424, 1964.
43. Graf, H.: Occlusal tooth contact patterns in mastication. *J Prosthet Dent, 13:*1055–66, 1963.

Chapter 14

Treatment Planning for Restorative Dentistry

WILLIAM F. MALONE, RINERT J. GERHARD AND JAMES T. OZIMEK

DIAGNOSTIC AIDS

THERE ARE a number of diagnostic aids which are employed to enable the dentist to prepare a comprehensive treatment plan.

Radiographic Surveys

The purpose of these is to inform the dentist of what is absent rather than what is present (see Ch. 6). There are five types of surveys commonly employed:

1. Full-mouth periapical study with bite-wing radiographs (20 views).
2. A quadrant survey (7 to 10 views).
3. Bite wings x-rays (2 to 4 views).
4. A Panorex type survey.
5. Simple periapical views (2 views or more).

Radiographs are taken and reviewed for the purpose of facilitating the identification of any diagnostic problem. They also aid in the development of a proper sequence of treatment as related to present or impending emergency situations seen in the oral cavity. The most common errors in radiographic surveys are (a) mistaking normal radiopacities and radiolucencies, (b) the omission of radiographs and (c) the failure of the development of a logical sequence for reviewing all types of radiographs.

Diagnostic Casts

The preparation of diagnostic casts and their placement in an arbitrary centric jaw relationship is done to mimic functional relationships of the mandible to the maxilla. This procedure is usually accomplished to determine prematurities and other miscellaneous occlusal relationships. The diagnostic casts can be used for the following information:

1. To review the teeth and relationship to each other in their given arch position.
2. The interocclusal relationship of the mandible to the maxilla.
3. The relationship of the gingival tissues to the clinical portions of the crown.
4. Improper tooth contour due to fractured restorations and caries.
5. The location of occlusal prematurities during centric closure.
6. The determination of the most effective functional prosthesis and its anticipated esthetics as related to the patient's plane of occlusion (Fig. 14-1).
7. The duplication of the initial set of diagnostic casts will also aid in (a) patient education to demonstrate function and the anticipated cosmetic results, (b) the prefabrication of preformed temporary restorations when fixed prosthodontics is contemplated and (c) the making of custom trays for various types of impression techniques.

Diagnostic casts are invaluable to the dentist as they enable him to review the case while the patient is not present in the operatory. This will save precious chair

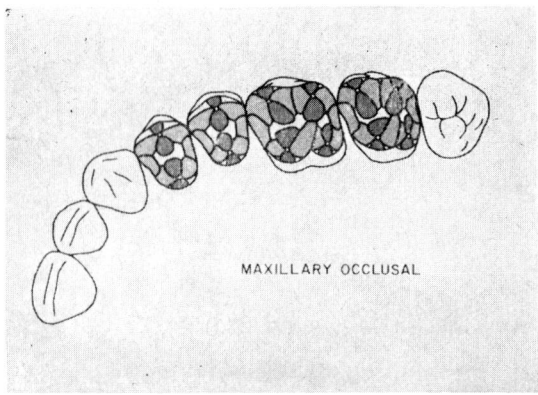

Figure 14-1. Programmed "wax-ups" on diagnostic casts are utilized to develop an ideal plane of occlusion on the upper arch while restoring the lower arch. This is a superior method of establishing an appropriate occlusion for a patient.

time and also demonstrate to the patient that forethought and organization preceded the actual implementation of the dental treatment. Diagnostic casts for study are usually prepared for cases of extensive restorative work, orthodontic treatment, occlusal discrepancies, the assessment of growth and development patterns and abnormal mineralization patterns. They are not indicated for every patient.

Photographs

Photographs (preferably the slide type) can be projected to illustrate to the patients the complexity of their dental problems. They can also illustrate deficiencies due to genetic influences or possibly the mode of treatment which will be employed. Photographs are also a superb modality for recording the progress of a patient's treatment, whether it be for extensive restorative work, orthodontic treatment or possible corrective measures for facial dimension alterations. In addition, a photograph is a valuable means of keeping records for the purpose of illustrating to the patient his former appearance when some disapproval is expressed by him as to the final outcome of extensive work. These records are definitely a means of defending a dentist's approach to treatment if litigation should occur.

TREATMENT OF ROUTINE INTRAORAL PROBLEMS ON AN EMERGENCY BASIS

Restorative dentistry is predominantly concerned with the replacement of tooth structure; that is, fillings, crowns and, at times, bridges. However, the modern concept of restorative dentistry is not as restrictive as it has been in the past. The basic philosophy is concerned not only with obtaining and maintaining oral health but also preventing dental disease, dystrophies, dysfunctions and all disorders affecting the total patient.

Restorative dentistry includes the diagnosis, prevention and treatment of diseases, developmental defects or traumatic injury to the hard tissue of the entire dentition.

The following conditions necessitate restorative dentistry:

1. Destruction of tooth structure by the carious process.

2. Poor relationship or positioning of teeth. This condition may result from entrapment and impaction of food between the teeth, deterioration of the supporting structures and fracture of the teeth subjected to abnormal stresses. Improper restoration of teeth may also lead to bizarre relationships.

3. Abrasion and attrition (Fig. 14-2).

4. Erosion.

5. Developmental defects, such as hypoplasia or abnormal forms in general.

6. Fracture, due to trauma.

Treatment Planning for Restorative Dentistry

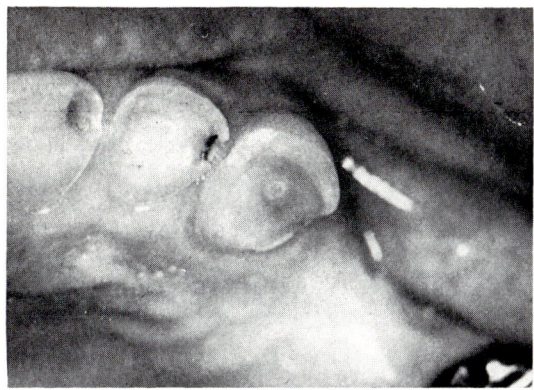

Figure 14-2. Abrasion of the anterior teeth resulting in exposure of the left canine. Cases of this nature are difficult to restore.

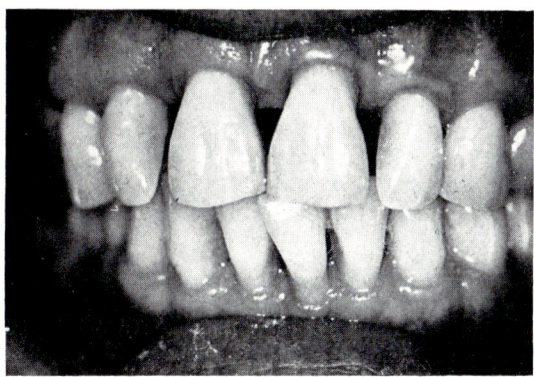

Figure 14-3. Cases in which anterior teeth have been treated by periodontal surgery are rarely esthetic. Prevention in the form of early analysis of cardinal symptoms is a more acceptable approach.

Soft Tissue Disorders

This is one type of emergency which can be drastically reduced by the recognition of insidious symptoms by the dentist. Frequently emergency treatment represents treatment at the terminal stage (Fig. 14-3). Alleviation of symptoms and palliative measures are indicated until a periodontist can institute effective long-term treatment.

Swelling in a pontic or abutment area of a bridge can be relieved by the reduction of redundant tissue and placement of a surgical pack. Equilibration may be required where soft tissue response reflects balancing side prematurities. Acute necrotizing gingivitis should be treated locally with gentle prophylaxis, saline rinses and peroxide treatment in addition to antibiotic therapy. The prognosis of future restorative work in these mouths is extremely poor. Therefore, imaginative prosthodontic procedures should be limited to patients who have a proven acceptable level of oral hygiene.

Carious Involvement

The conditions which usually require attention due to pulpitis are (a) carious invasion, (b) deep cavity preparation and (c) traumatic injury to the tooth itself.

A cresol derivative in combination with a zinc oxide and eugenol (ZOE) base is employed by some operators with a good deal of success. A type of steroid compound is also used, containing 1% soluble prednisolone, 24% solution of cresatin, 25% p-chlorophenol and 50% USP gum camphor. One theory as to the mode of action is that it prevents the liberation of lysosomes from the mast cells, thereby preventing dissolution of the undifferentiated mesenchymal tissue in the area or lysis of the odontoblastic cells. An indication for therapy is an impending acute pulpitis.

There is some question whether a single application of a corticosteroid is sufficient or if replenishment is necessary after approximately ten to fifteen days. The research on the success of this anti-inflammatory drug still remains somewhat obscure as duplication of results from one investigator to another leaves a good deal to be desired. The use of calcium hydroxide, ZOE and liners is always a more conservative approach.

One material that merits mention is the interim caries control medication by Caulk called "I.R.M.". This material when mixed to a puttylike consistency is a superb emergency medicament that will resist the destructive properties of the oral cavity for sufficient time to evaluate the affected tooth.

Trauma

The severity of the trauma and the age of the patient usually distinguish the manner of treatment to be employed, for example
1. Pulp capping (younger patients).
2. Pulpotomy (younger patients).
3. Endodontic treatment.
4. Extraction and debridement.
5. Replantation, etcetera.

The following treatment is usually followed in most of the above instances after a brief history of the trauma and the usual medical and dental history.
1. Give adequate local anesthesia.
2. Cleanse the entire area with saline solution concomitantly performing a digital evaluation.
3. Isolate the fractured tooth with rubber dam.
4. Place the indicated pulpal recovery agent:
a. *Pulp capping:* calcium hydroxide, a copal liner and a zinc oxide and eugenol dressing.
b. *Pulpotomy:* formocresol and ZOE.
c. *Pulpal extirpation* (large exposure): a eugenol cotton pellet placed with ZOE and protective cap.
5. Place a stainless steel bandage with a sedative cement within the limits of functional protrusive movements, which means it will be slightly shorter and more protrusive than the normal arch position. This is particularly important in the young patient as the canines have yet to assume their proper arch position.

If the tooth has been fractured beyond the limits of treatment or has been displaced to the point of endangering vital structures, remove it. In the case of avulsion an attempt should be made to place a sterile root canal treatment with gutta percha and sealer before replantation. Stabilization of these teeth can be accomplished by orthodontic or surgical intermaxillary fixation wire size 0.030 to 0.040. Acrylic material can be painted on the wire to further strengthen the improvised splint.

After a suitable period of time has elapsed, evaluation of a pulpal condition of the tooth should be made. If it is found to be deficient, initiate root canal therapy or remove it. When the tooth is asymptomatic, place an acrylic and cast gold coping transitional crown with a sedative-type cement used as a luting agent.

PRECISE TREATMENT PLANNING

Caries Control

Most cases can be handled in the following manner:
1. The use of diagnostic aids which are increased in refinement as the severity of the clinical situation increases.
2. Evaluation and prerestorative treatment of the supporting structures.
3. Occlusal relationships checked and equilibrated (Fig. 14-4).
4. Caries control with amalgam restorations (possible pin buildups) and endodontic treatment initiated concomitantly. Badly broken-down molars and canines have preference after alleviation of pain symptoms. Adaptic or other anterior restorative materials are used as a caries control material until crowns can be placed to enhance esthetics.
5. The placement of restorations or prostheses.

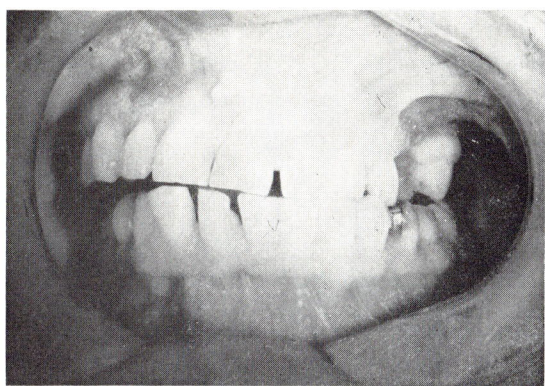

Figure 14-4. Left working mandibular relationship which illustrates group protection. Note that the right balancing side is not in contact.

The following sequence can be employed in the majority of cases with widely divergent time schedules after the caries control program has been completed. One suggestion to the patient with a higher DMF rate is the placement of one crown on a lower molar to illustrate the rationale of maintaining the integrity of the dentition at a maximum level of efficiency. Other crowns will follow and the economic aspects of this type of dental care will not appear overwhelming.

Logical Sequence of Treatment

Rule #1—Develop a logical direction of treatment based upon the evaluation of pertinent diagnostic tools.

Rule #2—Treat the patient in an organized chronological sequence to implement a provisional diagnosis.

Rule #3—Develop a proper sequence of implementation based upon a patient's right to select the direction of treatment; implement the tentative treatment plan with flexibility so that alternate treatment plans may be adapted because of adverse clinical situations which may arise.

Treatment planning is most important. One such sequence can be described as follows:

I. *Patients with a full complement of teeth.*
   A. *Operative.*
      1. Prophylaxis.
      2. Restorative dentistry.
   B. *Operative and orthodontics.*
      1. Prophylaxis.
      2. Restorative dentistry.
      3. Orthodontic treatment.
   C. *Endodontics, operative and periodontics.*
      1. Initial scaling.
      2. Caries control procedures.
      3. Endodontics.
      4. Periodontics.
      5. Restorative dentistry.
   D. *Surgery, endodontics, periodontics, operative, fixed partial prosthodontics or removable partial prosthodontics.*
      1. Initial scaling.
      2. Surgery.
      3. Caries control procedures.
      4. Endodontics.
      5. Periodontics.
      6. Restorative dentistry.
      7. Fixed partial denture prosthodontics.
      8. Removable partial denture prosthodontics.
II. *Patients with a partial complement of teeth.*
   A. *Surgery, endodontics, operative, fixed and removable prosthodontics.*
      1. Initial scaling.
      2. Surgery.
      3. Caries control procedures.
      4. Endodontics.
      5. Restorative dentistry.
      6. Prosthodontics.
   B. *Surgery, endodontics, operative, fixed and removable prosthodontics where periodontics will occupy the major part of the operator's time.*
      1. Root planing.
      2. Surgery.
      3. Concomitant caries control and periodontal surgery.
      4. Endodontics.
      5. Periodontal prosthodontics.
   C. *Prosthodontics only.*

1. Fixed partial denture prosthodontics.
2. Removable partial denture prosthodontics.
3. Possibly implantology with fixed partial prosthodontics.
III. *Edentulous patients.*
   A. *Surgery and prosthodontics.*
      1. Surgery.
      2. Prosthodontics.
   B. *Prosthodontics only.*
      1. Prosthodontics.
      2. Implantology.
      3. Maxillofacial prosthodontics.

This categorization will aid in the determination of the final course in treatment and will be a guide during preliminary mouth examination.

Operative Dentistry

The diagnosis portion of operative dentistry usually is relegated to the selection of the type of restorative material to be used in a given patient. This is usually dependent upon (a) the age of the patient, (b) the DMF rate and profile of supporting tissues of the patient, (c) the dental education level of the patient (oral hygiene, etcetera), (d) the ability of the operator and familiarity with various methods of restoration and (e) the financial resources of the patient.

Amalgam restorations are the most widely used (and abused) type of restorative material. They are used extensively because of ease of manipulation, relative economy in comparison with other materials, adequate resistance to masticatory forces and possible insertion in relatively inaccessible areas; that is, in cervical caries or in the distal lingual surfaces of mandibular molars.

Anterior Restorative Materials

There have been continued attempts to develop an adequate restorative material which will be acceptable and still not be considered a semipermanent restoration. This is understandable because these materials have been notorious in their deficiencies:

1. The deleterious effects to pulpal vitality, either by low pH or caustic ingredients.
2. The fact that they are soluble in oral environments and discolor.
3. Lack of resistance to masticatory stresses.
4. Their esthetic deterioration; that is, in mouthbreathers.
5. Marginal percolation in some anterior restorations; that is, acrylics.
6. Poor finish of polished surfaces.

The ideal or even a somewhat acceptable material has yet to be perfected to the point that it will satisfy requirements of consideration for placement in the category of permanent restorative materials. When the presently available materials are used, however, the following is a necessity. They are usually indicated for esthetic reasons for less extensive lesions of the proximals of the anterior teeth or possibly the gingival areas. The following steps are necessary:

1. Minimal cavity preparation but adequate retention and resistance form.
2. Rubber dam isolation.
3. Adequate pulpal protection; that is, liners and bases commensurate with the dictates of the materials.
4. Full coverage if an incisal angle is involved before insufficient tooth structure becomes a problem.

Even with the use of pins, the anterior restorative materials available are usually inadequate for incisal restoration. Acrylics, which percolate excessively, are the only lasting restorative materials which withstand incisal forces of mastication.

Composite materials have shown the capabilities to eventually replace all metal restorations. This statement is not intended to be a generality but time will prove it valid. There are definite improvements which must be realized before these materials can be employed to greater advantages. One obvious problem is the lack of attention by the manufacturers to insure that all these materials are radiopaque. Another ever-present problem is the toxic qualities of the material. They are usually compared to silicate cements which were never acceptable. However, the composites apparently are proving more resistant to wear, less soluble in the oral environment and color stable. The incorporation of fluoride might assist in their acceptance as a caries control material.

Gold Restorations

It is not proposed to belabor the fact that cohesive gold is a superior form of restorative dentistry. Foil is a time-proven material. However, the manner in which it is taught requires a definite amount of review. To state that foil is an excellent restorative material for treatment in patients with cervical erosion and proximally in anterior incisors when a crown is being placed on an adjacent tooth is redundant. Indications for foil can be summarized in two categories; it should be

(a) placed *only* in mouths with proven superior hygiene or low DMF rates or (b) used to augment a treatment plan.

Cast gold procedures are used primarily to impart strength to the teeth that have lost sufficient structure to withstand normal forces of mastication. Additional advantages are excellent contact points and superior tissue tolerance. Inlays should *not* be placed in mouths with poor oral hygiene. Gold has little therapeutic value. Cast gold work has been made efficient due to improved cutting instruments and better impression materials. The cavity preparation design has undergone a distinct change. Because gold inlays are much stronger than amalgam restorations, they can be employed effectively terminating with a knife edge. A gingival bevel is also indicated as a finish line. A slight modified proximal slice can be employed which will not involve more dentinal tubules than with an ordinary butt joint finished inlay preparation. The finished bevel is in a "clear area" and easy to laminate (Fig. 14-5). Modified slices are usually indicated on all the molars and on the distal of the premolars with slight modification on the mesial proximal of the premolars to prevent a display of gold. The cementing media of an inlay should be regarded as a luting agent with some sealing properties but its adhesiveness should not be expected to retain the casting in the cavity.

There are many cavity preparations of diverse types available for varying clinical situations for particular patients. Unless these are known by the individual operator, it is impossible to make the most effective selection. Constant reference to texts, periodicals and review literature will acquaint him with the materials and preparations available. For example, the recent advent of cast gold pins (horizontal pins,

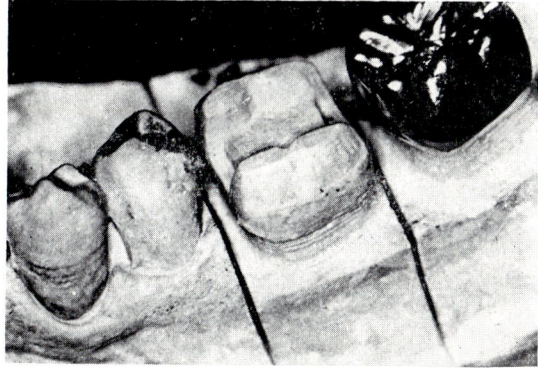

Figure 14-5. There are current treatment trends which have increased occlusal surface coverage. For example, MODBL castings on the mandibular molar.

vertical pins and nonparallel and parallel techniques) can definitely conserve tooth structure. A preparation which involves a considerable amount of dentinal tubules is not a conservative cavity. Hence, as stated before, a mesial-occlusal (MO) inlay which broadly exposes the axial, gingival and pulpal floors of the cavity in a moderate to relatively deep preparation places a tooth in jeopardy. An MO inlay does not cover that much surface of the tooth externally. A three-fourths crown preparation which covers more tooth surface has only two retentive grooves which may be the only two points where dentinal tubule involvement is necessary and more conservative.

It is logical that conservation of tooth structure and maintenance of gingival integrity is fundamental. One way of doing this is by the use of pins. Full coverage is used more extensively where the margins are tucked gently underneath the soft tissue; however, a good deal of dentinal tubules and predictable biological response is noted with the use of radical reduction of tooth structure. Full coverage may still be necessary in a high decayed, missing, and filled (DMF) rate patient. However, in a caries-resistant mouth with adequate periodontal health a less radical method that will still maintain the restorations is desirable. Therefore, occlusal rehabilitation does not necessarily depend solely upon full coverage as a retentive factor but utilizes cast pins to augment both conventional type preparations and strict pin ledge type preparations.

Pins: Indications and Contraindications

Indications:
1. Cosmetic considerations are of prime importance.
2. Relatively caries-free dentition.
3. As additional retention on abutment teeth with short coronal anatomy.
4. Splinting for periodontal cases. (Pins have never been proven superior to full or partial veneer crowns.)

Contraindications:
1. Patient with a high caries index.
2. Long span fixed prosthesis.
3. Teeth that have a short clinical crown.
4. Patients under twenty years of age.

Pins have caught the imagination of dentistry but have never enjoyed the extensive use which certain gifted clinicians predicted. One deterrent has been the lack of properly designed research to confirm their claims of superiority (for example, the effect of pins after placement in respect to stress, the pulpal damage and retentive properties). Another problem is the lack of uniformity when placing the pin holes. The diversification of instrumentation has also contributed to the confusion of the dentist. The Ney technique when employed as an indirect-direct method with a "template" for placement of predetermined retentive holes assists in eliminating an "air of bewilderment" regarding clinical and laboratory implementation.

It is our opinion that with reduced caries for the populace and refinement of present techniques, pins will enjoy comprehensive and expanded usage by the entire profession. The lack of universal acceptance of pin restorations illustrates a definite need for courses in academic institutions which will enhance imaginative methods such as pins. Pins are not new but the methods of implementation are.

Fixed Partial Dentures

Fixed prosthodontics is the ideal manner in which to restore a tooth or teeth which were lost because of unavoidable circumstances (Fig. 14-6). The more critical areas

Treatment Planning for Restorative Dentistry

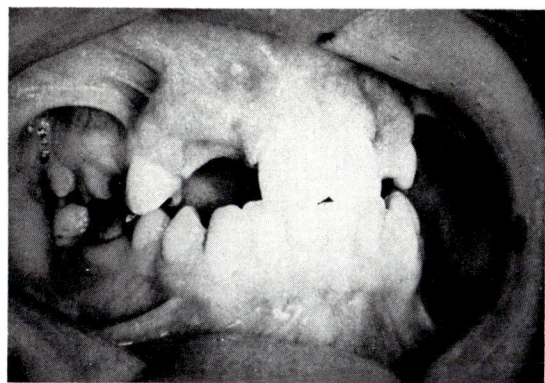

Figure 14-6. Esthetics remain the most reliable incentive for dental services. Dental education programs for patients that stress this premise are usually successful. The fixed partial denture is the most desirable.

of bridge construction are not the obvious problems of fabrication but rather careful planning before the preparation of the abutment teeth. The following reasons are the common causes of failure in fixed prosthodontics:

1. Disregard of Ante's law [1] and the subsequent excessive span coverage. (Ante's law is the average measurement of the square millimeters of the intended abutment of the lost teeth versus that of the intended abutment teeth. If the sum of the square millimeters of the periodontal ligaments of the lost teeth is comparable to the square millimeters of the intended abutments the prosthesis is a valid approach.)
Note: These rules can be amended if the long span bridge has a removable prosthesis as an antagonist.

2. Failure to anticipate occlusal forces. Disclusion should be used when any doubt of occlusal pattern exists. (This is the use of the canines to immediately disengage the dentition during lateral excursion) (Fig. 14-7, A, B).

3. Attempting to utilize fixed prosthodontics (molar mechanics) to rectify a gross skeletal discrepancy.

4. The use of inlays as retainers on abutment teeth. In our opinion they are contraindicated unless augmented with pin retention.

5. Selection of fixed prosthodontics for the splinting of severely involved periodontal teeth. Diagnostic indecision

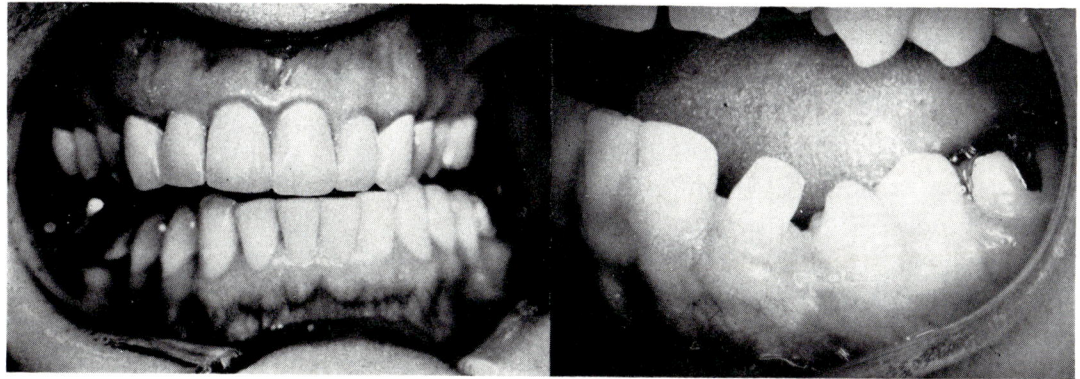

Figure 14-7. (A) A patient with a class II (Angle) relationship illustrating disclusion during left lateral mandibular excursions. The lingual slope of the canine is responsible for immediate Bennett movements. Care must be exercised when the lingual surface of the maxillary canine is developed. (B) A missing canine can result in esthetic problems, premature bone loss and ineffective mastication. Early orthodontic treatment is indicated with subsequent restorative splinting techniques.

merely reflects poorly upon the restorative dentist and the periodontist.

6. Inadequate embrasures, poor pontic design and lack of morphological contours. *Note:* Stein pontic design has been shown to possess superior tissue tolerance and electrosurgical reduction of tissue adjacent to the intended abutment extends the longevity of the prosthesis.

Gingival Termination

An academic dilemma in regard to gingival finish line has been the subject of many research papers because it is a substantial determinant for the longevity of a fixed prosthesis. It is the consideration of how and where the gingival marginal termination can be more appropriately placed. A discussion of this point is pertinent to the design of a prosthesis used to augment periodontal treatment. The following crucial factors are not only complex but will also require mature clinical judgment by the dentist.

1. *The DMF rate of the patient.* Usually the terminal gingival margin is tucked under the free margin of the gingival tissue. A test for acceptable gingival margin depth is gentle pressure from an air syringe that will retract the tissue and enable the operator to view the terminal margin. With a low DMF rate, an operator's latitude is much greater and the gingival margin can terminate slightly above the tissue. As a general rule, however, it is tucked gently underneath the soft tissue in the younger age groups where the caries susceptibility rate is known to be high.

2. *The age of the patient.* In younger patients, the margin should be placed under the free margin of the soft tissue. In older patients where recession of the soft tissue has taken place, the margins can be placed above the tissue unless there is the reduced root-crown ratio where the soft tissue remains high as in a younger individual. Gingival response is less predictable in this age group after various manipulations during restorative procedures.

3. *The present or projected oral hygiene.* Poor oral hygiene leaves little latitude in the termination of the margin. It is usually placed below the crest of the soft tissue except in geriatric fixed prosthodontics where the margin is placed above the tissue where the gingival crest height has a lower attachment.

4. *Periodontal cases.* Almost universally, it can be stated that all forms of retainers and pontics should be kept away from the tissue. The only exception to this rule is an anterior cosmetic compromise. It also follows that the gingival termination of the crown should follow the crest contour height of the tissue along the entire circumference of the tooth enabling the restoration to support the tissue and prevent lymphatic stagnation and eventual gingival cyanosis. Studies which attempt to adapt universal rules to all clinical situations are ludicrous.

Types of Occlusion

There are three main types of occlusion which can be noted upon examination of the patient. This is merely a guideline, not an inflexible listing, because a combination of these groups will be seen daily in dental practice.

1. *Balanced occlusion* usually refers to bilateral balance seen in complete denture service and bilaterally free and partial dentures. A certain segment of our populace with a natural dentition also have a bilaterally balanced occlusion. They are in the percentages of less than 12 percent and they are usually past the age of fifty and possess well-developed mandibular musculature. If these patients are asymptomatic and possess well-defined bone support, re-

storative work should assume the same occlusal pattern. Equilibration or occlusal treatment, whether it be at the pre, during or post restorative phase, has unparalleled pitfalls. This is due to the years of attrition (possibly abrasion) which assisted in developing the meticulous contact of the teeth during function.

2. *Canine protection* is associated with the younger patients (seventeen to twenty-six years) in the natural dentition. Bilateral canine rise is commonly seen in class II malocclusions, micrognathic mandibles and variations in vertical overlap and horizontal overjet of the anterior teeth. Any clinician who consistently has his patient move from centric closure position with his teeth in contact during routine examination will note the tremendous influence of the canine in immediate disengagement (immediate Bennett) of the dentition and continued influence as the canine controls (progressive Bennett) movement during further lateral excursions.

3. *Group protection* refers to the position and interdigitation of the buccal cusps of the mandibular arch meeting the buccal cusps of the maxillary arch during lateral protrusive excursions of the mandible. The contact on the working side involves the canine, premolars and sometimes the mesial buccal cusp of the upper molar. Balancing side contacts are usually nonexistent.

Common-Sense Occlusal Treatment

1. *Note the edentulous areas in the oral cavity.* There may be gross discrepancies in the plane of occlusion due to supereruption or migration of an antagonist. The tooth involved must be placed in proper arch position or removed before any prosthesis is fabricated.

2. *Remove malpositioned third molars.* They are generally poor abutments due to inconsistent root formation and lack of bone support. Poor oral hygiene is encouraged with their unpredictable arch position and they are commonly a cause of malocclusion.

3. *Keep the marginal ridges of the anticipated restorations commensurate with the remaining dentition if the plane of occlusion is acceptable.* If there is contact in a more retruded mandibular position (seen in about 90 percent of patients) before maximum intercuspation, the distal to mesial slide will be smooth and not cause periodontal destruction.

4. *Maintain the occlusal vertical dimension of the patient.* Violation of existing vertical dimension is the most common cause of failure of all extensive restorative work. If quadrant work is anticipated, posterior occlusal stops should be maintained so the original asymptomatic neuromusculature complex will not be jeopardized by a compulsive urge to complete treatment of a neglected oral cavity in a matter of weeks.

The following are two common ways to maintain the vertical dimension:

a. Restore all four second molars first and wait for an appropriate period of time before a full mouth approach, or leave the untouched second molars as a vertical occlusal reference.

b. Place restorations in alternate quadrants and wait until they feel "natural," for example, upper right quadrant followed by the lower left quadrant, lower right quadrant and finally anteriors maintaining, if possible, the sanctity of the canine.

5. *Use dental materials where they are indicated.* An ideal esthetic situation would result from porcelain jackets on the four maxillary incisors with porcelain fused to metal crowns (porcelain placed over the incisal edge of the canines and buccal surfaces) on the premolars and complete gold

on the molars. A complete rehabilitation with porcelain fused to metal crowns with all porcelain occlusal surfaces should be a rare restorative technique. A complete and immediate disengagement of posterior occlusion where the significance of Fischer's angle * is questionable could be one such occasion. A removable prosthesis with porcelain teeth as an antagonist is another indication.

Equilibration

There are two general methods a clinician can follow when equilibrating a dentition. One method starts with

1. Centric relation disharmony.
2. Nonfunctional prematurities (balancing side).
3. Functional prematurities (working side).
4. Nonfunctional inclines (including eccentric habits).
5. Correct posterior prematurities in protrusive.

The second method which is considered more applicable to the treatment of the natural dentition is accomplished in this order:

1. Correct incisal relationship during protrusive movements.
2. Review the canine relations from tip to tip to centric relation (working side to centric position). The idling side (balancing) should not be in contact while the working side is in the upper canine tip to lower canine tip position.
3. The opposite lateral excursion is then checked.
4. Centric relation is checked in the midmost, uppermost and distalmost mandibular position.

The rationale of the second method assumes a more practical nature when one must locate prematurities in a natural dentition. Most dentists are at a distinct disadvantage if they must determine a subtle prematurity with all the teeth in or near maximum intercuspation. The problem increases when the patient possesses a difference between maximum intercuspation and the most posterior retruded contact position during centric closure. The method of checking the lateral protrusive position first and gradually testing the occlusion toward centric relation occlusion is considered adequate for maintenance of supportive structures and is more comprehensive for the majority of dentists.

Methods of Occlusion Treatment

There are two principle methods utilized:

1. *Pankey-Mann-Schyler technique* which utilizes a horizontal component of mandibular freedom for complete oral treatment. This is accomplished with a Broadrick analyzer and incorporation of the theories of Monson's sphere, modified curve of Spee and Bonwill's triangle. It has strong reference to the sanctity of the canine function in particular and generally to the vertical and incisal guidance tables. The chief attraction of the method is the intellectual activity which precedes the reduction of teeth and a programmed hiatus between maxillary and mandibular treatment.

2. *Gnathological approach* (a poor term but a method of identification). This usually infers the incorporation of a refined manner of recording the terminal hinge axis as a primary premise and the coordinated placement of cusps by means of the drip-wax technique. The cuspal height and breadth is dictated primarily by the condylar movements. Both methods mentioned are applicable divergent concepts merely

---

* The angle shown between the protrusive movement and orbiting condyle in the midsaggital plane illustrated on the vertical recording plate of a pantagraphic tracing.

implying that an intellectual evaluation should proceed the placement of any restorative material. There should be a distinct visualization of how the final product will perform and appear. This is of paramount importance and cannot be underestimated.

Rehabilitation

Because of the advent of high-speed instrumentation, accurate impression techniques and increased comprehension of mandibular movements (because of the various gnathological approaches which seemingly mimic the three-dimensional behavior of the temporomandibular joint), oral rehabilitation has become a reality. The dentition of a particular patient can be restored to acceptable function.

The following are the Indications for Oral Rehabilitation:

1. Malposed teeth with a treatable periodontal condition.
2. Advanced abrasion causing loss of vertical dimension.
3. Temporomandibular joint disturbances caused at times by overclosure because of loss of teeth and occlusal disharmony.

Note: The symptoms of temporomandibular joint disturbances must be eliminated before any adequate treatment is initiated. Temporomandibular joint registration with an articulator from a patient with temporomandibular joint dysfunction will merely result in an abnormal reading not reliable enough to utilize as a treatment index (*see* p. 131).

4. A patient with large amalgam restorations with insufficient tooth structure to withstand the normal forces of mastication.
5. Acquired and hereditary deformities, such as amelogenesis imperfecta and dentinogenesis imperfecta (Fig. 14-8, A and B).
6. Esthetic demands of the patient.

Note the common causes of failure in oral rehabilitation:

1. Alterations of vertical dimension either beyond the limits of normal rest position or overclosure beyond the areas and position of functional efficiency.
2. Attempts to establish simultaneous contact of all teeth in all eccentric excursions of the mandible in each rehabilitation case, regardless of the dictates of the occlusion under consideration.
3. Employment of materials not suited for use in a particular case; for example, an all porcelain occlusal surface case which

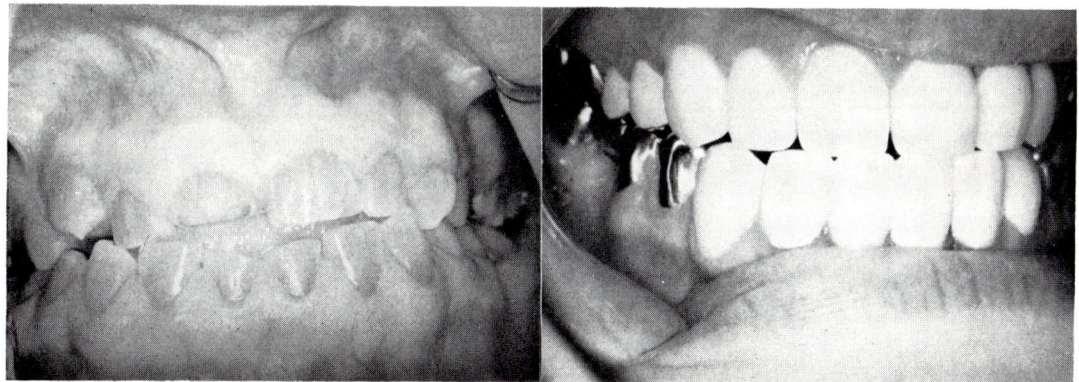

Figure 14-8. (A) Dentinogenesis imperfecta (opalescent dentine) which illustrates a true loss in vertical dimension in an 18-year-old female patient. (B) Treatment with restorative dentistry (two-year postoperatively).

is very difficult to equilibrate. Realization of the limitation of the restorative materials effective for a particular individual is necessary before initiating any treatment.

Note conditions, stated by Brecker,[2] that are known for their associated clinical difficulties when anticipating an oral rehabilitation in any given patient:

1. Occlusion of different levels.
2. Occlusion with an excessive vertical overlap.
3. Occlusion with a horizontal overlap (overjet).
4. Occlusion with a prognathous mandible.
5. Occlusion with mobile teeth.
6. Occlusion influenced by wear due to bruxism.
7. Occlusion with an anterior or posterior crossbite.
8. Occlusion with abnormal tongue and swallowing habits.
9. Occlusion treated previously.
10. Abnormal functional occlusion of convenience.

The conclusion is that the anatomical area of the oral cavity cannot be reduced to a simple entity but must be related to the patient's entire occlusion, his esthetics and comfort. One can remedy but seldom correct Mother Nature. The increments which spell a successful oral rehabilitation are scholarly diagnosis, logical sequence according to relative importance, built-in flexibility and meticulous implementation utilizing the first of these three steps as a guideline to the patient's needs.

Precision Attachments

There has been a subtle evolution in the approach to removable prosthodontics. More semiprecision attachments are being employed on abutment teeth by the dentist. The attachments are usually designed to afford maximum retention and maintain the proximal retentive guide plane.

There are some thoughts which should precede the construction of a prosthesis:

1. Will the patient accept the prosthesis and utilize it in the manner it was intended? What is the projected hygiene of the patient?
2. Should it be a fixed prosthesis? How long is the span?
3. What is the condition of the abutment teeth—caries, periodontal involvement or extensive old restorations?
4. What will be the design of the prosthesis?
5. What are the psychological, dental education and economical profiles of the patient?

Ideally the integrity of the anterior quadrants should be maintained to preserve esthetics and stabilize the posterior teeth. Resistance to lateral displacing forces are provided by rigid bracing components of the remaining teeth and supporting mucosa. Prefabricated attachments are available to join a removable prosthesis to a fixed restoration.

If the clinician is unaware of the existence of the various types of attachments, it is certain that he will never employ them. A dentist with an insatiable desire to remain current will not only be an asset to his patients but will enjoy the versatility of his profession.

Note the following classification of attachments for fixed removable prosthesis:

1. *Intracoronal attachments* (paralleled abutment preparations).
   a. Schatzmann.
   b. Ney-Chayes.
   c. Sterns .031, .028, .070.
   d. C & L.
2. *Extracoronal attachments* (nonparalleled abutment preparation).

a. Dalbo (vertical displacement).
  b. Chismani (expensive and versatile).
  c. Ceka (reasonable and selective).
  d. Scott (ridge lap modified).
3. *Stud attachments* (postcrown type with reduced crown-root ratio).
  a. Ceka (Fig. 14-9).
  b. Gerber.
  c. Dalbo.
4. *Bar attachments* (substructure with denture bases).
  a. Andrews bridge (lost alveolar bone).
  b. Baker bar (universal application and economical).
  c. Dolder bar (nonvital teeth).
  d. Boitel bar (screw bar retention).
  e. Ackerman (distal cams for esthetics).
5. *Auxiliary attachments.*
  a. Teleseal (periodontal cases).
  b. Telescope crowns with customed screws (tooth-supporting dentures).
  c. Ipsoclip.
  d. Frictional clip.

These attachments can take the dreariness out of partial dentures. Economical accommodations can be made so that a partial can be constructed and the additional cost of the attachment merely added to the service fee for a conventionally clasped partial.

Periodontal Prosthesis

This term is somewhat overdone but has captured the attention of the profession because of its "herodontic approach." Admittedly the integrity of the tissue remains an undeniable primary premise, but not to the point of subjugating all other disciplines. Most dentists would rather prevent the "piers at low tide look" than treat a patient who has had massive tissue removal to correct a periodontal problem. A number of these cases would possess better esthetics with a six tooth anterior fixed prosthesis with an improved incisal guidance than the use of a parallel horizontal pin splint augmented with nonparallel pins to ensure retention. The latter's prognosis is unreliable and the esthetics undesirable.

There are indications for pin splints, but not to the exclusion of common sense. The utilization of splinting to assist or complete periodontal therapy is not done as a substitute for inadequate occlusal treatment. Programmed short-time retention of poor abutment teeth is inappropriate. Careful appraisal of teeth with a reliable prognosis will lend stature to both disciplines. Exceptions to this rule can be rendered on an individual patient basis. Periodontal treatment without the supporting restorative work will fail. The trend in splinting teeth is a rational one but must be tempered with proper selection of the abutment teeth and removal of poorly supported teeth.

The use of telescopic crowns as a substructure and splints of porcelain fused to metal crowns or acrylic veneer crowns an-

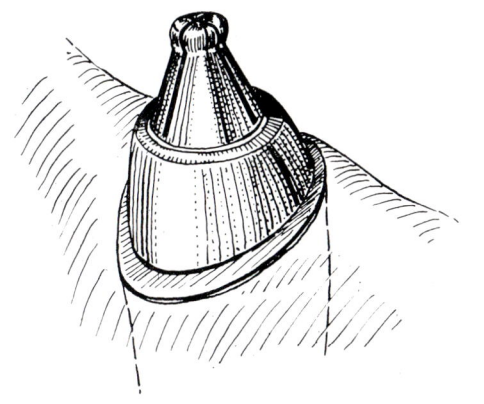

Figure 14-9. Precision substructure (Ceka attachment) for a tooth-supported denture. The tooth has been treated endodontically.

teriorly (full gold posteriorly for proper occlusal relationships) has shown a tremendous potential. The principal advantage is the reduced crown-root ratio. There are a few disadvantages to telescopic-type prosthodontics with periodontal patients.

1. The poor hygiene of the patients does not always improve. Cervical caries is a reality.
2. Impressions of periodontally treated teeth tear and distort.
3. The prognosis of the splints is not always predictable.
4. Additional expenses for refined restorative work restrict innovative procedures.
5. Maintenance of vertical dimension during substructure construction is difficult.

Note: There is a distinct difference in design of telescopic crowns for fixed and removable prosthodontics.

One way of treating a borderline case is the use of provisional or transitional splints which would assist the treatment team in determining the prognosis of a difficult case. The provisional splints are usually fabricated with gold cores and stabilizing bars with acrylic processed to them. An occlusal posterior stop of gold can be used to establish some form of occlusal tripodization with the margins terminating well above tissue.

Cases which show a great deal of difference in size between the maxilla and mandible (skeletal problems) or early loss of teeth with no replacement are only treated successfully by prevention.

Adult orthodontics with periodontal cases have a guarded prognosis. Only in cases of early tooth loss where teeth are moved discriminately into the bony defect on younger patients is there any measure of success. A generalized negative bone profile regardless of age will fail magnificently with minor tooth movement. Orthodontic treatment of cases with congenital defects, for example mineralization defects in combination with periodontics and restorative dentistry, can provide excellent clinical results.

Tooth-Supported Dentures and Retentive Clip Bar

Teeth previously considered inadequate for support because of extensive caries, poor periodontal prognosis and poor arch distribution or position can, at times, be rendered useful.[3] The relative ease of tooth preparation and relatively short chair-time makes these procedures feasible (Fig. 14-10).

Innovative treatment is specifically indicated for a patient who demonstrates (a) excessive loss of supporting bone regardless of etiology; (b) a widely divergent maxillomandibular relationship; (c) unfavorable anatomical position of muscle attachments and a large tongue which would directly reduce the stability of a conventional prosthesis; (d) anticipated lack of psychological adaptation to the acceptance of conventional complete denture service, for

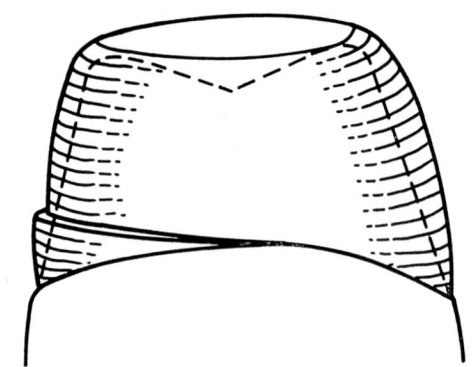

Figure 14-10. Telescopic crowns for tooth-supported dentures. This type of telescopic crown differs from the telescopic crown used in fixed prosthodontics.

example, a patient with a history of poor partial denture adaptation; (e) history of poor tissue tolerance to normal occlusal forces; and (f) a systemic condition in which extractions would present a risk to the patient.

There are two main contraindications to these forms of treatment: (a) systemic or psychological complications which contraindicate any restorative treatment and (b) patient disapproval of the treatment plan for economic reasons.

After the usual diagnostic aids have been reviewed and the course and sequence of treatment decided by the dentist, the patient must be informed of the advantage of salvaging the remaining teeth. This is not difficult for the construction of a lower stabilizing bar where the increased cost is minimal, but to save multiple teeth with poor prognosis at a definite increase in financial expenditure requires patient education. This is particularly true if the patient has had a functional retentive upper denture. These patients project this retentive quality of the upper denture to the anticipated lower denture.

One advantage for patients when using tooth-supported dentures with telescopic crowns is the flexibility incorporated in the event that a supporting tooth is lost. Another factor which patients appreciate is the preservation of the residual ridge. Most patients are willing to endure any reasonable procedure which will prevent insidious bone loss. Most patients are also receptive to the rationale that the prosthesis will be more stable than conventional restorative treatments. A large number of the teeth used to support lower dentures need endodontic, periodontic and restorative treatment which makes the approach involved. A reduced crown-root ratio is necessary to ensure a measure of predictable success.

Technical Implementation

All teeth to be used for any additional support should be evaluated periodontally and their vitality preserved, if possible. The sole exception to the preservation of vitality is the intentional reduction of crown-root ratio which lowers the fulcrum on a given tooth and commonly necessitates devitalization of a given tooth. A dowel, gold core and amalgam pins or combination of these can be utilized to connect the coronal and radicular portion of the tooth before preparation. Preparation of the coronal portion is performed in the usual manner utilizing a knife-edge gingival termination. Adequate gingival dilation is necessary before impression materials are used. Electrosurgery is a superior modality to accomplish this, due to the accessibility of the electrode points.

Occasionally the only remaining teeth with adequate bone support are two lower vital canines (Fig. 14-11, A and B). A stabilizing clip bar with distal cams can be employed if the antagonist is a complete denture. Maximum esthetics can be realized with this design. The affluence of the enlarged middle class is demanding more service and more imaginative means to save their existing dentition. Patients who earlier in life had clinical conditions that dictated orthodontics, endodontics and periodontic treatment but were unable to undertake treatment are now presenting themselves for belated treatment of complex restorative problems. The remaining dentition is far from desirable but is receptive to treatment when the dentist engages in an innovative approach to treatment with the patient's permission. Clip bars can also be employed in combination with Ceka, Dalbo, Thompson attachments and other more imaginative retentive devices which preserve the basal bone. Dolder bars

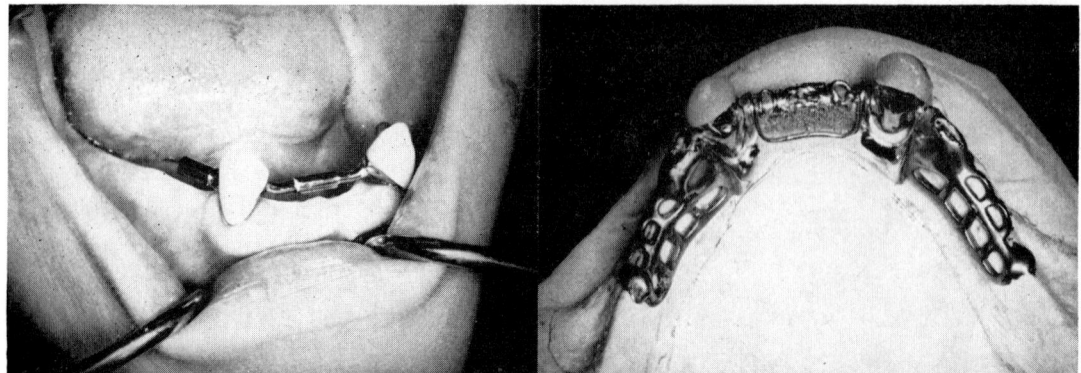

Figure 14-11. (A) A clip bar attachment to stabilize the mandibular canines. The internal clip can be processed directly to the denture base. (B) The metal framework for the superstructure of a clip bar attachment. This refinement is required when additional support is required.

are another form of clip bar with the abutment teeth usually having been treated endodontically.

Implantology

The profession has turned its head away from this field far too long. The improved technics have made this procedure worthy of consideration. There are obvious problems:

1. The people who need implants have insufficient bone to support an implant.
2. The oral cavity is less than ideal for maintaining an area free of epithelial invagination.
3. Implantology has been performed and insufficient attention was given to the manner in which the superstructure was fabricated.

The indications for implants are diverse but the contraindications are more apparent:

1. Systemic disease; for example, collagen disturbances.
2. Insufficient bone to support implants.
3. Anatomical limitations.
4. Patients who lack education and economic resources.
5. Psychologically unfit patients.

Classification according to tooth distribution:

1. Fully edentulous areas.
2. Bilaterally free-end edentulous areas.
3. Unilateral free-end.
4. Relay type for the use of a pier between long span abutments.
5. Fixation and transfixation of periodontally involved teeth.

The first category is more dramatic but the remaining groups approach the more ideal restorative clinical situation. The following are the types of implants employed:

1. Blade implants-intrabony.
2. Tripod pin-intrabony (Scialom).
3. Screw pin-endosseous.
4. Mattress type-subperiosteal (Chercheue).
5. Polymer (Hobish).
6. Intramucosal inserts.
7. Transosseous.
8. Endosseous endodontic stabilizer.
9. Ramus implant.

The blade implants have shown the most versatile and rational results. However, it must be understood the objective of the dental profession is to maintain a healthy dentition. It is futile to expend 150 hours of treatment and not spend fifteen minutes to inform the patient of improved methods of oral hygiene. A natural trend is towards less removable prosthodontics if we are to realize the anticipated effect of an efficient preventive dentistry program.

REFERENCES

1. Ante, I. H.: The fundamental principles, design and construction of fixed and partial prosthesis. *J Mich State Dent Soc,* 17:187, 1935.
2. Brecker, S. C.: Practical oral rehabilitation. *J Pros Dent,* Nov.–Dec., 1959, p. 1001.
3. Malone, W. F., Gerhard, R. J., Ensing, H., Morganelli Joseph L.: Imaginative prosthodontics. *J Am Acad Gen Dent,* June, 1970, p. 23.

Selected Reading

1. Preiskel, H. W.: *Precision Attachment in Dentistry.* St. Louis, Mosby, 1968.
2. Myers, G. E.: *Textbook of Crown and Bridge Prosthodontics.* St. Louis, Mosby, 1969.
3. Kerr, D. A., Ash, M. A., and Millard, H. D.: *Oral Diagnosis,* 2nd ed. St. Louis, Mosby, 1965.
4. Tocchini, J. J.: *Restorative Dentistry.* New York, McGraw-Hill, 1967.
5. Tylman, S. D.: *Theory and Practice of Crown and Bridge Prosthodontics.* St. Louis, Mosby, 1970.
6. Skinner, E. W., and Phillips, R. W.: *The Science of Dental Materials.* Philadelphia, W. B. Saunders, 1967.
7. Wilson, W. H., and Lang, R. L.: *Practical Crown and Bridge Prosthodontics.* New York, McGraw-Hill, 1962.
8. Bassett, R. W., Ingraham, R., and Koser, R.: *An Atlas of Cast Gold Procedures.* Los Angeles, Uni-Tro College Press, 1964.
9. Linkow, L., and Chercheue, R.: *Theories and Techniques of Oral Implantology.* St. Louis, Mosby, 1970, vols. I and II.
10. Oringer, M. J.: *Electrosurgery in Denistry.* Philadelphia, W. B. Saunders, 1962.
11. McElroy, D. L., and Malone, W. F.: *Handbook of Oral Diagnosis and Treatment Planning.* Baltimore, Williams & Wilkins, 1969.
12. Schultz, L. C., Charbeneau, L. C., and Doerr, R. E.: *Operative Dentistry.* Philadelphia, Lea & Febiger, 1966.
13. Sturdevant, C. M., Barton, R. E., and Brauer, J. C.: *The Art and Science of Operative Dentistry.* New York, McGraw-Hill, 1968.
14. Gilmore, H. W.: *Operative Dentistry.* St. Louis, Mosby, 1969.
15. Huffman, R.: *Procedures of Occlusal Treatment—A Teaching Atlas of Oral Morphology.* Anaheim, Denar Corporation, 1969.

Chapter 15

Endodontic Diagnosis and Treatment Planning

EDWARD E. BEVERIDGE [*]

DECISIONS OF DIAGNOSIS

For much too long a period of time, and in too many minds, diagnosis has been thought of as a passive, "once only" hurdle to surmount before the dentist can "get in and get to work." In essence, however, diagnosis should be an active, continual process executed with enthusiasm, curiosity and the greatest degree of thoroughness and skill.

Hopefully, the goal of every dentist is to achieve and maintain optimal dental health for his patient. The fulfillment of this objective is best determined by the positive affirmation of a number of critical questions. This systematic sequential questioning and answering can appropriately be thought of as the *decisions of diagnosis*. Following this must be the planning, sequencing, pricing and arranging of the agreed upon treatment (treatment planning). Treatment is begun, progress evaluated, altered, if necessary, and ultimately completed. *The process of maintenance and continual reappraisal (diagnosis) should be perpetual, periodic and performed with purpose!*

The decisions of diagnosis can be collated into three basic groups. These are the patient-related factors, the technical factors and the dentist-related factors. While for literary purposes we must list these various components of these factors in some order, it should be clearly evident that the measurement of these criteria are usually not necessarily observed in the same order. Regardless of the sequence of these decisions, however, complete and competent diagnosis from patient to patient or from time to time or from dentist to dentist demands that all of the criteria be evaluated.

Patient-Related Factors

The patient-related factors can be summated in six broad categories:

1. The general *systemic health* (to include extraoral and intraoral soft and hard tissue diseases not related to teeth).

2. The *educational level*—an estimation of the patient's degree of desire and knowledge of the value of saving teeth.

3. The *psychological status* of the patient; that is, will he be a management problem?

4. Does the patient have adequate *time* to enable him to have the necessary treatment completed?

5. Does he have adequate access to *financial resources* that enable him to obtain the desired treatment?

6. An assessment of the *patient's* acceptance of the dentist and his staff's *personality* and environment.

The history and extraoral examination, as they are generally taught and practiced, to a large extent aid in the answering of

[*] Deceased.

questions related to the general systemic health and the psychological assessment of the patient. Though certain elements of the extraoral examination such as lymphadenopathy, lacerations and extraoral fistula may be indicative of tooth-related problems, they are basically considered under the general systemic health. It is not within the scope of this chapter to deal in depth with all the criteria and procedures of history taking and extraoral examination. (See Chaps. 1 and 2). Those criteria directly relevant to pulpless teeth will be considered later in this chapter.

Technical Factors

The technical factors are basically tooth related and should be evaluated from a perspective based upon the relative value of their degree of importance in the retention of the tooth. Or, to look upon it in another way, what are the most limiting tooth-related factors which will predictably affect the retention of a tooth? The order of criteria strongly directs the sequence that one should follow as the intraoral examination is conducted and simultaneously correlated with radiographic interpretation.

These questions must, therefore, be answered affirmatively before one can progress to the next most limiting element. If the answer to any of the questions is negative, then generally the tooth should be extracted.

1. *Is the tooth strategic now or might it be in the future?* For example, a poorly aligned, partially erupted, short-rooted third molar need not be given any further consideration in its retention. Its fate is obvious.

2. *Is the periodontium healthy or through treatment could it be returned to a state of health that the patient could maintain?* Any tooth, whether it is to receive a simple plastic filling or complex cast restoration, whether it is to be orthodontically moved or serve as a bridge abutment, a retainer for a precision attachment partial or an abutment in an overdenture, depends upon a healthy attachment apparatus for its retention. This high priority criterion, therefore, demands the use of a periodontal probe and a mouth mirror in *every* intraoral examination, *except* those performed in *edentulous persons*. Figures 15-1, A and B, typify the type of periodontal pathosis that could be determined only by use of the periodontal probe and might otherwise be interpreted as a periapical lesion.

3. *Is the tooth free of a vertical fracture?* Though no valid clinical research findings are available either pro or con, it is the experience of most that a vertical fracture of a single-rooted tooth which extends the length of the root ends in the extraction of the tooth because of the ultimate development of a chronic, untreatable, unmaintainable periodontal defect. In multirooted teeth, if a vertical fracture extends into the trifurcation or bifurcation, then consideration could be given to the possibility of hemisectioning.

4. *Is the tooth free from any other root defects?* This would include such things as anomalously short roots, internal or external resorption, perforations and horizontal fractures. The treatability of these conditions varies and will be considered later.

5. *Is the tooth restorable to function?* In most instances this question is easily and quickly answered. On occasion, the answer must be derived after investigation. (*See* #4 under TREATMENT OR DIAGNOSIS section.) In an increasing number of situations our traditional concept of function which required that clinical crowns be restored to full occlusion must be ardently reviewed in light of the success of tooth borne "overdentures" and root burial

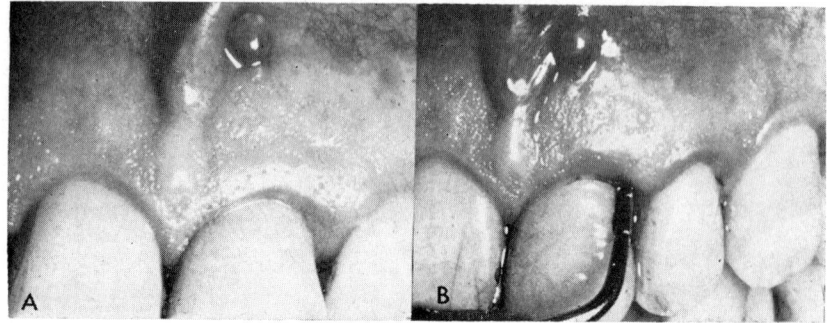

Figure 15-1. (A) Suspected periapical abscess because of fistula. (B) Periodontal lesion detected only by use of periodontal probe. The central incisor was vital.

techniques. As seen in Figure 15-2, the involved teeth are performing a highly functional role in the preservation of the alveolar process providing resistance to lateral displacement and contributing to retention of the denture.

6. *Is the pulp healthy or, if not, can the tooth be treated endodontically?* It may seem paradoxical that in an educational experience devoted to endodontics the health of the pulp or the likelihood of being able to treat a tooth endodontically is the least critical tooth-related factor. This is the case, however, because endodontic therapy is a highly predictable, successful (90 to 95 percent) form of treatment for the retention of a tooth.[1]

Dentist-Related Factors

The dentist related factors can be assessed in five categories:
The dentist must ask and answer the following questions of himself:

1. Is he *able* to perform the treatment indicated?

2. Does he *want* to perform that type of treatment?

3. Does he have an adequate amount of *time* in his schedule?

4. Are his *fees* adequate that he can afford to take the time to do the indicated treatment well?

5. Are his and his staff's *personalities* compatible with that of the patient?

These factors are self-explanatory and need no elaboration.

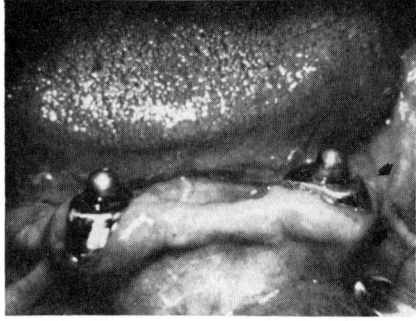

Figure 15-2. Two mandibular cuspids have been retained by endodontic therapy and restored with attachments that provide retention of a full lower denture. Note the retention of the alveolar process associated with the cuspids in contrast to the resorption of that in the area of the former premolars and molars.

TREATMENT OR DIAGNOSIS?

It is hoped that the reader will accept the contention that a complete and thorough diagnosis must include the best possible assessment of the above named factors and that these should be determined prior to the formulation of a meaningful treatment plan. This will markedly reduce the all too frequent compromises and alterations that must be made in treatment plans as one gets into treatment. A more complex case, or one which includes a greater number of variable tooth-, patient- or dentist-related factors demands that the dentist either derive a greater number of contingencies in his treatment plan, dependent upon the response to various steps of treatment, or more logically, that he answer as many of these questions as possible as *part of the diagnosis*. This suggests, therefore, that some acts of treatment actually be considered as acts of diagnosis. These would include an example in the various categories:

1. *Periodontal health.* If an acute periodontal abscess exists, one may have to incise, drain and currette and wait for healing of the area before an affirmative answer can be given to this question. At other times, a flap may need to be laid in order to assess the predictability of a return of the area to health or whether a root amputation or hemisection is indicated or feasible.

2. *The vertical fracture.* How can we tell the extent of the vertical fracture? Most often this can only be answered by the removal of caries, previous restorations and

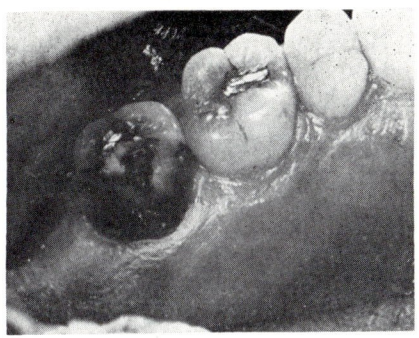

Figure 15-4. In this instance following hemisection it was concluded that periodontal health could not be maintained and that restoration would be either extremely difficult, or impossible.

the following out of a fracture line with either fissure burs or a diamond stone. As one follows one of these vertical fractures, he must continue to ask himself the other questions. Can I provide a final environment that the patient can maintain in good periodontal health? Secondly, can I place a restoration which will return the tooth to function? Thirdly, if the fracture involves the pulp, can I do the endodontic therapy? In multirooted teeth, particularly maxillary molars with the fracture running from mesial to distal, a hemisection can be considered. Figure 15-3 shows one instance where this approach was successful while Figure 15-4 exemplifies negative answers to the questions of a healthy environment and restorability.

3. *The root defects.* As an example, many cases of external resorption or perforations can be repaired if their location is accessible to repair through surgical procedures. This usually can only be answered by laying a flap and visualizing the defect (see Fig. 15-5, A and B).

4. *Can the tooth be restored?* This frequently can only be answered by the removal of previous restorations and caries while continually and affirmatively answering to one's satisfaction that he will be able to get a good impression of the finish

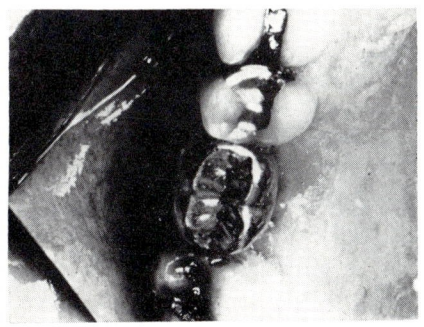

Figure 15-3. A maxillary first molar where hemisection was possible. The lingual root was removed following a vertical fracture into the trifurcation. (Reproduced by permission of John I. Ingle, D.D.S., and Lea & Febiger Company, from *Endodontics*, 1965.)

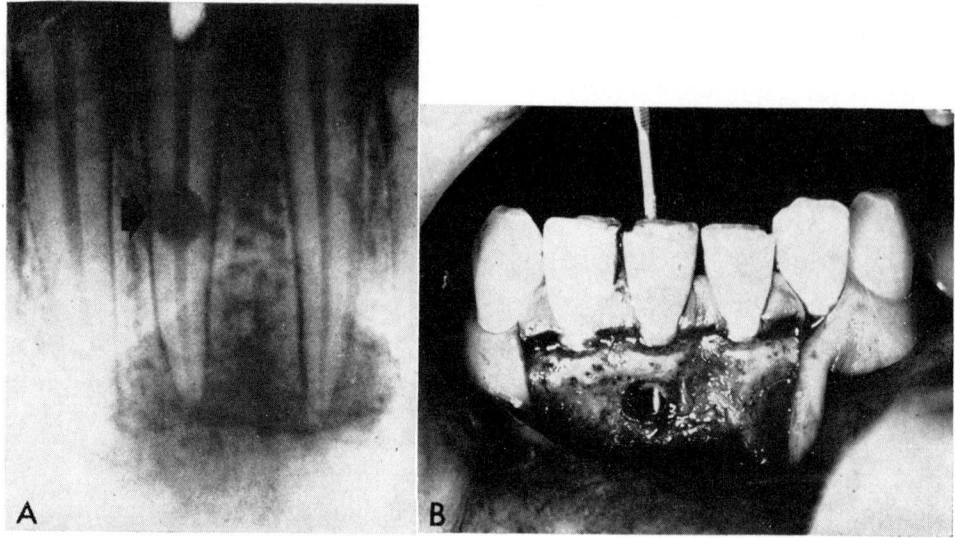

Figure 15-5. (A) Radiograph reveals resorption. (B) A flap has been laid and the defect visualized showing it to be repairable.

line and leave a periodontal environment which the patient will be able to maintain in good health.

5. *Can endodontic therapy be performed?* Many times the radiographic appearance of a tooth needing endodontic therapy is such that there is reasonable doubt that there is a patent, negotiable root canal. In these days of highly refined restorative procedures, oftentimes the fate of an entire case may depend upon the successful endodontic treatment of a single tooth. It is necessary to determine as part of the diagnosis prior to any treatment plan that this highly strategic tooth could be counted upon as a successful abutment. This would, therefore, demand that the tooth be opened and the canals negotiated.

In many communities of this country today there is cooperation between varied specialists to a degree that the American public has never before enjoyed. This cooperation is not without its disadvantages, however. An endodontist evaluating a tooth in question as to restorability may, for example, overestimate the capability of the referring restorative dentist. Therefore, the question of whether a tooth can be restored must properly, in this case, be answered by the professional who must restore the tooth. In other cases the ability to successfully treat a periodontal condition must be determined by the periodontist and whether a pulpless tooth can have the root canal filled must be answered by the endodontist.

SPECIFIC PROBLEMS RELATIVE TO THE PULPALLY OR PERIAPICALLY DISEASED TOOTH

It is the intent of this segment that the dentist upon completion will know which questions to *ask* during the taking of this history, what to *look* for during the examination, how to *conduct* testing procedures, and lastly, how to *correlate* these various findings. It is proposed not to devote much time and space to the diagnosis of what probably represents well over one-half of the problems arising from pulpal or periapical disease. The wide open cavity to the pulp, the draining fistula and the tooth, which is obviously fractured into the pulp chamber, are all sure giveaways, offering little challenge to diagnostic acumen. Therefore, the reader's attention will be directed to those criteria of history, examination and testing which are involved in the less readily diagnosable conditions relevant to pulpal and periapical disease.

Chronic Pulpitis

The most frequent condition confronting the general dentist and endodontist alike, which is difficult to diagnose, is chronic pulpitis. Dentistry, as a whole, has been guilty of allowing the public to suffer unnecessarily the pain of chronic pulpitis because of our inadequate diagnosis and decision-making. The "wait-and-see" lack of treatment in the sort of case shown in Figure 15-6 is greatly overused, often abused and is a sham for inadequate diagnostic aptitude. In this case, there is clearly chronic, apical, sclerosing osteitis associated with the mandibular first molar. This is the result of longstanding pulpitis.

The diagnosis of chronic diseases of the pulp can be extremely difficult. Seltzer and

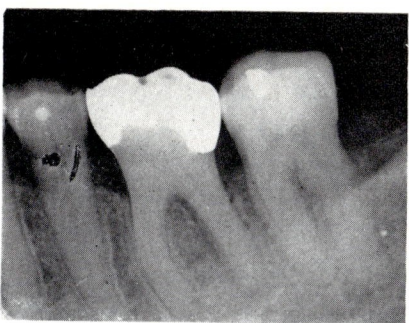

Figure 15-7. A mandibular first molar showing marked reduction in the diameter of the pulp canals due to the calcific degeneration as a component of chronic pulpitis.

Bender[2] have clearly shown that our present testing modalities are less than 30 percent accurate in predicting the actual histologic condition of the pulp. Lawson and Mitchell[3] have also shown that actual degenerative and inflammatory conditions can exist and be painless so it is small wonder that so many people suffer with undiagnosed and untreated pulpitis.

Chronic pulpitis is most often associated with the tooth which has had one or more restorations in it for some period of time. Often there is evidence or history of a pulp cap.

The pain is generally dull in nature, occasionally sharp, responsive often to extremes of heat and cold, and at times nagging to the point of keeping the patient awake at night. Radiographic examination generally does not reveal radiolucencies around the apices of the teeth but instead may show a condensing osteitis or increased radiopacity of the bone surrounding the apices. Another common finding associated with chronic pulpitis is the marked diminution of the diameter of the pulp canals (Fig. 15-7) as a result of calcific degeneration. Often comparison of the tooth in question with its contralateral fellow reveals this reduction in pulp canal radiolucency.

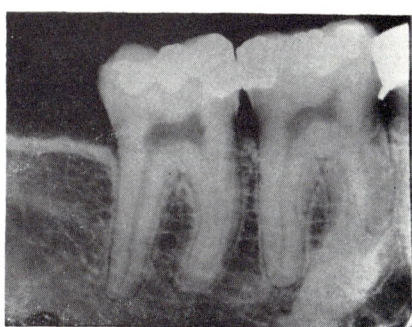

Figure 15-6. A mandibular first molar with a long-term history of pain demonstrating chronic pulpitis and resultant periapical osseous sclerosis. (Reproduced by permission of John I. Ingle, D.D.S., and Lea & Febiger Company, from *Endodontics*, 1965.)

With the advent of high-speed tooth reduction techniques and the increased utilization of full crown coverage, more and more cases of pulpitis are being seen and they are very difficult to diagnose because the full crown prevents the employment of the usual modalities of testing.

Vertical Fractures and Enamel Invagination

With the increasing age of our population and the increased retention of teeth by the profession, we are coming into an era where more people have more teeth at an older age. With this comes the price of an increasing number of teeth suffering from vertical fractures running from the crown into the root. The history of pain is often the only clue to the vertical fracture, being elicited by heat, cold, biting on objects and giving varied and unreliable results to testing. Unless the vertical fracture happens to be in the plane parallel with the central beam of an x-ray, radiographic diagnosis is generally negative.

A large number of the vertical fractures seem to be associated with overextended class I alloys and class I cast gold inlays where the underlying supportive dentine has been lost in the area of the supplemental grooves which cross over the proximal, marginal ridges of enamel. Cameron,[4]

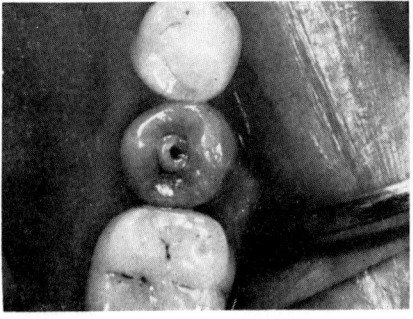

Figure 15-8. A Japanese male with occlusal enamel invagination of the mandibular second premolar.

Richey et al.[5] and others have presented excellent discussions dealing with the cracked-tooth syndrome for those who wish to pursue the subject in depth.

Lingual and occlusal enamel invaginations, particularly of maxillary lateral incisors and mandibular premolars, should always be considered when searching for the etiology of unexplained pulpal and periapcial disease. These are oftentimes found bilaterally and are relatively common amongst Orientals, Alaskan Indians and Western American Indians. (Fig. 15-8).

Occlusion

One of the key factors associated with teeth which either already have vertical fractures or are potential candidates is the occlusion. Thoughtful correction of exaggerated cusp to fossae relationships may frequently prevent fracture from taking place.

Occlusion also becomes of great concern in cases where a recent restoration has been placed with a centric prematurity or placed under excessive load during function or balance movements. The acute apical periodontitis from a tooth in hyperocclusion together with the insult of preparation and cementation of a new crown can often be confused with that of a tooth suffering pulpal disease. Misinterpretation could easily lead to needless endodontic therapy where only occlusal adjustment is required.

The new crown left in hyperocclusion on a recently completed endodontically treated tooth can also retard healing and once again only relieving the occlusal discrepancy will allow a periapical lesion to go ahead and heal normally.

Ingle[6] and Natkin and Ingle[7] clearly have given evidence that the occlusal trauma induced by bruxing can lead to periapical osteoporosis and even pulpal death. This has been seen not only in female adolescents but also in adult females and males as old as thirty-two years of age.

Malocclusion can be a primary factor in a fourth situation where radiographic interpretation suggests a periapical condition where as a result of the occlusion the problem is one of a periodontal nature. Figure 15-9, A and B, suggest a rather classical periapical lesion as the result of pulpal death, but careful evaluation, however, suggests that the fistula over the left central incisor is in keeping with the tentative impression formed from the radiograph. The astute observer, however, will note a severe occlusal relationship, the maxillary overbite being so severe that the four mandibular incisors are completely out of view when in centric relationship.

Figure 15-9, C, shows the lingual palatal tissues on the maxilla revealing an indentation in the palatal mucosa and gingival tissues made by the incisal edge of the mandibular incisal teeth. Without recognizing the compound problem in this case, one would not have placed a silver point through the gingival sulcus on the lingual aspect of the left central incisor as shown in Figure 15-9, D, which fully demonstrates that the etiology of this condition is the occlusion and that we are dealing with a periodontal abscess and not a periapical abscess. Pulp testing confirmed the diagnosis as it indicated the tooth to be vital.

Palpation

One of the important aspects of diagnosis is that of palpation, a step often neglected. Palpation should be done with the

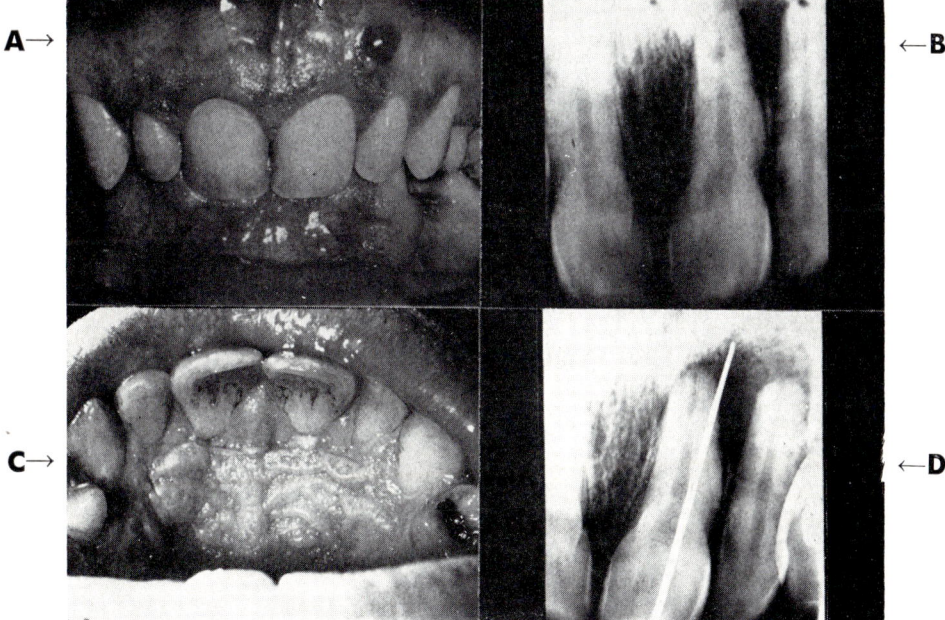

Figure 15-9. (A) Apparent typical fistula related to periapical lesion; note extreme overbite. (B) Radiograph suggesting periapical lesion associated with maxillary left central incisor. (C) Palatal view showing traumatized gingival tissue from mandibular incisors when in centric occlusion. (D) The radiograph demonstrates a silver point placed through gingival sulcus confirming periodontal lesion. Tooth tested vital. (Reproduced by permission of John I. Ingle, D.D.S., and Lea & Febiger Company, from *Endodontics*, 1965.)

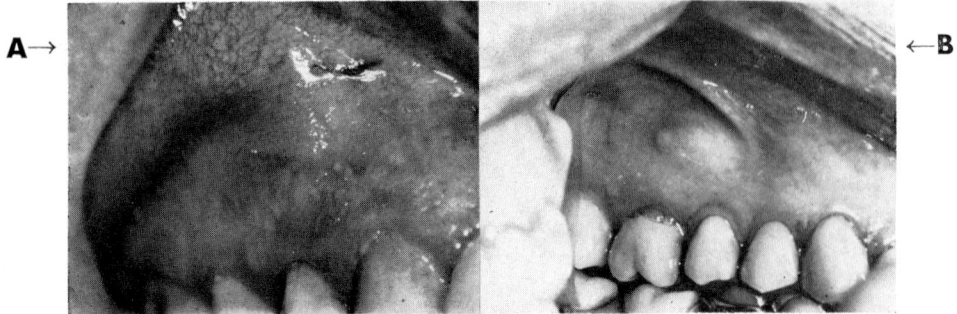

Figure 15-10. (A) This enlargement on palpation proved to be soft, painful and fluctuant. This was a swelling associated with an abscess. (B) This enlargement on palpation proved to be hard and painless and the overlying tissue was thin and blanched readily. The adjacent teeth were pain free and the vitality normal. It was thought that this was an exostosis.

index finger comparing bilateral structures or areas. Consistency of swelling or enlargement should be noted as to whether or not it is indurated, fluctuant, spongy, painful or pain free. Figure 15-10, A, demonstrates an instance where palpation revealed the area to be soft, fluctuant and painful. When the raised area seen in Figure 15-10, B, was palpated the lesion was hard and painless and the overlying tissue was thin and blanched easily. In collaboration with the history, testing and radiographic interpretation, palpation, therefore, confirmed that in Figure 15-10, A, the diagnosis was an acute apical abscess and Figure 15-10, B, was an exotosis similar to that which is often found lingual to mandibular premolars, torus mandibularis.

When using palpation, the relationship of the swelling to the alveolar process should be assessed; that is, whether or not the swelling seems superficial to and detached from the alveolar process or is apparently directly extended and attached to the alveolar process. This could be an important feature where tumors are present.

In patients when surgery is anticipated, palpation is valuable in estimating the relationship of the root and the overlying bone. This is of particular significance in flap design. Careful palpation can lead to recognition that a root end or root prominence has either very thin or even no bone covering it. Failure to recognize such a problem and then employing an inadequate or improper flap could lead to a dehiscence following surgery (Fig. 15-11).

Radiographic Interpretation

Space allocation does not permit an in depth study of radiographic interpretation as it applies to diagnosis and treatment planning of pulpal and periapical disease.

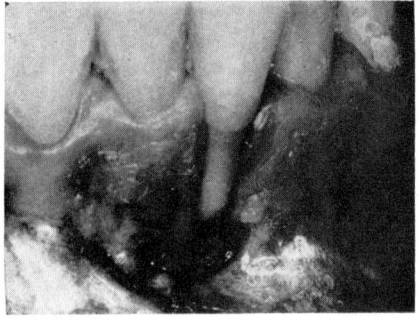

Figure 15-11. A mandibular central incisor which had a retrofilling reveals a dehiscence following poor flap design. (Reproduced by permission of John I. Ingle, D.D.S., and Lea & Febiger Company, from *Endodontics*, 1965.)

The entire subject is covered in Chapter 6.

The author would be remiss, however, not to include a number of conditions which can resemble periapical disease as a result of pulpal death. The successful and proper treatment for these conditions in these patients requires the employment of all of the available techniques of diagnosis and the greatest amount of concern and skill on the part of the clinician. For example, Figure 15-12 shows the early or "osteolytic" phase of a cementoma. Failure to diagnose this case properly could easily lead to unnecessary endodontic therapy or even to extraction. Figure 15-13 shows a

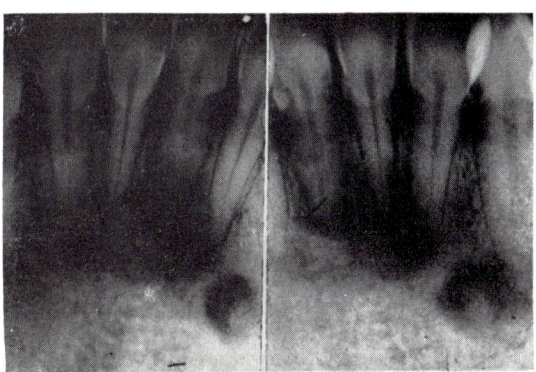

Figure 15-12. Periapical radiolucency which could be mistaken for periapical abscesses as a result of pulp death. Testing, however, showed this to be a first stage cementoma ("osteolytic" phase). (Reproduced by permission of Dr. Albert Abrams.)

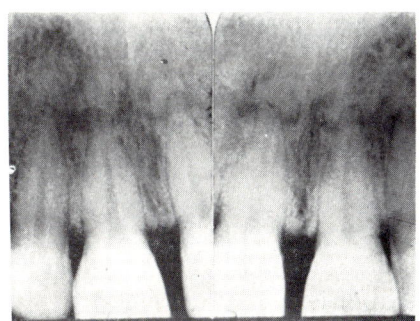

Figure 15-13. Radiographs of mature cementomas in 30-year-old female. (Reproduced by permission of Dr. Albert Abrams.)

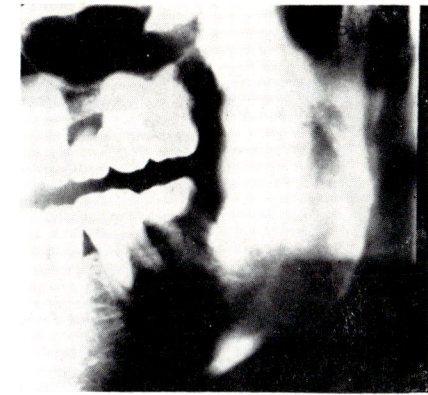

Figure 15-14. Metastatic renal carcinoma which could easily be mistaken for a cyst associated with the mandibular first molar. (Reproduced by permission of Dr. James Taylor and Dr. Albert Abrams.)

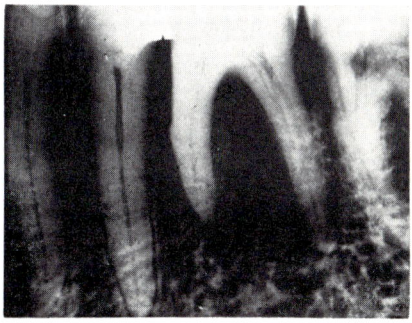

Figure 15-15. Squamous cell carcinoma which could easily be mistaken for a periapical or periodontal abscess. The teeth checked vital. (Reproduced by permission of Dr. Albert Abrams.)

mature cementoma, and again, failure to diagnose this condition could lead again either to unnecessary endodontic therapy or extraction. This is likely if the clinician were to rely heavily or entirely upon radiographic interpretation.

Follicular cysts and a host of neoplasms could well be overlooked if the suggested detailed examination is not carried out. Such an example is seen in Figure 15-14. The hasty, snap decision based on this single radiograph could lead one in the direction of endodontic therapy or perhaps ex-

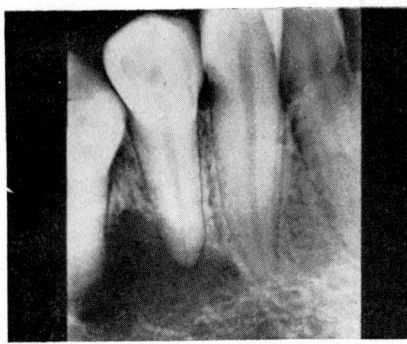

Figure 15-16. This periapical radiolucency resembles a periapical abscess but was diagnosed as a traumatic bone cyst of unknown etiology and does not require treatment. All teeth tested vital. (Reproduced by permission of Dr. John C. Wantulok.)

traction of the mandibular first molar depending upon the clinician's philosophy. Careful testing, examination and biopsy, however, showed this case to be a metastatic renal cell carcinoma; the tooth was vital. This situation demanded decisive treatment to treat the tumor, not time wasted in endodontic therapy or extraction and the usual waiting period for healing.

Another example in which it would be easy to make an error based purely on the radiograph is shown in Figure 15-15. Here a mandibular first molar with a somewhat unusual punched out lesion in the bifurcation would suggest that either periodontal or endodontic therapy, or both, should be instituted. However, careful testing and examination proved this tooth to be vital. A biopsy of the lesion showed a squamous cell carcinoma. Figure 15-16 is an example of a traumatic bone cyst. The teeth were vital and root canal therapy was not indicated.

PULP TESTING

The results of the interview and history are generally referred to as the *subjective findings;* the results of the patient's response to testing procedures is generally referred to as the *objective findings.* One should take great caution in avoiding the acceptance of subjective findings in lieu of objective test results. Granted, both must come from the patient, and thus, in the true sense, both are subjective. But as will be shown later, it is possible to at least crudely quantitate the patient's response to testing procedures. Though the patient's history is invaluable in establishing the diagnosis, the trap in accepting the patient's distinction of which tooth is causing the pain is that man lacks the accurate proprioceptive mechanisms to accurately discriminate the source of pain. This is borne out by the frequent occurrence of a patient suggesting, for example, that cold solutions elicit pain in the second mandibular molar when, in fact, testing and subsequent pulp removal showed that it was the first molar which was the offender, not the second. In this example, if one would have accepted the patient's discrimination, the wrong tooth could be entered, the pain problem would persist, and the patient would be faced with the treatment of two teeth instead of one.

On the other hand, the technology of our testing methods is still in the Dark Ages. Seltzer and Bender [2] have shown adequately that the relationship between test results and the actual histologic diagnosis of the pulp condition is less than 30 percent. One might ask then, Why use testing modalities at all? The best answer is that we have so little to go on in diagnosing pulpal and periapical disease that we must employ everything that we can to the best of our abilities.

One of the problems which makes the reliability of testing procedures and of subjective observations by the patient is that imposed by the patient's emotional and physical state. The person who has been in constant pain is certainly going to have a different threshold of pain than when he is well rested and free of pain. Therefore, test findings unquestionably will vary from one time to another and from one patient to another. This, then, puts in jeopardy the entire concept of "normal" pulp responses.

A second factor which confounds the *interpretation* of both subjective and objective findings is that of communication. What may be "++" to one patient at one time, may with the same stimulus actually produce a "+++" or "++++" reaction on the next visit. With a given stimulus, the hyperactive patient is apt to give a high reaction, whereas the stoic, placid individual may give no response at all. These problems suggest then a basic philosophical approach to the administering of test procedures and their interpretation.

Requisites of Testing

First, in any testing procedures, adequate controls must be utilized. If one is questioning the vitality, for example, of the maxillary cuspid, the best control to compare with would be a normal, uninvolved cuspid on the other side. Because of variations in bulk, thickness of the enamel, size of the pulp, length of pulp canals and so forth, the maxillary lateral incisor certainly is not a very good control tooth for a maxillary cuspid. Nor is a bicuspid a good control for a molar. Therefore, in all instances, the best control tooth is the normal contralateral tooth. Lacking this, a comparable tooth in the opposite arch is a reasonable control. For example, if the right maxillary first molar is missing, then a lower first molar would be a reasonable control for the questionable maxillary left first molar. Similarly, a lower cuspid is approximately equal in bulk, etcetera to the maxillary cuspid. As mentioned before, since man lacks the proprioceptive acuity to always distinguish between the adjoining teeth, the adjacent teeth should always be tested. Therefore, the minimum number of teeth which is acceptable to interpret responses to testing should be (a) the tooth in question, (b) the normal contralateral or opposing tooth and (c) the two adjacent teeth.

As nearly as possible, any test stimulation should be standardized either in terms of quantity of stimulus, length of time it is applied, the quality of stimulus, and hopefully, all three standards would be applied.

Because of the emotional and physical factors mentioned before, the variation of pain threshold, the relation to environment, even with the best controlled requisites of testing, the results can only be interpreted basically for that patient for that day. Unfortunately, there are no set standards of range of reaction to the vitalometer or to heat or to cold. These "normals" are personal and will vary from time to time within the same patient.

Modalities of Testing

The *electric vitalometer* is probably the most widely used and most easily interpreted method of testing presently available. A number of battery-operated types have been utilized in the last few years but it is the feeling of many that their constancy of stimulus is affected by the deterioration of the batteries. Many people still favor the cord operated vitalometer. The most reasonably reliable result from vitalometer testing is when no response is observed on all surfaces of the tooth in question on a number of repeated testings. This, invariably, is a reflection of a nonvital necrotic pulp. All other readings are relative as described earlier and should not be relied upon solely as the basis for diagnosis.

Cold and heat can be useful in pulp testing; however, the problem exists with both modalities of arriving at a standardized degree of stimulus. In the case of cold, the author prefers to utilize direct ethyl chloride spray using a *quantitation of time* of application and *duration of pain* felt by the patient. In the use of heat, the author also prefers to standardize the *length of time* taken for heating a spatula and the *length of time* it takes the patient to respond to pain and the *duration* of it. The technique of using heat and cold is given elsewhere in detail by this author.[8] This "crude" quantitation of heat and cold is useful particularly in the detection of the tooth with chronic pulpitis when the duration of perception of stimulus is greatly attenuated compared to "normal" contralateral and adjacent teeth.

Percussion is a useful modality in determining the presence of inflammation in the periodontal membrane space. There is a high degree of reliability in interpreting painful reaction to percussion as being an extension of the disease process influencing the periodontal membrane space. Caution must be exercised, however, as this could be due to no more than a new crown or filling in hyperocclusion.

The *test cavity* can, on occasions, be employed, particularly in instances where full crown restorations make the employment of the other modalities impractical or impossible. It is done without local anesthetic and the perception of pain by the patient upon entering the dentine is suggestive that the tooth possesses some degree of vitality.

The *anesthetic test* employs the injection of local anesthetic solutions and is particularly useful in cases of referred pain. Where pain is thought to be present in the maxillary arch but the dentist suspects it is a lower tooth, selective use of anesthetic in the maxilla, which does not eliminate the pain, then strongly confirms that the etiology is lying in the mandibular segment.

Recent research by Howell, Duell and Mullaney[9] and also Kopel and Crissey[10] suggests that the use of *thermographic crystals* may be useful in identifying a tooth with a nonvital pulp. However, Goldberg[11] has demonstrated relatively similar temperatures on the labial surfaces of vital teeth as compared to nonvital teeth. This whole area of measurement of temperature as the reflection of pulp vitality is one of the new horizons which, hopefully, will lead to more sophisticated diagnostic tools.

Interpretation

The interpretation of the hundreds of combinations of test results along with findings from history and examination would be beyond the scope of this chapter. Excellent selections can be found elsewhere in the standard endodontic textbooks.[1] The one aspect of interpretation that bears stressing here is that in youngsters innervation apparently has not developed in the normal tooth up to the age of approximately twelve years, and therefore, they do not respond in "normal" fashion to the vitalometer, heat and cold. In fact, experience shows that children who have suffered no traumatic injuries, no caries, etcetera, do not perceive any discomfort to these modalities of testing. This makes the diagnosis of pulp conditions in teeth of youngsters up to the age of twelve to fourteen extremely difficult and strong reliance must, therefore, be placed on radiographic interpretation, color of the crown, presence of fistula, etcetera.

THE INTERRELATIONSHIP OF PULPAL, PERIAPICAL AND SYSTEMIC DISEASES

Fundamental to the success of any service profession is a group of basic attitudes and concepts. Following is a partial list which might be considered "core" to dentistry as a whole and endodontics in particular.

Attitudes and Concepts of Endodontic Therapy

1. A full complement of natural teeth with adequate supportive structures is a superior mechanism of oral physiological function and emotional oral image.

2. With increasing life expectancy, more people will have increased need for lasting, efficient physiological oral systems.

3. Each tooth lost places an increased share of masticatory load on the remaining teeth.

4. There is a high degree of expectancy that any edentulous person will be a dental cripple to some degree or another.

5. In teeth which have adequate root length development, the pulp is not essential for the maintenance of the tooth as a functional member of the masticatory organ. Well-treated pulpless teeth, properly restored, have a life expectancy equal to teeth that are not pulpless.

6. With rare exceptions, general systemic health is not a limiting factor in the performance and expected success of endodontic therapy.

7. Pulpless teeth that have received adequate endodontic therapy are *not* foci of infection.

8. The age of the patient is not a limiting factor in the success of endodontic therapy.

9. The number of pulpless teeth in a given person is not a limiting factor in the success of endodontic therapy. There is no limit to the number of pulpless teeth that can be treated for a patient.

10. Because of basic psychological and physiological needs and improved public dental health education, an ever-increasing segment of the public desires and demands the saving of the natural teeth.

With these basic attitudes and concepts as a background and with all tooth-related factors being favorable to support the endodontic therapy and retention of the tooth, there is little to favor the extraction of a tooth where some medical problem exists with three exceptions. Whether to extract or retain, with these exceptions, then should be based upon the other patient-related and the dentist-related factors.

As a general rule, when a patient is afflicted with some systemic condition, the extraction of a tooth, compared with endodontic therapy, is more traumatic, both physiologically and psychologically.

The three unequivocal conditions which demand extraction in favor over endodontic therapy are (a) where teeth are associated with a neoplasm which requires radical resection (b) where an avulsed tooth is in the fracture line of the mandible or maxilla and (c) the nonvital tooth, in the line of fracture of the maxilla or mandible.

As in all things involving mankind, there exists a "gray zone." The literature up to this time tends to favor the extraction of any teeth which will be within an area receiving radiation therapy. The supporters of this philosophy contend that this lessens the likelihood of osteoradionecrosis and subsequent "radiation caries." However, on a physiologic basis, it would seem logical that if enough time were available to allow healing to take place following the endodontic therapy, that teeth so treated would remain in health following radiation therapy. Certainly following radiation therapy the exposed area has been amply demonstrated to possess decreased ability to repair.

TREATMENT PLANNING COMPLICATIONS DUE TO SYSTEMIC CONDITIONS

State of Fatigue

Perhaps the most frequently encountered complication is that of the fatigued patient who has been in intense pain, running a fever and suffering loss of sleep for a number of days and who exhibits malaise. In this condition he is usually not capable of making rational, value judgments, and treatment planning and treatment should be limited to getting the patient out of his painful and fatigued state. This should always involve, where identifiable, opening the involved tooth, placing medication and putting the patient on analgesic and antibiotic therapy as indicated. Usually, with the relief of pain derived from the local anesthesia and therapy, and as a result of his fatigue, he is then able to get some sleep and on the next visit is in a more rational frame of mind to make good, decisive judgments as to his further treatment.

Psychological Complications

Another frequently encountered complication is the result of psychological disturbances. Probably the vast majority of patients seeking dental and particularly endodontic treatment present with a lesion of *fear*. To overcome their fear requires careful evaluation and prudent treatment planning and treatment. A wide range of treatment techniques are available to the astute clinician. They range from TLC (tender loving care), hypnosis, sedatives, tranquilizers, nitrous oxide-oxygen analgesia and in the most extreme cases, occasionally, general anesthesia.

Other psychological and neurological problems can be encountered in patients who are mentally retarded or suffering from cerebral palsy or epilepsy. Frequently, various forms of the above-mentioned adjunctive patient management solutions are required.

On rare occasions, patients who suffer from claustrophobia are encountered and the utilization of the rubber dam becomes a problem. Again, other modalities of treating this patient must be employed.

Drug Complications

An endodontist's or general practitioner's hands are frequently tied in the management of pain or infectious problems by the increasing number of patients who report either low tolerance or an allergic reaction to the wide variety of anesthetics, analgesics and antibiotics. Their complications run the gamut from simple gastritis to nausea, diarrhea, dizziness, rashes and of course, in the extreme, anaphylactic shock ending in death to such agents as penicillin. The ever broadening options available in drug therapy have been helpful in maneuvering around these idiosyncratic drug reactions, but it is suggested that in the face of positive history regarding the reactions to these drugs that close cooperation be maintained with the patient's physician.

A constant problem is the patient who presents with an alleged or proven allergic reaction to local anesthetic. Fortunately, for the patient who presents with a chronic apical periodontitis or necrotic pulp, most endodontic therapy can be completed painlessly without the necessity of relying upon local anesthetic. Where there is either acute or chronic pulpitis, however, and anesthesia is necessary for painless therapy, then the dentist must follow one of two courses. He must either undertake, preferably in cooperation with an allergist or other physician, skin testing to determine whether or not the alleged reaction to anesthetic is truly one that is allergic in nature or whether it is psychologic in nature. Oftentimes, people report having had "an allergic reaction" to Novocain® when in fact they suffered emotional shock. The other course of action is to elect a means of controlling the pain which negates the use of local anesthetic. This can be done through premedication with either sedatives or tranquilizers and the use of nitrous oxide-oxygen analgesia in some cases, and in others it may require an intravenous barbiturate or some type of general anesthetic.

The complications involved in the general anesthetic approach are obvious to the general practitioner, who is neither trained nor equipped to give general anesthesia. Oftentimes, the logistics of taking the patient to a hospital or a trained anesthetist or oral surgeon skilled in the use of these techniques is cumbersome. Regardless of the inconvenience, however, one should not undertake what could be a life-threatening use of the local anesthetic merely for his *own* convenience.

Patients on systemic corticosteroid therapy could well present a problem with an acute apical or pulpal condition. The management of the infection could be problematical and must be the dentist's responsibility and be shared with the physician who has prescribed the steroid therapy.

Pregnancy

It is suggested by most obstetricians and pediatricians that any extensive dental treatment be avoided during the first trimester of pregnancy. However, if a pregnant woman presents with a painful tooth during the first trimester, emergency treatment must be done. It is suggested that collaboration be established with the attending physician. Certainly, all elective surgical and conservative procedures should be withheld until well within the second or third semester.

Hormonal influences often affect healing capabilities during any portion of the pregnancy. Therefore, every effort should be made to treat pulpless teeth conservatively, delaying perhaps even avoiding surgery until postpartum.

All too often the new mother finds herself too busy to worry about dental work started while still pregnant. This has met with disastrous results in some cases. Proper cooperative timing and sequencing of treatment can avoid these catastrophes.

Diabetes

The diabetic patient was at one time thought to be a contraindication for having endodontic therapy done. Figure 15-17, A, shows the case of a 68-year-old woman at the time of completion of endodontic therapy. Prior to the time of therapy she had suffered a stroke, myocardial infarction and was uncontrolled in her diabetic condition. Figure 15-17, B, shows the complete healing following a two-year period.

In the case of the uncontrolled or marginally controlled diabetic, elective surgical procedures should be waived in favor of conservative, nonsurgical treatment. At least the conservative portion of the treatment can be carried out until such time as the patient's diabetic condition can be brought into control. In some acute pulpal or periapical conditions, it may be indicated to prophylactically place the patient

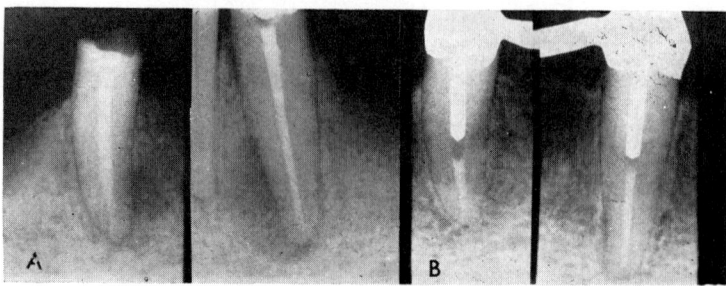

Figure 15-17. (A) Mandibular right and left cuspid at time of completion of endodontic therapy in 68-year-old female with uncontrolled diabetes, history of stroke and myocardial infarction. (B) Healing following two-year period in spite of a continued uncontrolled diabetes condition. Restorations support an overdenture.

on antibiotic therapy to aid in the control of potential infection.

Reduced Intermaxillary Opening

Patients presenting with problems which prevent them from presenting the dentist with a workable intermaxillary opening must often be treatment planned and treated differently from the normal. A patient may be in this condition as a result of trismus following injury of a ligament or muscle following an inferior alveolar nerve block or as a result of temporomandibular joint dysfunction from a variety of causes. Some patients may have suffered fractures of either the mandible or maxilla and are held by intermaxillary wiring. If this type of patient presents with an emergency pulpal or periapical problem, it may require modification of normal procedures in order to relieve the pain of that condition. As an example, where a patient has a limited intermaxillary opening, access could be made into the pulp chamber of a mandibular molar through the buccal surface. This is not recommended as a regular procedure but in the interest of saving the tooth and allaying pain until the patient attains the normal intermaxillary opening, this would be an acceptable procedure. The main effort of the dentist and oral surgeon or medical specialist involved should be directed towards maintaining comfort and treating the patient's problem which prevents the normal intermaxillary opening.

Blood Dyscrasias

Hemophilia presents a dangerous problem when pulpal or periapical disease occurs. Certainly, elective surgical procedures must be avoided. Close cooperation with a hematologist or other physician must be maintained. In this particular condition, endodontic therapy offers very reasonable advantage over extraction in that seldom is there massive bleeding involved with pulpectomy or normal endodontic procedures. Dealing as we are at the apical foramen with a small number of small arterioles and in such a confined area as the tooth and periapical structures, pressure and time are in our favor to avert any serious bleeding problem. On the other hand, the extraction of the same tooth would present a wide area of cortical bone and severed periodontal ligament vessels which present a difficult problem to obtain clotting in the case of hemophiliacs.

The patient with leukemia and his attendant bleeding and healing problems can be a challenge to all of the health profession. As in the situation of the hemophiliac, it often is desirable that the endodontic therapy be initiated if only to bring relief of pain in the terminal patient to avert the great problems that could be encountered following extraction.

Other Diseases Influencing Endodontic Treatment

Actinomycosis can inhibit normal healing following endodontic therapy or may even present a problem during the therapy with continuous weeping from the periapical tissues.[12] Following a reasonable period of time and after the assurance of thorough biomechanical cleaning and shaping, if the canal continues to weep, one should consider the possibility of this condition. Microscopic and microbiologic investigation of the exudate is indicated.

In patients with pemphigus, thoughtful consideration should be given before entertaining surgical procedures, particularly those which might be elective. Depending upon the degree and state of the condition at that time, the rubber dam may well accelerate the tissue slough.[13]

As in the declining leukemic patient, terminal cancer patients with pulpal or periapical pain of any type, the humane course of treatment may be that of pulp extirpation, medication and sedation rather than extraction. In these situations, completion of the root canal filling may not be necessary.

Conclusion

With the exception of the patient suffering with a neoplasm involving teeth or a fracture of the mandible or maxilla in which the teeth in the line of fracture are nonvital or avulsed, there are no systemic conditions where it is beneficial for the patient to have an extraction in preference to endodontic therapy. Endodontic therapy, on most occasions, is less traumatic, more physiological, demands less of recuperative and reparative powers of the body and is more beneficial to the patient psychologically.

RECORDS

Perhaps in rebellion to the voluminous paperwork required in the dental school and the Armed Forces, most practitioners are inept record keepers. It is indeed a shame that so many practitioners, having seen so many criteria in the evaluation of a patient's mouth, record so few of them. Certainly, it would be out of the question to make notes of all of the *normal* findings in the mouth; but, certainly, the presence or absence of certain *pathologic conditions* demand proper annotation on the records.

As practice associations, group practice and military installation clinics become larger and more men work cooperatively, the patient is apt to get short shrift, moving from one dentist to another if proper records have not been kept. Many is the time that the dentist has been handicapped when handling an emergency for his associate by not having adequate information relative to the condition of that patient prior to treatment. Many of these factors have definite bearing on the emergency treatment to be given at that time. How many malpractice suits have been lost by both physicians and dentists because they have not kept adequate records of the history, the examination and of the treatment given? An important point which was learned through listening to the patient or looking at him, or testing him, deserves to be recorded. Not only for the patient's benefit in the future treatment, particularly if an associate must step in, but also to protect the dentist in this era of increasing malpractice suits. Also, the third party intermediary financing agencies will continue to demand greater and greater amounts of record keeping.

PUTTING IT ALL TOGETHER

The biggest challenge facing dentists and dental education today is the sharpening and perfection of our collective diagnostic acumen. Diagnosis has been and always will be the most difficult phase of dental education. How to restore teeth, how to make bridges and dentures, and so forth, is the easy part. Some even propose that the dentist of the future will spend the majority of his time in diagnosis with skilled technicians taking over the technical duties of fillings, dentures, etcetera.

Putting it all together is a lifetime experience. Apparently, this is what somebody had in mind when they called it "the practice of dentistry." We are but given the simplest of tools to begin this practice when we leave our dental school. We must continue to learn. We must learn from our good and our bad experiences. We must be willing to share our difficult problems with men of various expertise.

In this chapter, an attempt has been made to suggest an orderly, systematic approach to this problem solving called "diagnosis and treatment planning." The challenge is here. A possible solution has been offered. Are you willing to accept the challenge and strive for perfection for the betterment of your patient, for the pride in yourself and for the advancement of our profession?

REFERENCES

1. Ingle, J. I.: *Endodontics*. Philadelphia, Lea & Febiger, 1965.
2. Seltzer, S., Bender, I. B., and Ziontz, M.: The dynamics of pulp inflammation: Correlations between diagnostic data and actual histologic findings in the pulp. *Oral Surg*, 16:846, 1963.
3. Lawson, B. F., and Mitchell, D.: Pharmacologic treatment of painful pulpitis. *Oral Surg*, 17:47, 1964.
4. Cameron, G.: The cracked tooth syndrome. *JADA*, 68:405, 1964.
5. Ritchey, B., Meldenhall, R., and Orban, B.: Pulpitis resulting from incomplete tooth fracture. *Oral Surg*, 10:665, 1957.
6. Ingle, J. I.: Alveolar osteoporosis and pulpal death associated with compulsive bruxism. *Oral Surg*, 13:1371, 1960.
7. Natkin, E., and Ingle, J. I.: A further report on alveolar osteoporosis and pulpal death associated with compulsive bruxism. *J Am Soc Periodont*, 1:260, 1963.
8. Goldman, H. M., Forrest, S. P., Byrd, B. L., McDonald, R. E., and Beveridge, E. E.: *Current Therapy in Dentistry*. St. Louis, Mosby, 1968, vol. 3.
9. Howell, R. N., Duell, R., and Mullaney, T.: The determination of pulp vitality by means of using thermographic cholesteric liquid. *Oral Surg*, 29:763, 1970.
10. Kopel, H. M., and Crissey, J.: Application of cholesteric liquid crystals in dental thermography, preliminary report. International Association for Dental Research. P. 51, 1970 (abstract).
11. Goldberg, M.: Temperature Measurement of Vital and Nonvital Incisors in Humans. M. S. Thesis, University of Washington, 1965.
12. Riley, D. P., and Howell, F. V.: Personal communication. 1970.
13. Shklar, G., and McCarthy, P. L.: The oral manifestations of benign mucous membrane pemphigus (mucous membrane pemphigoid). *Oral Surg*, 12:950, 1959.

Chapter 16

Case Presentation

WILLIAM F. MALONE, RINERT J. GERHARD AND JAMES T. OZIMEK

CASE PRESENTATION usually refers to the conference that takes place between the patient and his dentist concerning the number of appointments which will be necessary to complete treatment and the estimated cost. There is a variety of circumstances which affect each patient individually and which must be discussed. The methods of communication between patients will also vary and the amount of dental education must be assessed by the dentist in presenting the case to the patient. In too many instances, this presentation is performed in a hurried manner or omitted entirely in some cases where explanation would have saved the dentist future problems in communication, either to clarify economic problems or to estimate the final esthetic result of treatment. The tremendous variety of patients with esthetic problems and the obvious limitations of dental treatment must be related to the patient in a customized clear manner.

There are usually five principles of case presentation which should be rigidly adhered to:

1. *Obtain and evaluate the patient's awareness of the complexity of his dental problem.* Relate to the patient the benefit of treatment and the penalty of neglect of his clinical problems. Estimate and discuss freely the frequency of appointments and the manner in which the clinical problem will be solved and how. The frequency (time expenditure), the cost and how the treatment will be accomplished is what the patient will be interested in. Explain how the estimated cost of the treatment is arrived at and relate the usual fee for the anticipated services. Demonstrate the aim and the goals of your treatment in simple clear-cut terms and underscore the importance of the maintenance of the completed work.

2. *Flexibility in the treatment.* The dentist should convey to the patient in an honest manner a feeling of thoroughness or carefully executed treatment for the given clinical situation. However, in any treatment plan there are definite restrictions in the economic status of the patient which will demand a certain amount of imaginative thinking and flexibility.

One of the better ways of presenting the treatment plan would be by a demonstration with a series of examples illustrating the normal and abnormal and how it is commonly corrected. Illustrations with other patients' models is one manner in which to communicate with the patient in a visual manner. For example, prediagnostic and postdiagnostic casts and possibly 35-mm slides are projected so the patient can inquire as to costs, frequency and number of appointments needed to accomplish the proposed treatment. The patient can then determine whether it is applicable both to his clinical situation and economic status. For the success of any extensive restorative case, an imaginative approach such as precision attachments, implantology and periodontal prosthesis will to a great extent depend upon the dentist's ability to communicate to the patient. A lack of understanding or communication between the patient and his dentist at this time whether it be with fees, the final cosmetic result or general restorative procedures will result in failure of any case regardless of the ability of the dentist.

3. *Dental patient education level.* There are varying techniques of educating the dental patient. The most effective mode of illustrating to patients is usually by means of visual aids whether purchased commercially or constructed by the dentist to illustrate the modes of treatment he anticipates. There are certain basic treatment procedures that can be understood by a large percentage of population. It should be remembered there are no instant techniques to convey to the patient's immediate acceptance of a given treatment plan other than an honest sincere approach by the dentist. Gimmicks are not the answer and the patient who has some amount of forethought and ability to analyze situations will subconsciously indict the dentist for commercializing the health professions.

4. *The development of patient education.* The object of this is to create a sincere relationship where the dentist will not need forced methods of commercializing dental treatment which is sorely needed.

It is true that patients because of financial limitations or possibly anatomical limitations will not be able to be the recipient of what we would label as ideal treatment. However, the dentist must always present an ideal arrangement for total comprehensive patient care and settle a good portion of the time for the practical. However, there are times when the ideal and the practical are synonymous.

5. *Consent of the patient.* It is of paramount importance to prevent embarrassing situations that will result from lack of forethought either in the actual design of proposed treatment or lack of imagination and versatility in the approach to any case. The patient should be allowed to exercise the privilege of choice of treatment related to his social and/or economic background.

Chapter 17

Oral Diagnosis and Treatment Planning in Removable Prosthodontics

RUSSELL H. LEE AND ROBERT M. SOMMERFELD

THE HISTORY

THE MEDICAL HISTORY and examination are important procedures in patient evaluation and will have a direct bearing on the prognosis of the complete denture patient. However, the physical and psychological understanding of the patient must be made at the interview. The interview should have two basic objectives. First, the doctor can evaluate the patient both emotionally and physically. Second, it is at this time that the doctor and the patient develop a rapport. If both of these objectives are not fulfilled, then the prognosis of successful complete denture prosthodontics is doubtful.[1]

Where should this initial meeting between doctor and patient take place? Many men feel that the initial interview should be conducted in the operatory in surroundings familiar to the patient. On the other hand, others feel that this setting threatens the patient and believe that a private office is the appropriate setting for this type of consultation. Either setting can be utilized successfully, if mutual trust between patient and dentist has been established. At this interview the chief complaint of the existing denture can be brought into the open.

What is the problem with the dentures? It is at the interview that this problem is discussed. The dentist must establish whether function, comfort, esthetics or retention of the denture is the problem.

THE ORAL EXAMINATION

Once the interview has been completed, the next logical step is to examine the patient. This examination should be systematic and include all associated structures of the stomatognathic system. Radiographs should be taken and include a Panorex and/or intraoral films. These films should be an integral part of any examination. It is on these films that any existing bony pathology, foreign bodies, retained root tips or unerupted third molars can be seen and examined. It is at the time of the oral examination that the prognosis of complete service should be determined. Also at this time, corrective surgery, if required, can be determined prior to construction of the complete denture. The type of impression procedure to be utilized should be determined. It is at this time that the limitations of the denture bearing area can be determined.

Soft Tissue

The anatomic form and integrity of the maxillary and mandibular edentulous ridges including the hard and soft tissues must be examined. This has a direct bearing on the type of impression procedure utilized. Also it has a direct bearing on the retention and stability of the complete denture. For example if flabby areas exist on the maxillary ridge, it may be advisable to relieve this section of the impression tray and place holes into the tray in order to capture this tissue at rest. Bilateral undercut areas of the maxillary tuberosity must be removed (*see* Ch. 19). These undercuts will prevent the securing of an accurate border seal in this region. Also the undercut areas or sharpness of the mylohyoid line on the mandibular ridge must be considered before any impression procedure. This area can be a constant source of irritation due to the thin mucosal covering. The integrity of the retromolar pad area and the masseter area must be observed. The retromolar pads must be included in all impressions. Flabby tissue in the maxillary and mandibular anterior area must be observed and examined. If this tissue is excessive or redundant, corrective surgery either by electrosurgery or by the scalpel must be utilized before complete denture construction is started. Tissue conditioners can be utilized to see if the tissue will respond prior to any surgery.

Maxillary Tuberosity

The intermaxillary space between ridges can be examined at this time. Protruberant localized areas especially around the maxillary tuberosity area must be evaluated to see if there is adequate interarch space. If there is insufficient interarch space then maxillary tuberosity reductions must be done surgically to provide the necessary room.

The area of the vibrating line should be examined. It is at this time that the amount of compressibility of this tissue can be determined for the postdam.

Tori

Maxillary tori that do not interfere with the posterior palatal seal area may not have to be removed if they are not lobulated or greatly undercut. However, if they do extend or come close to extending onto the vibrating line, then these tori will have to be surgically removed in order to achieve an adequate seal in the posterior area of the denture. Lingual tori on the mandibular ridge will have to be removed if adequate comfort for the lower denture is to be achieved. The mucosa over these areas is thin and tightly stretched. This will be a constant source of irritation for the lower denture unless removed or the denture base is greatly relieved (*see* Ch. 19).

Muscle and Frenum Attachments

The location of muscle attachments have a direct effect upon the retention and stability of the denture. If the denture base is overextended into the muscle attachment area, the seal of the denture could be temporarily broken with muscle activity while speaking, masticating and swallowing. The position of the muscle attachments also indicates the length of the denture flanges and the area of basal seat coverage which can be achieved during the impression procedure.

It is sometimes not necessary to remove a maxillary labial frenum due to the tissue drape of the lip. The drape will seal the border of the denture even though the frenum extends onto the crest of the ridge. Buccal frena which have their attachment on the crest of the ridge must be surgically removed.

Diagnostic Aids

1. *The old denture.* The old denture that the patient is wearing may be of significant importance in determining the chief complaint of the patient. First, one must de-

termine if these dentures are adequate or inadequate. If the denture cannot be improved upon, it is advisable not to start treatment with this patient. If gross inadequacies of the old denture are evident, these should be noted and corrected prior to the construction of new dentures. This may involve the correction of the vertical dimension, the correction of the occlusion, the extension of the peripheral borders to the correct areas, and possibly the correction of the seal area around the posterior border of the maxillary denture. If we can correct these inadequacies of the old denture and obtain a favorable response from the patient, the acceptance of the new dentures and the prognosis for the new denture will be greatly improved.

2. *Radiographs.* It is only on Panorex and/or intraoral films that foreign bodies, retained root tips, unerupted third molars, retained teeth, cysts and tumors can be viewed. These films will be an aid to determine whether or not these structures should be removed. If the patient is elderly and has deeply embedded ratined root tips or third molars and has not experienced any problem with them and if there is no observable pathology around these structures, it may be indicated, due to health reasons, to leave these structures embedded in the tissues.[2] Also, if third molars are present in younger individuals who are to receive complete dentures, it may be advisable not to remove these third molars until they start to erupt into the denture. This will help to preserve the alveolar process which remains around these structures.[3]

3. *Diagnostic casts.* These diagnostic casts can be taken at the time of the oral examination and can be a great aid in planning in any preprosthetic surgery. Also, they serve as a permanent preextraction record for immediate denture service.

TREATMENT PLANNING

Preprosthetic Surgery

General Considerations

The success and prognosis of complete denture prosthodontics can be directly related to the surgical preparation of the mouth prior to complete dentures. The retention and stability of complete dentures cannot be obtained without proper preprosthetic surgery. Therefore, the diagnosis of any abnormal oral condition is of utmost importance. Before any diagnosis can be rendered for an edentulous patient, the dentist must have a concept of the shape and form of the ideal maxillary and mandibular edentulous arches. The maxillary residual ridge should be broad and well rounded, with no excessive undercuts in the tuberosity or labial flange area; the frenum attachment should be below the crest of the ridge and have a dense tissue covering. The mandibular residual ridge should be broad and well rounded with no excessive undercuts on the mylohyoid area, and the retromolar pad area should be preserved; the frenum attachment should be below the crest of the ridge and have a dense tissue covering. In general, only those undercuts which directly interfere with denture insertion and removal should be removed.

Small bony spicules or projections which could develop into future "denture sore spots" should be surgically removed prior to complete denture service. All foreign bodies, cysts, tumors, pathologically involved root tips and impacted third molars should be removed. If impacted or retained teeth are present in young individuals, it may be better not to disturb the eruption potential of these teeth and preserve the alveolar process around these teeth.

Pendulous hyperplastic tissue (epulis fissuratum and papillary hyperplasia) which does not respond to conservative therapy should be surgically removed (see Ch. 19).

It is possible to remove slight anterior undercuts by compressing the buccal or lingual surface, or both, of a socket without the removal of any bone. Whether this procedure preserves alveolar height or not is not known.

In general, it is acceptable to have an anterior undercut if it extends from cuspid and still allows insertion of the denture.

The Maxilla

It is possible to preserve all anterior undercuts provided that none exist in the posterior region. If posterior undercuts are present and no anterior undercuts, then preserve the posterior undercuts.

Palatal tori are removed if they have marked undercuts, impinge on the postdam area or are excessively large. Most palatal tori will not interfere with complete denture service.

Labial and buccal frena will require surgery if they encroach onto the crest of the residual ridge and are broad.

Large protuberant tuberosities will have to be reduced if they encroach upon the vertical dimension. As a rule of thumb, have enough clearance for the denture bases plus 2 to 4 mm of free way space between the dentures.[4]

The Mandible

If no bilateral posterior undercuts exist in the retromylohyoid area, then one can preserve any anterior undercut.

Mandibular tori should be removed prior to complete denture service. The mucosa covering these tori is thin and because of its location is always prone to irritation. Also, it is difficult to complete the lingual seal around the mandibular denture with tori present.

Buccal frena which are broad and encroach upon the crest of the ridge should be surgically removed (see Ch. 19).

Vestibuloplasty procedures should be carried out on selected patients and only when all conventional techniques have failed. It is questionable to utilize this procedure if the patient is not attempting to wear adequate existing dentures. If the procedure is carried out, one must be prepared for some regression of sulcus height. Laney believes that the skin graft helps prevent proliferation of connective tissues which can cause obliteration of the sulcus (see Ch. 19).[5]

The existing mandibular denture can be modified and extended with autopolymerizing acrylic resins at the time of surgery and be utilized as the splint to hold the skin graft immobile.

NONSURGICAL TISSUE CONDITIONING

The ability of oral tissues to support dentures is greatly dependent on many physical and psychological factors. Included among these are (a) the health of the oral tissues, which is affected by the general health of the individual; (b) the mental attitude of the patient towards prosthetic treatment; (c) the size, shape and relationship of the jaws; and (d) the degree of irritation imposed by the artificial appliances.

Retention, stability and adequate function in any given complete denture case cannot always be assured, but when the health of the oral tissues is restored prior to prosthetic treatment, the prognosis becomes more favorable. The oral tissues are constantly exposed to irritation by mechanical, thermal and bacterial agents. The lips, tongue and oral cavity are particularly sensitive to nutritional disturbances and dietary disorders. Atrophic or degenerative oral mucosal changes are an indication of the state of all body mucosal tissues and may be the result of an underlying metabolic deficiency.

In edentulous patients, biting with anterior teeth and vigorous chewing with the posterior teeth should be minimized to prevent dislodgment of the denture and subsequent injury to supporting tissues. Foods must be soft or reduced to small sizes by proper cutting, grating or crushing. Mechanical factors associated with a denture placed on soft tissues prevent adequate chewing of hard foods without discomfort to the patient, thus restricting the diet of the edentulous patient.

The edentulous patient must take care not to jeopardize his future nutrition because of the use of a denture and a change in diet.[6] It should be pointed out that the edentulous condition may have been caused, in part, by poor nutrition and that giving more attention to a proper diet may result in better general health and possibly a longer life span (see Ch. 21).[7]

The family physician should also be alerted to oral and physical disorders recognized by the dentist. The proper vitamin and mineral supplements to the patient's diet will improve the status of the oral tissue for the reception of prosthetic appliances.

Just as dietary supplementation may be an advantage in clinical treatment, so will mechanical correction of the old denture prove to be valuable prior to fabrication of a new prosthesis. The old denture should be checked for incorrect occlusal vertical dimension, incorrect centric occlusion and

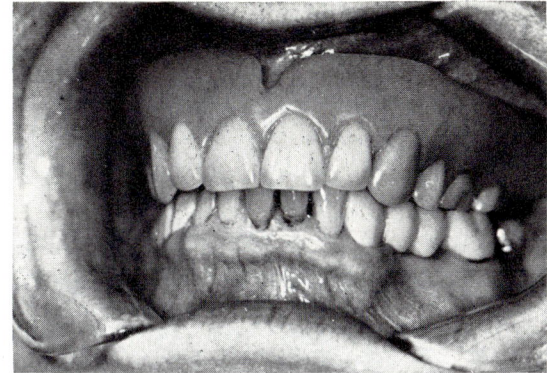

Figure 17-1. Correction of occlusion as an aid to tissue treatment prior to new maxillary denture impressions.

overextension of the border areas due to extensive resorption of the residual alveolar ridges. A soft and flabby, sometimes fibrous mucosa referred to as epulis fissuratum, is commonly associated with the labial borders of ill-fitting dentures. A tissue treatment material is advisable to line the denture and mechanically reduce the proliferated tissue.[8]

Tissue treatment materials were introduced to cushion abused tissues and to restore them to a healthy condition prior to the fabrication of new dentures. When properly used these materials provide comfort to the patient and allow him to wear the appliance during the period of tissue recovery.

The old denture must be prepared by correcting any gross areas of faulty occlusion or vertical dimension and trimming away gross undercuts from the denture's tissue surface (Fig. 17-1). Prepare the tissue treatment material according to the manufacturer's directions and apply it evenly to the old denture. Insert the denture and have the patient close lightly into centric relation. After several minutes the denture is removed from the patient's mouth and the excess material is trimmed from the borders with a scissors or hot

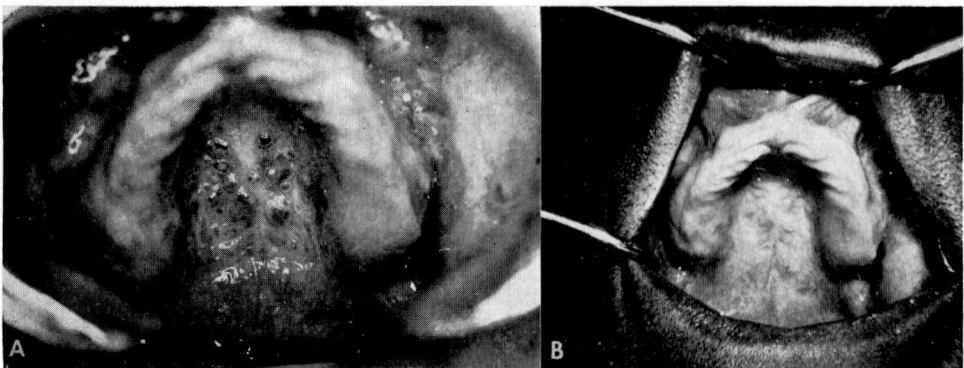

Figure 17-2. (A) Inflammatory papillary hyperplasia. (B) Improved tissue of patient in A ten days after tissue treatment.

spatula. The same procedure is then repeated with the opposing denture.

The restoration of tissue to sound tone and color cannot be accomplished overnight. The number of treatments required depend on how badly the tissues were abused and the systemic health of the patient. Recovery may require anywhere from several weeks to several months of continued dietary supplementation and repeated tissue treatments. Tissue treatments should be repeated every four to five days as the material becomes too firm to be responsive to tissue movement (Fig. 17-2, A and B). The tissue treatment is finished when the tissue appears normal and the patient is comfortable. Dietary supplementation is continued with the cooperation of the patient's physician. The temporary lined dentures may be worn while new dentures are being constructed. Preparation of the patient and the edentulous oral tissue for clinical prosthetic treatment should be the rule of practice in full denture service.

*SPECIAL REMOVABLE PROSTHESES

The prosthodontist may be called upon to aid in the treatment of patients with unusual prosthetic requirements. These patients, in general, have either congenital or acquired deformities of the oral cavity. These deformities are generally induced by accident, neglect, disease or by a disturbance of normal development. As in all normal cases a history, examination, diagnosis, prognosis and treatment plan for constructing the prosthesis should be as comprehensive as possible.

Success is largely dependent upon a systematic approach to the basic principles applied to the construction of dentures for ordinary types of cases. Deviations, however, will require a compromise treatment in most instances. The final treatment plan for many of these cases will be the result of a coordinated effort and consultation with other medical and dental specialists.

Acquired Deformities

Most acquired dental deformities are the result of treatment for oral tumors or trauma. Radiation therapy and surgery remain as the only effective tools for treatment of squamous cell carcinoma of the upper alimentary tract. The use of radioisotopes, cobalt and linear accelerators have

* Cases 1 through 7. See Figures 17-3A,B, 17-4, 17-5A,B,C, 17-6A,B, 17-7, 17-8A,B,C, 17-9A,B.

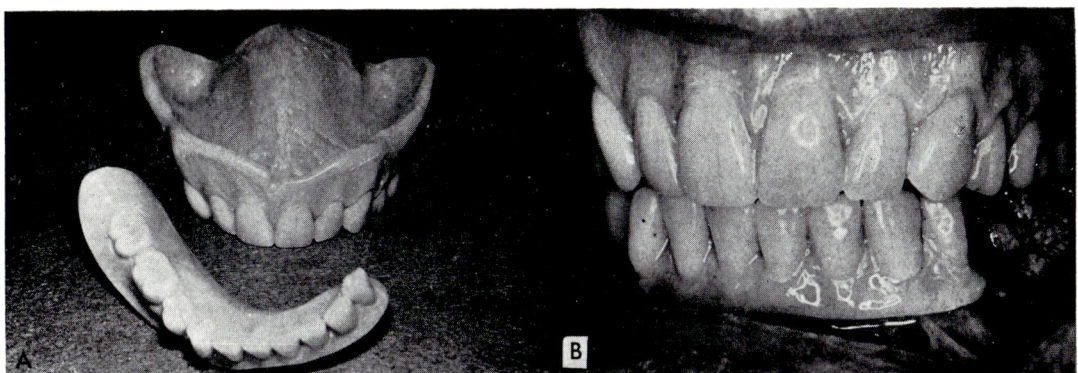

Figure 17-3. Case 1. (A) Maxillary and mandibular prostheses for a patient who has undergone partial resection of the mandible due to a malignant lesion. (B) Prostheses *in situ*.

become increasingly sophisticated; however, large doses of irradiation can adversely affect the oral tissues from the standpoint of prosthetic rehabilitation.

The oral mucous membrane may be considered slightly more sensitive to radiation than skin. As radiation treatment is initiated, one may observe a reddening of the mucosa as the level of radiation reaches 1200 to 1500 rads. At about 2500 rads, white patches appear on the mucous membrane of the lips, cheeks and tongue. This, according to Edgerton et al.[10] may represent an overgrowth of *C albicans* and a sloughing of the mucosa. Progressive treatment to the 3500 rad level initiates severe irritation and frequent epithelial sloughing. The patient will generally complain of a sensitivity to spicy foods and extremes in temperature. The lips and corners of the mouth become ulcerated and angular cheilitis is usually present as the radiation level reaches 5500 rads. An early and rapid swelling of the major salivary glands in the line of irradiation, followed by a marked glandular atrophy and xerostomia develops after the fourth to sixth week of oral irradiation.

The severe change in the oral environment of irradiated patients in many instances will lead to a rapid decalcification of tooth structure. The teeth in the line of irradiation should be extracted as early as possible prior to the onset of treatment and with the least possible trauma to the supporting bone. The other teeth, though not in the direct line of radiation, should be treated with topical application of 10% sodium fluoride solutions. The remaining teeth are more prone to decay than those in a normal oral environment (see p. 74).

Following irradiation, the construction of a dental prosthesis should be delayed for six to eighteen months depending on the

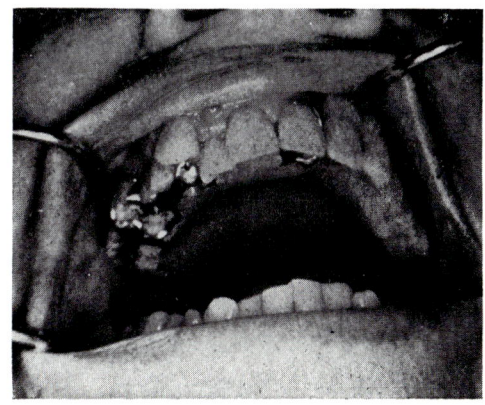

Figure 17-4. Case 2. Maxillary prosthesis for a patient who has undergone partial maxillary resection.

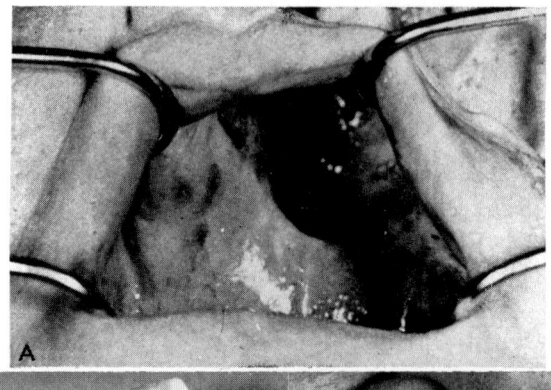
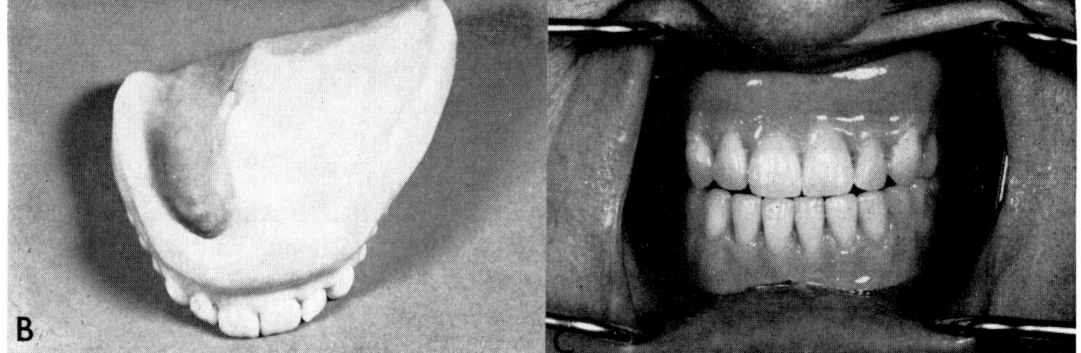

Figure 17-5. Case 3. (A) Edentulous patient following partial maxillectomy. (B) Maxillary prosthesis for this patient. (C) Maxillary and mandibular prostheses *in situ*.

amount of irradiation and the condition of the oral mucosa. The technique used must be as nonirritating and atraumatic to the tissue as possible. Longlasting, resilient materials are generally considered for those patients.

Patients who have lost a portion of their oral anatomy due to traumatic injury or surgical removal of pathological tissue present similar prosthetic challenges. Complete rehabilitation of these patients includes surgical, dental, social, vocational and emotional treatment. When large portions of the maxilla are missing, the patient is usually unable to ingest food without great difficulty. Normal tongue movement will force the bolus of food through the defect. Speech is also affected with loss of portions of the maxilla. Reestablishing normal palatal contour is very important for these patients. The occlusion may be arranged so that the teeth articulate on the unaffected side. The teeth should be out of occlusion on the side of the defect to avoid irritation to the underlying postsurgical scar tissue.

The loss of function which results from a partial loss of the mandible depends mainly on the area of the jaw removed and whether or not intraoral mucosa must be sacrificed. Patients with a unilateral resection posterior to the area of the first premolar have almost no disturbance in mandibular function and experience minimal facial disfigurement. The movement of the mandible is not restricted, but on wide opening there will be a five to seven mm shift of the jaw toward the resected side. When the mandible is removed at the midline, there is a medial sag of the soft tis-

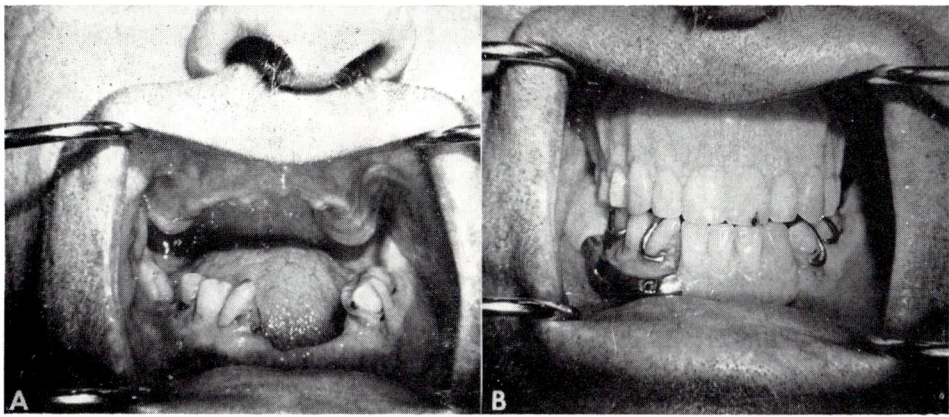

Figure 17-6. Case 4. (A) Patient with malaligned dental arches due to a traumatic injury. (B) The maxillary and mandibular prostheses *in situ*, the latter utilizing a labial bar as the major connector.

sues causing abnormal facial appearance contributing to impaired occlusal relationship and reduction of available tongue space.

Mastication is restricted by the greater deviation of the jaw to the side of the defect. After some months, speech becomes relatively normal, but mastication will remain a difficult problem. Centric position for these patients should be established at a vertical relation allowing three to 4 mm of interocclusal distance. This greater interocclusal distance gives the patient more tongue space to produce the proper phonetic sounds. Nonanatomical teeth are used to provide a more equal distribution of forces during mastication. A resilient lining material is also recommended to further cushion the compromised postsurgical tissue of the mandible.

Congenital Deformities

There are a number of congenital defects which may result in abnormal maxillomandibular relationships. Of these the most common oral congenital defect is the cleft of the lip and/or palate. One of every eight hundred live births exhibit this deformity. There are approximately five thousand children born in the United States each year with clefts.

Palatal clefts vary greatly in extent from those involving the soft palate only to those continuing into the hard palate and including the alveolus in the premaxillary area either unilaterally or bilaterally. The cleft palate patient relies upon contributions from the pedodontist, oral surgeon, orthodontist, prosthodontist, pediatrician, plastic surgeon, otolaryngologist and speech therapist for maintaining the proper long-

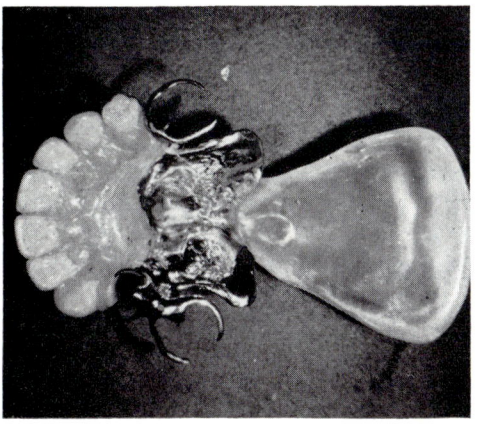

Figure 17-7. Case 5. Partial denture with obturator for a patient with an unrepaired cleft of the alveolus and palate.

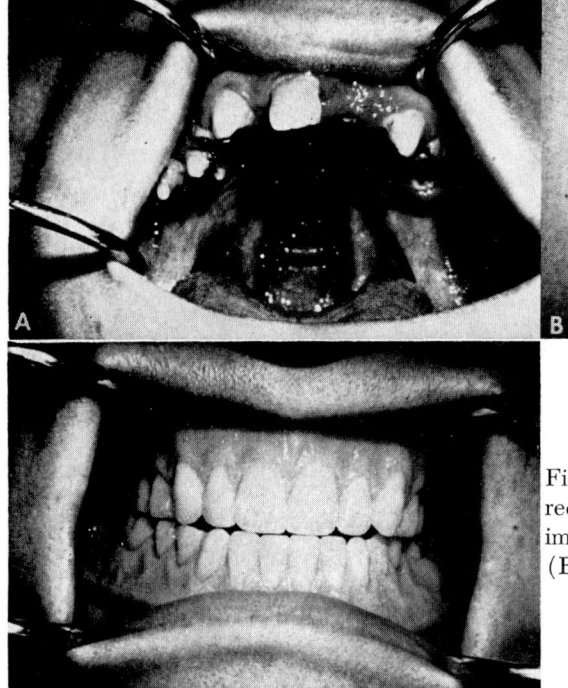

Figure 17-8. Case 6. (A) This cleft palate patient required extraction of all the remaining teeth and immediate maxillary and mandibular dentures. (B) Maxillary prosthesis. (C) Dentures *in situ*.

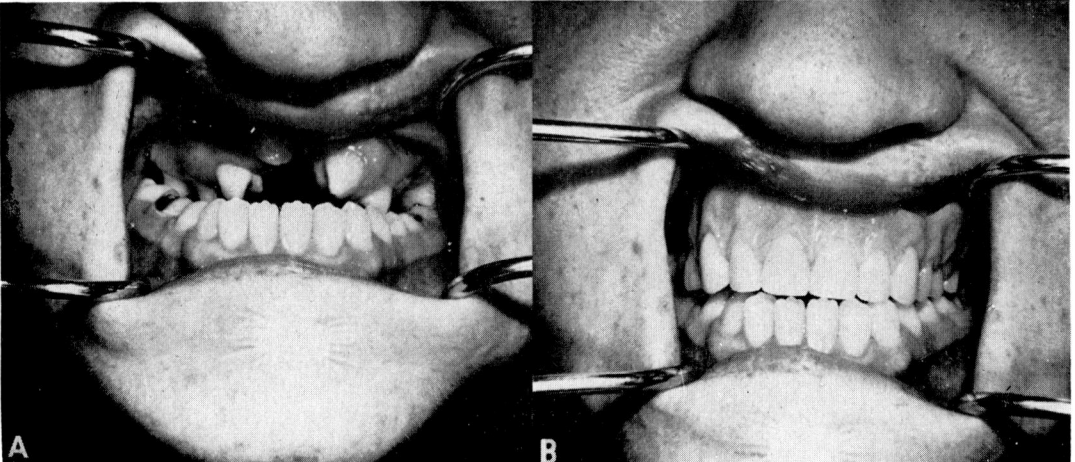

Figure 17-9. Case 7. (A) Cleft palate patient with reduced vertical dimension of occlusion and malaligned dental arches. (B) Maxillary overlay prosthesis for this patient in situ.

term treatment plan during his or her lifetime.

A speech appliance or dental obturator is a prosthetic appliance used to close a congenital or acquired opening in the palate. Prosthetic treatment may begin in early infancy with the fabrication of positioning and feeding appliances. The prosthodontist is generally called upon to construct speech appliances. These appliances may simply replace one or two missing teeth during the deciduous and mixed dentition stages or may be either complete or partial dentures with an obturator to correct velopharyngeal incompetence.

The normal soft palate in conjunction with the lateral and posterior walls of the pharynx serves to regulate the air stream in an oral direction by closing off the nasal cavity during speech. The necessary impounding of the air stream to make a sudden release of oral breath for selected speech samples is not possible when there is inadequate velopharyngeal closure. This creates a nasal flow of air and the accompanying increased nasal resonance. It is the function of the obturator to redirect the flow of air through the oral cavity.

The obturator consists of three main portions: the palatal portion, which may also function to replace missing teeth and tissue; the velar portion, replacing missing tissue of the soft palate; and the pharyngeal portion, occluding the nasopharyngeal portion. The location of the pharyngeal portion is determined by the greatest constriction in the lumen of the nasopharyngeal portion. It is identified by a bulging of fibers from the superior and middle constrictor muscles of the pharynx. This bulging of tissue is located at the level of the first cervical vertebrate and is termed "Passavant's ridge."

Most clefts of the palate in the past have been surgically repaired with occasional failures due to unintelligible speech and interruption of maxillary growth centers. These patients generally exhibit a lack of maxillary growth both in a vertical and anterior projection. The result is an underdevelopment of the middle third of the face with a small maxilla and a mandible which appears larger when the teeth occlude. The excessive interocclusal distance which may result can be restored in the palatal portion of the prosthesis. There are many cases which will result in better growth patterns and more favorable speech results if treated with an obturator. Each case should be examined by all specialists concerned with the decision for proper management made by all members consulted.

With the refinement of radiotherapy and surgical techniques, more extensive treatment is being considered for persons with acquired and congenital deformities. Because of the advances in knowledge and materials, prosthodontics can aid in the reconstruction of these patients' functional parts with prosthetic restorations designed to return the patient to a relatively normal state.

REFERENCES

1. Koper, A.: The initial interview with complete denture patients: Its structure and strategy. *J Prosthet Dent*, 23:590, 1970.
2. Sharry, J. J.: *Complete Denture Prosthodontics*, 2nd ed. New York, McGraw-Hill, 1968, p. 158.
3. Laskin, D. M.: Indications and contraindications for removal of impacted third molars. *Dent Clin North Am*, 13:927, 1969.
4. Krol, A.: *Complete Denture Notes*. Stockton (Calif.), University of Pacific, School of Dentistry, 1968.
5. Laney, W. R., Turlington, E. G., and Devine, K. D.: Grafted skin as an oral prosthesis

bearing tissue. *J Prosthet Dent, 19:*69, 1968.
6. Nizel, A. E.: *The Science of Nutrition and Its Application to Clinical Dentistry.* Philadelphia, W. B. Saunders, 1966, pp. 421–426.
7. Roworthy, R. H.: *Nutrition and Dietetics in Dental Health.* University of Pennsylvania, 1947, p. 238.
8. Pendelton, E. C.: Preoperative treatment in full denture service. *Ill Dent J, 17:*6, 1948.
9. Gerhard, R. J.: Personal communication.
10. *Oral Care for Oral Cancer Patients.* Report of a conference held in Chicago, Illinois, June 1968. Public Health Service Publication No. 1958.

Chapter 18

Orthodontic Diagnosis

HOWARD ADUSS AND SAMUEL PRUZANSKY

THE CONCEPTS and tools employed in orthodontic diagnosis and the objectives of orthodontic treatment are germane to all of dental practice. This can be demonstrated by first considering the procedures involved in orthodontic diagnosis and second, the questions commonly asked by dentists and the consumers of orthodontic services.

THE DATA BASE

Orthodontic diagnosis is characterized by a well-defined data base.[1] In addition to a history and clinical examination, such data includes photographs, dental casts, cephalometric radiographs and panoramic and/or periapical x-ray films. Additional diagnosis studies, such as speech evaluations or tomography of the temporomandibular joint are dictated by specific patient needs (Figs. 18-1, 18-2, 18-3). The value of a well-defined data base is that it provides a standardized means for determining a treatment plan and a methodology for continuous monitoring of treatment and long-term results.

Diagnosis is not a single event in orthodontic practice but a continuous procedure to maintain quality control. In dealing with a growing and changing child, the need for such monitoring is self-evident. By this process, clinical intuition, or "flying by the seat of one's pants," gives way to a systematic guidance system.

THE HISTORY

As with every patient in a clinical setting, certain basic demographic characteristics are essential. For the child, birth weight and birth order are among the essential items to be considered. The fact that a child was premature or was a mature, low–birth-weight infant affords some insight into his developmental potential. While a record of the patient's systemic health and nutritional intake are significant in terms of his developmental progress, birth order may also yield information regarding the status of the child within the family constellation and reflect on his behavioral patterns. Habits, such as thumbsucking, are obviously significant (Fig. 18-4).

A history of disorders of the oropharynx or upper respiratory tract is meaningful in that abnormalities in this region can affect facial appearance as well as occlusion. For example, large faucial tonsils may alter tongue posture by displacing the tongue anteriorly and inferiorly. Obliga-

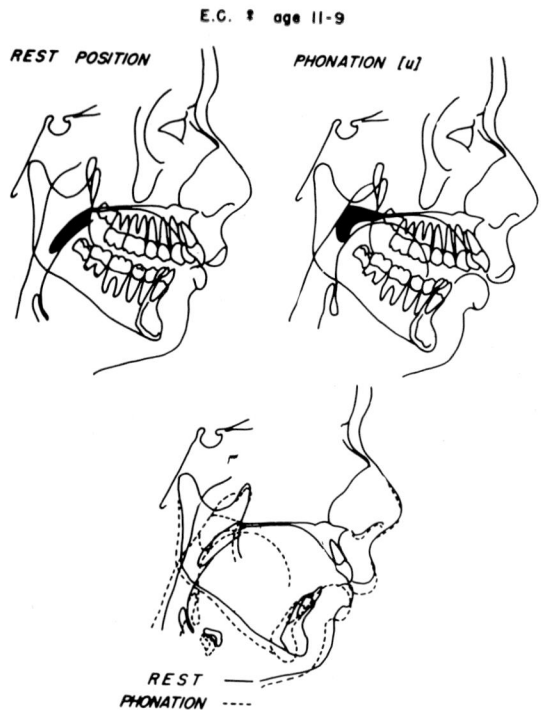

Figure 18-1. The functional pattern of a patient using labiodental substitutions for bilabial sounds during sustained phonation of the vowel /u/. During phonation, the lower lip is pressed against the mandibular incisors and is lingual to the maxillary incisors. The abnormal lip posture and hypermentalis activity result in a flattening of the mandibular incisor segment and accentuation of the maxillary incisor protrusion.

tory mouth-breathing, due to obstructive adenoids, may result in aberrant function of the orbicularis oris musculature with resultant deleterious effects on the dental arches (Fig. 18-5).

In the course of taking the history, it is often possible to determine the patient's motive for treatment. While this may not be an important consideration when dealing with a receptive and pliable youngster, with older adolescents or adult patients, motivation and acceptance of treatment with all of its inconveniences and imagined esthetic limitations, becomes critical.

Meeting with the parents of a child allows one to assess the degree of cooperation that can be expected during the treatment period and also to estimate the child's growth potential. In so doing, it may be valuable to avoid the embarrassment of discovering that the patient is an adopted child. A final consideration in the family history involves an evaluation of particular patterns of inheritance. Genetic histories are significant when dealing with congenitally missing teeth, supernumerary teeth and patients with unusual syndromes (Figs. 18-6 and 18-7).

THE CLINICAL EXAMINATION

The clinical examination begins by looking at the face and the facial musculature, not only in repose but in function. This includes the posture of the labial musculature at rest and in animated speech (Fig. 18-8). Given a patient with a marked overjet, one should consider how he performs the bilabial sounds such as the consonants b, p and the vowel /u/, (Fig. 18-9). If this is accomplished by approximation of the lips, then there is considerable forward projection of the mandible which in time may become a habit. If instead, there are labiodental substitutions for the bilabial sounds, then the associated hypermentalis activity may have an adverse effect on the incisors (Fig. 18-9).

Digital examination of the quality of the labial and buccal musculature is important as an estimate of tonicity. The presence of an abnormal median superior labial frenum can account for a diastema and displacement of the maxillary incisors. If in elevating the upper lip, the tissue between the incisors and the incisive papilla blanches, as a result of fibrous tension, then frenec-

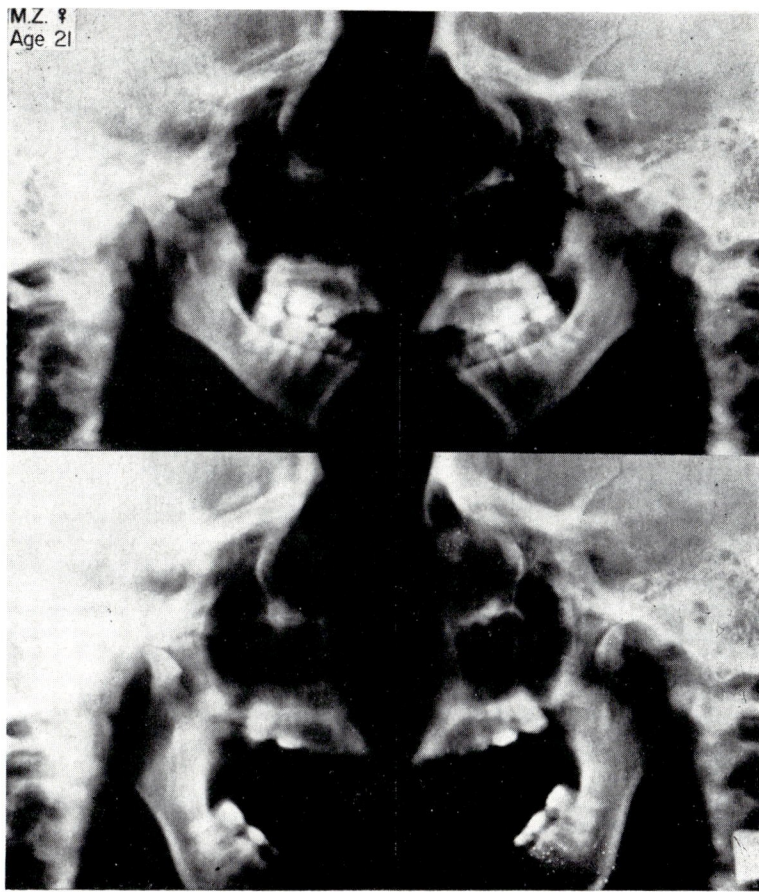

Figure 18-2. Pathologic flattening of the articular surface of the mandibular condyle associated with abnormal occlusal interferences and temporomandibular joint pain dysfunction syndrome.

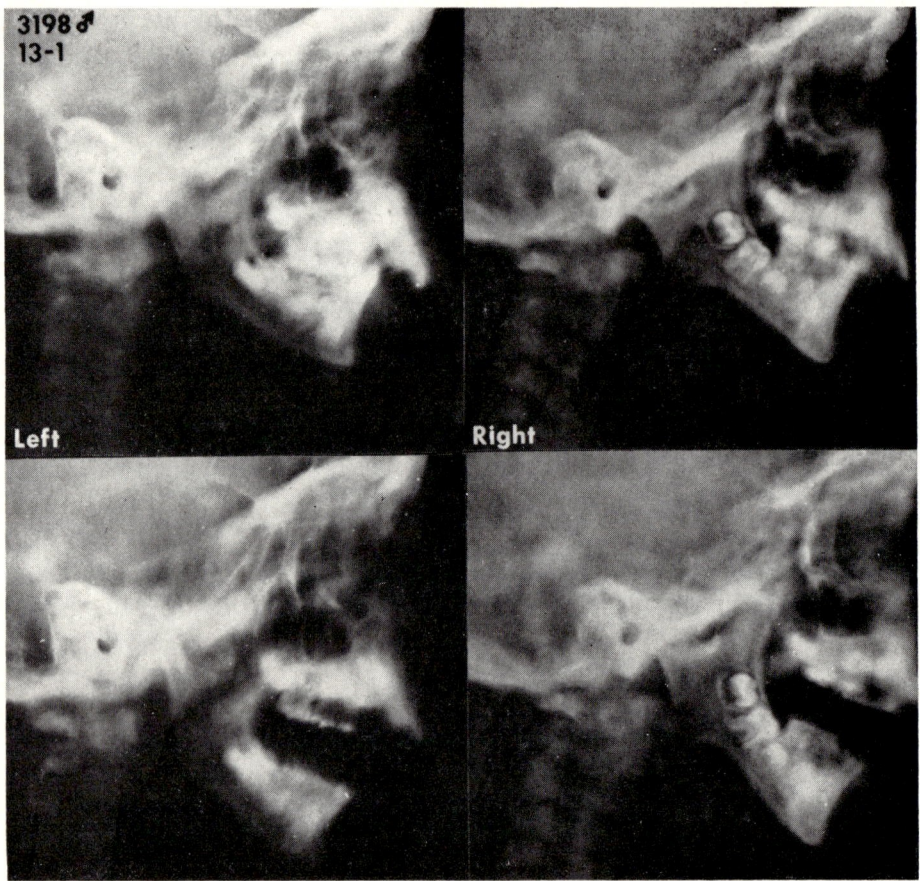

Figure 18-3. Tomograms of the temporomandibular joints of a boy with facial asymmetry (age: 13 years, 1 month). The configuration of the condyle on the right side, in the absence of temporal bone pathology, suggests there was an undiagnosed and unreduced condylar fracture at an earlier age.

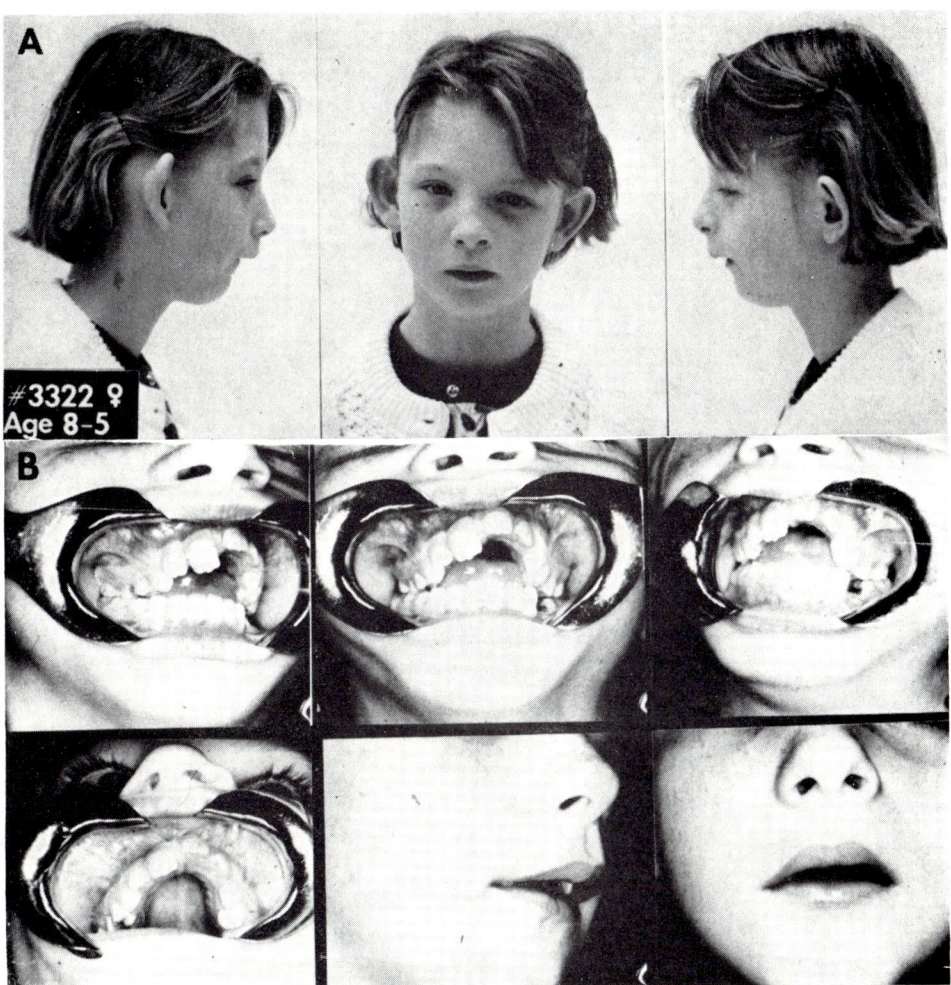

Figure 18-4. The effects of a persistent and intense thumbsucking habit. Note the anterior open-bite, asymmetric deflection of the maxillary incisors, and the gross labial imbalance.

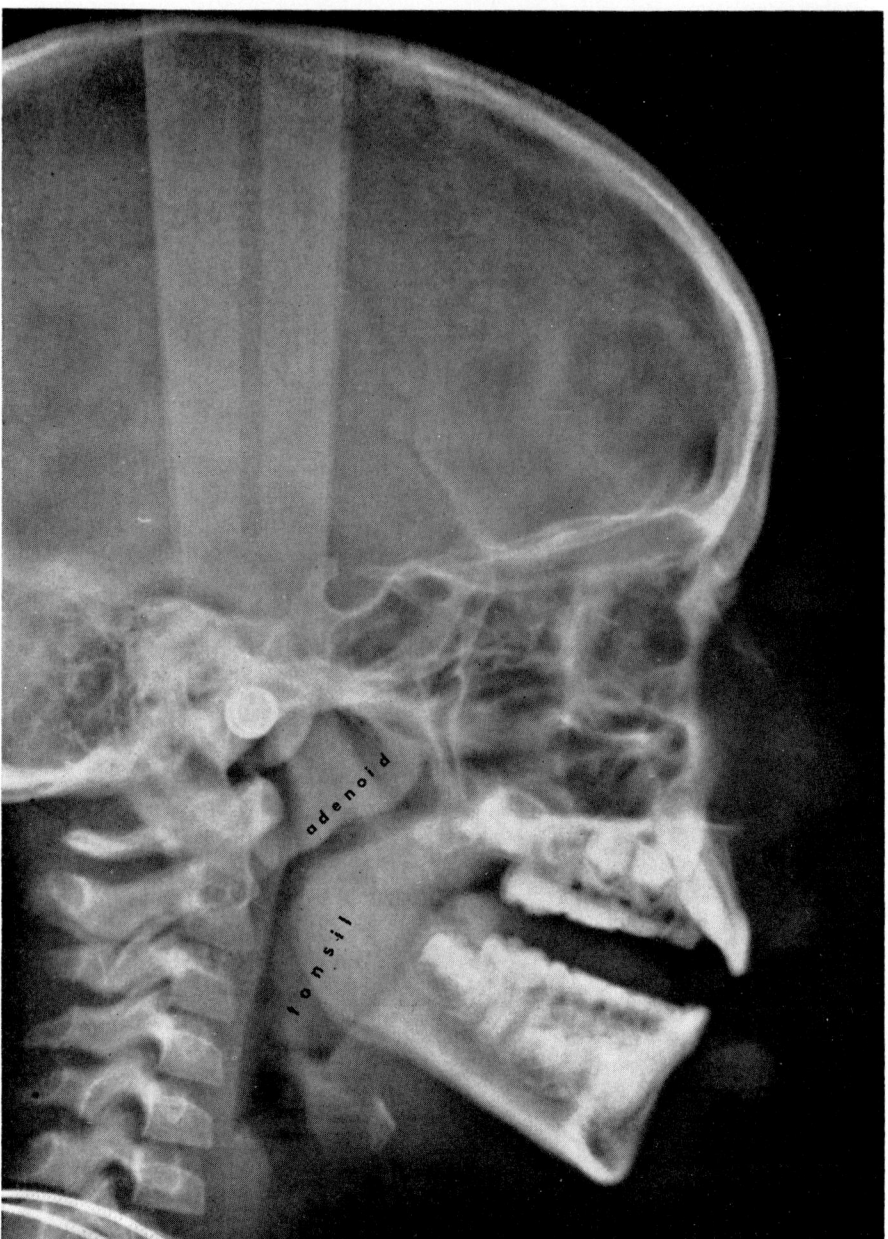

Figure 18-5. Lateral roentgencephalogram demonstrating a large adenoid mass and faucial tonsils. Obligatory mouth-breathing may result from occlusion of the nasopharynx by the enlarged adenoid. Large faucial tonsils may displace the tongue anteroinferiorly. Either condition may result in aberrant orbicularis oris function with deleterious effects on the dental arches.

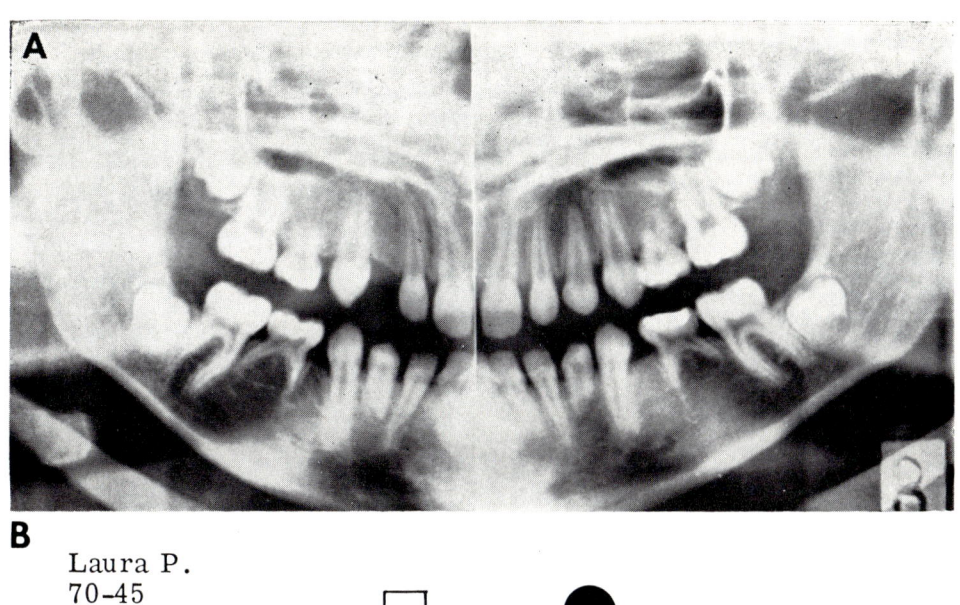
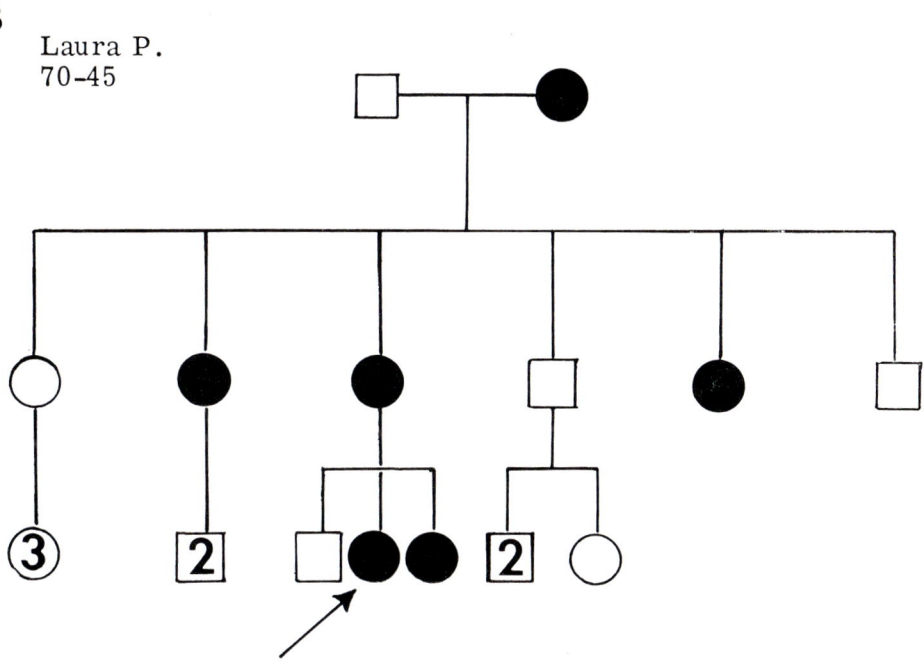

Figure 18-6. (A) Panorex radiograph depicting a pattern of oligodontia present in the females of a family. (B) The family pedigree. The oligodontia is probably transmitted as an autosomal dominant.

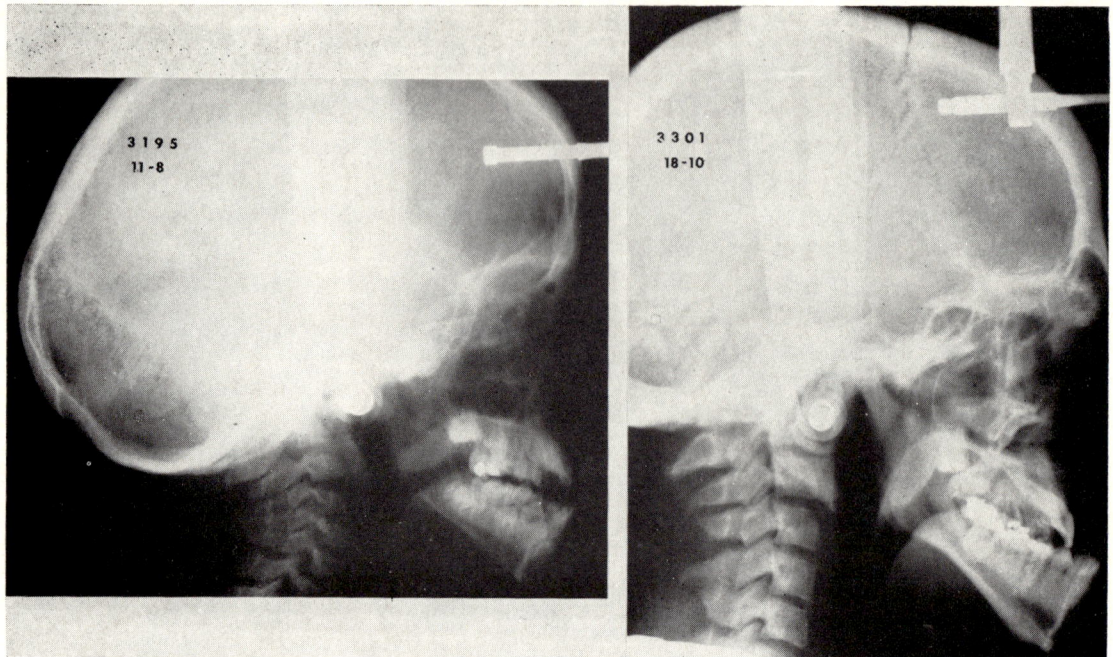

Figure 18-7. Lateral roentgencephalograms of two brothers with familial platybasia.

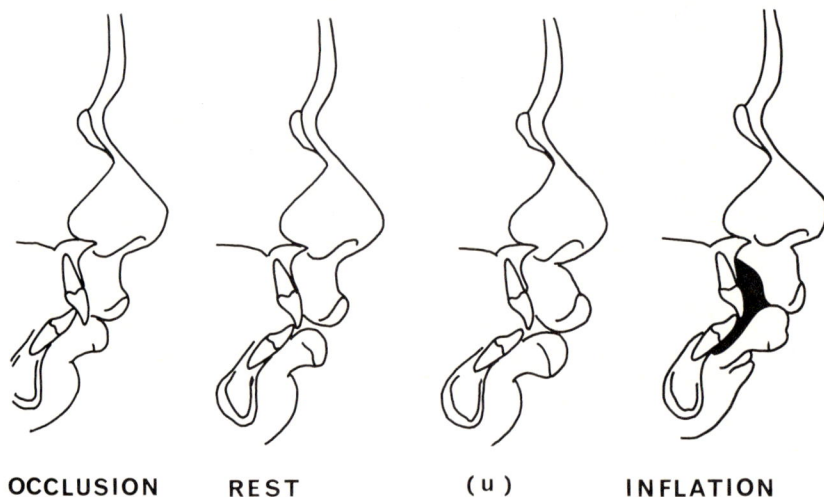

OCCLUSION   REST   (u)   INFLATION

Figure 18-8. Tracings of lateral roentgencephalograms demonstrating the various postures of the lips at rest and during function. Incisor overbite and overjet, as well as the position of the lips, are well within normal limits.

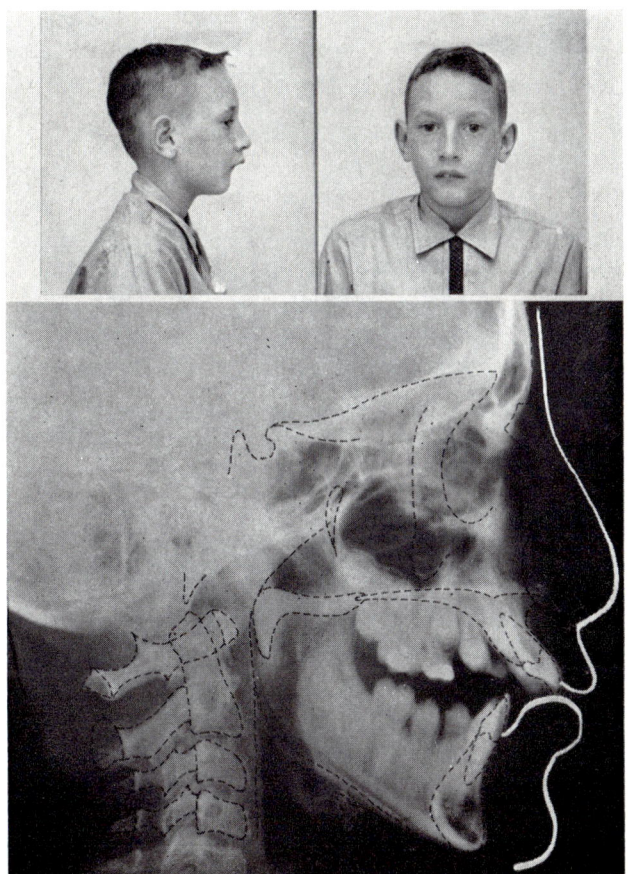

Figure 18-9. Abnormal labiodental substitution during phonation of the vowel sound /u/ due to marked maxillary overjet. Note how the lower lip curls lingual to the maxillary incisors.

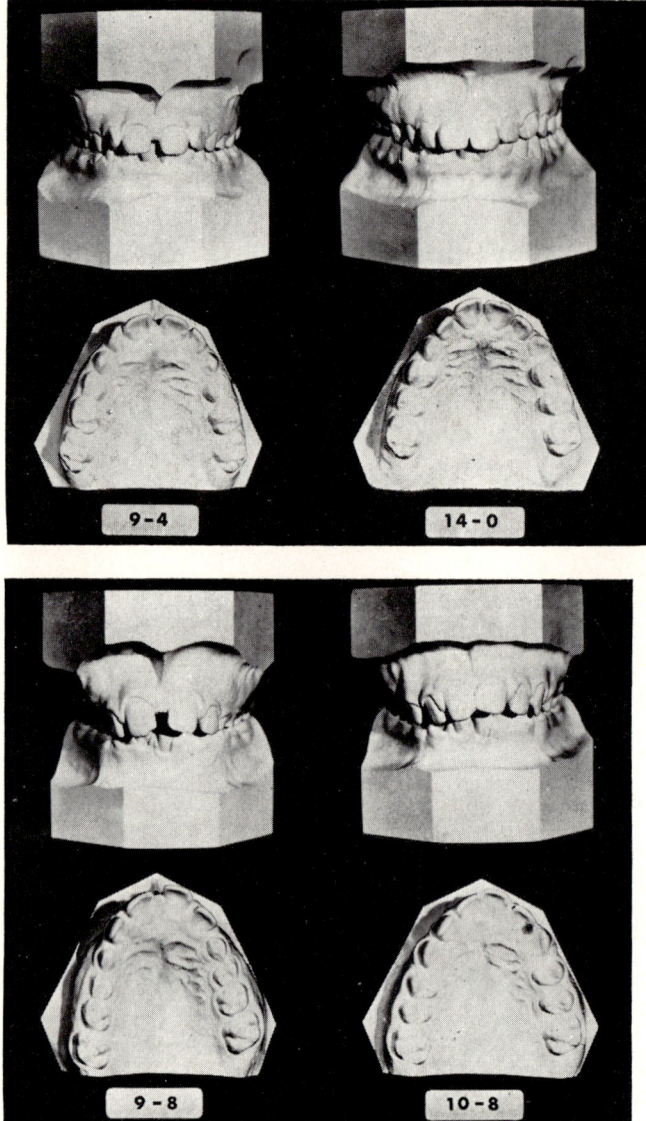

Figure 18-10 (Top) and Figure 18-11 (Bottom). Preoperative and postoperative dental casts demonstrating spontaneous correction of the diastema following resection of a fibrous median superior labial frenum. No appliances were utilized.

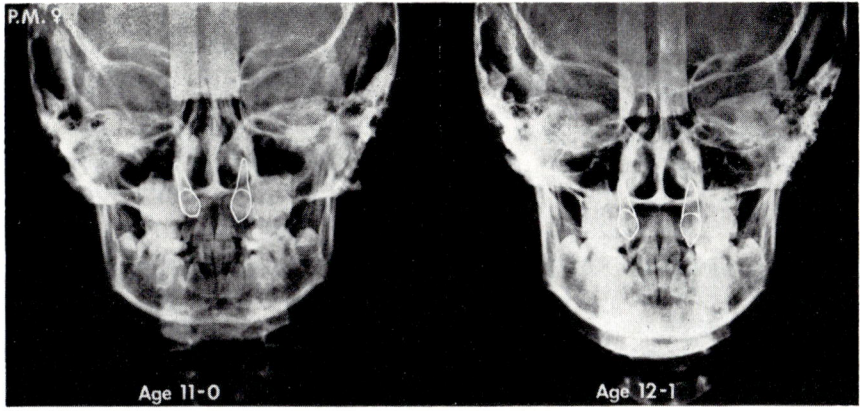

Figure 18-12. Clinical examination followed by radiographic confirmation at age eleven indicated that the maxillary canines were "off-course" in their eruption pattern and might be impacted. The deciduous canines were extracted as a preventive measure. One year later, the maxillary canines were in a more favorable alignment and ultimately erupted into proper position.

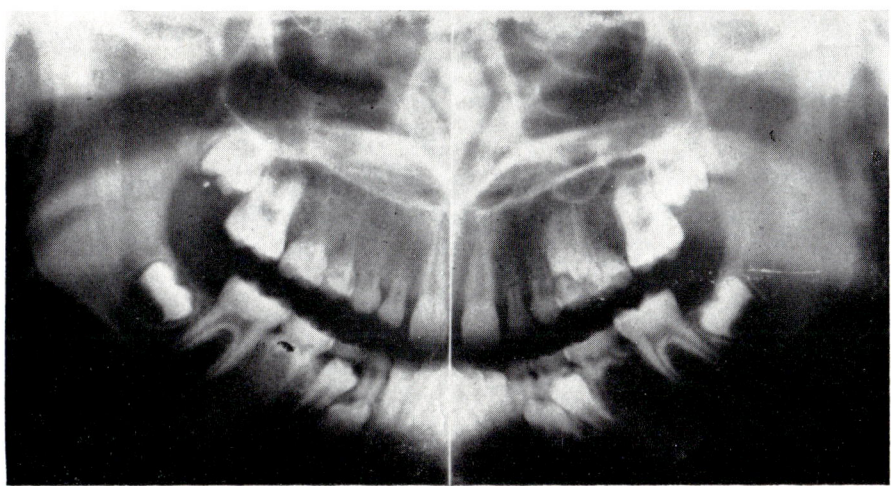

Figure 18-13. Oligodontia disclosed during the course of an examination to determine the cause of delayed eruption in a 12–5 year old boy.

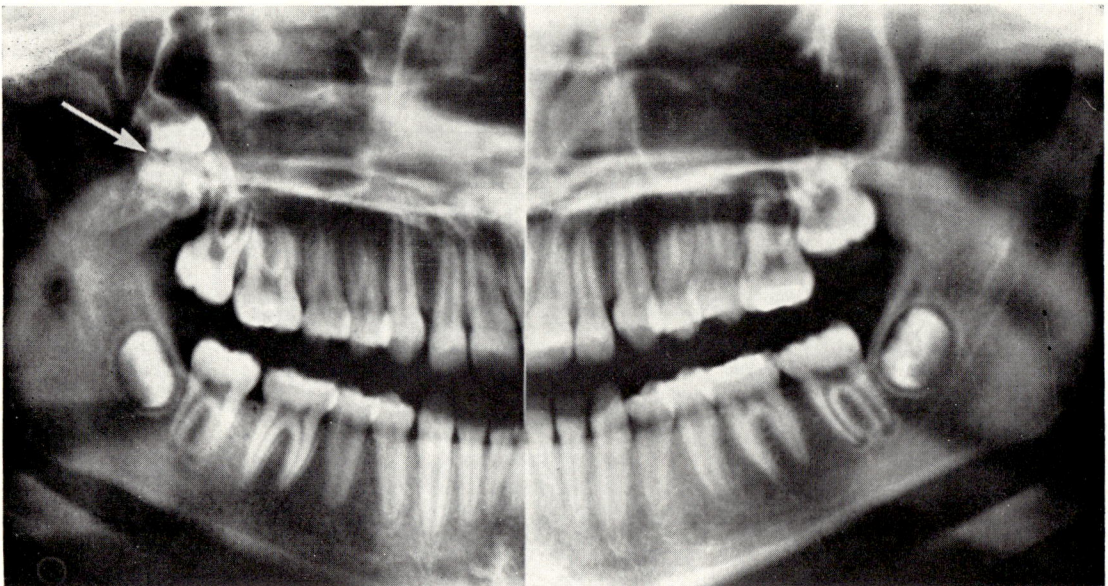

Figure 18-14. Odontogenic tumor disclosed during routine preoperative radiographic examination of a female patient age 12–3 years. The wide area covered by the panoramic radiograph allows early detection of a variety of pathologies which might go undiscovered with routine pedodontic radiography.

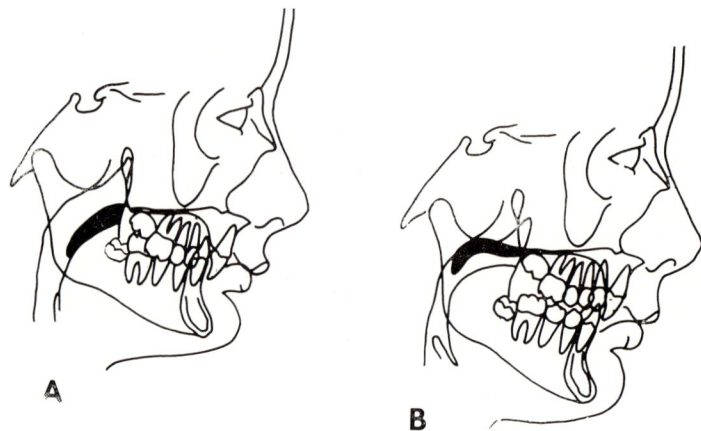

Figure 18-15. Functional analysis. Tracings of lateral roentgencephalograms demonstrate (A) in occlusion, the deep overbite and complete buccal crossbite and (B) at rest, the limited freeway space insufficient to clear the deep overbite.

tomy is indicated. Frenectomy, when performed in the mixed dentition and in the presence of sufficient tooth material, will result in spontaneous closure of the diastema (Figs. 18-10 and 18-11).

THE DENTITION

Methods for categorizing malocclusions have been proposed by many investigators. The Angle classification, based on the relation of upper and lower first molars, remains a standard index, albeit a limited one, in characterizing occlusal disharmony. This classification, as well as others, may be found in standard orthodontic texts and will not be considered in this chapter. It should be noted, however, that a computerized system has recently been developed for classifying malocclusions which may ultimately prove useful in clinical practice.[2]

The disciplined clinician soon learns the value of identifying and counting the teeth in each arch. The process should be repeated when reviewing radiographs of the dental arches.

When examining a patient in the mixed dentition, it is wise to palpate for unerupted canines. Failure to locate the telltale elevation in the maxilla or mandible may suggest an eruption path that is off-course and will lead to canine impaction. If detected early, it may be possible to realign the eruption path by selective extraction of deciduous teeth (Fig. 18-12).

Attention should be given to abnormalities in number, size, shape and position of individual teeth. Failure of teeth to erupt in a sequence that is in harmony with the remainder of the dentition is often indicative of some localized pathology and warrants radiographic evaluation (Fig. 18-13).

In the preschool age period, one of the most common reasons for referral to an orthodontist is the presence of a crossbite occlusion. This may be limited to the incisor segment and/or one or both buccal segments. The question arises, Why should

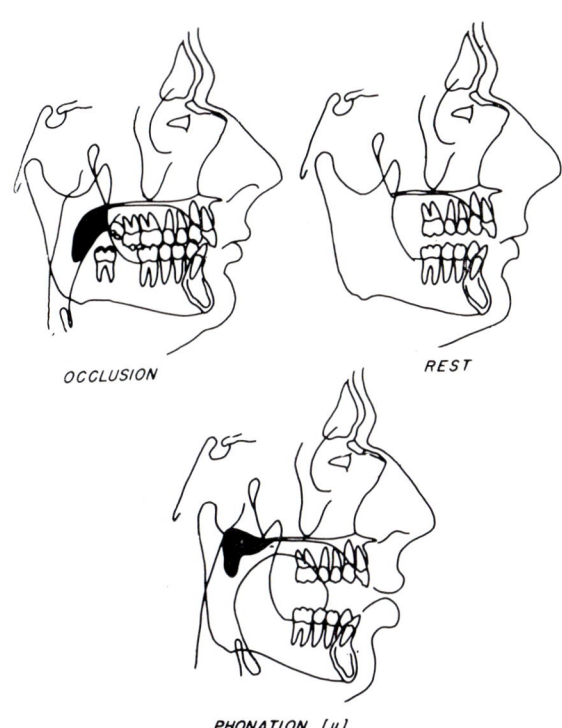

Figure 18-16. Functional analysis of the variation in freeway space, at rest and during phonation of the vowel /u/. These differences are characteristic of patients with a "square" type of mandible.

this be corrected in a dentition which is to be exfoliated?

Functional analysis through direct clinical observation will provide the answer to this question. By looking at the relationship of the lower midline to that of the upper, as the mandible moves from rest to occlusion, it will be observed that the lower midline shifts from a symmetrical relationship toward the side of the crossbite as the teeth come into occlusion. The shift in jaw posture clearly suggests that a crossbite is a significant orthopedic problem that may affect temporomandibular joint function, jaw growth and subsequent tooth eruption.

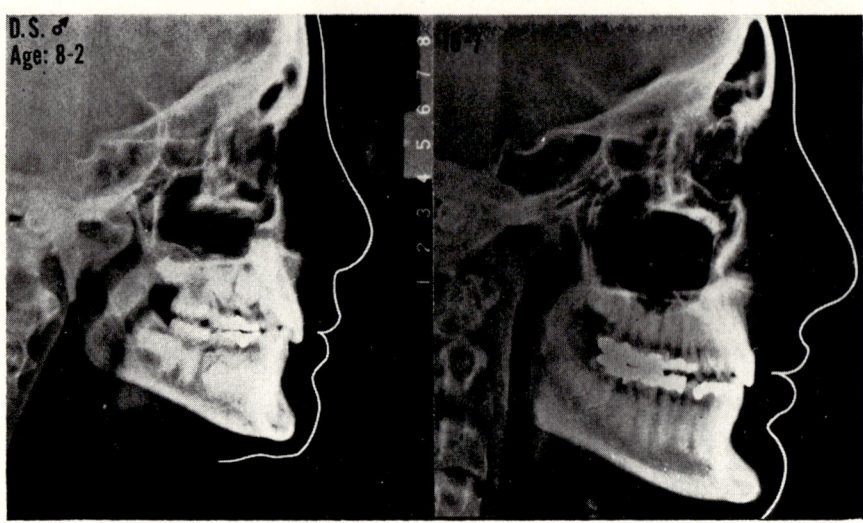

Figure 18-17. Serial lateral roentgencephalograms, at ages 8–2 and 16–7 years, demonstrating the postpubertal development of a prominent chin. The effect of this type of change must be considered in relating the incisors to the apical base and the soft tissue profile.

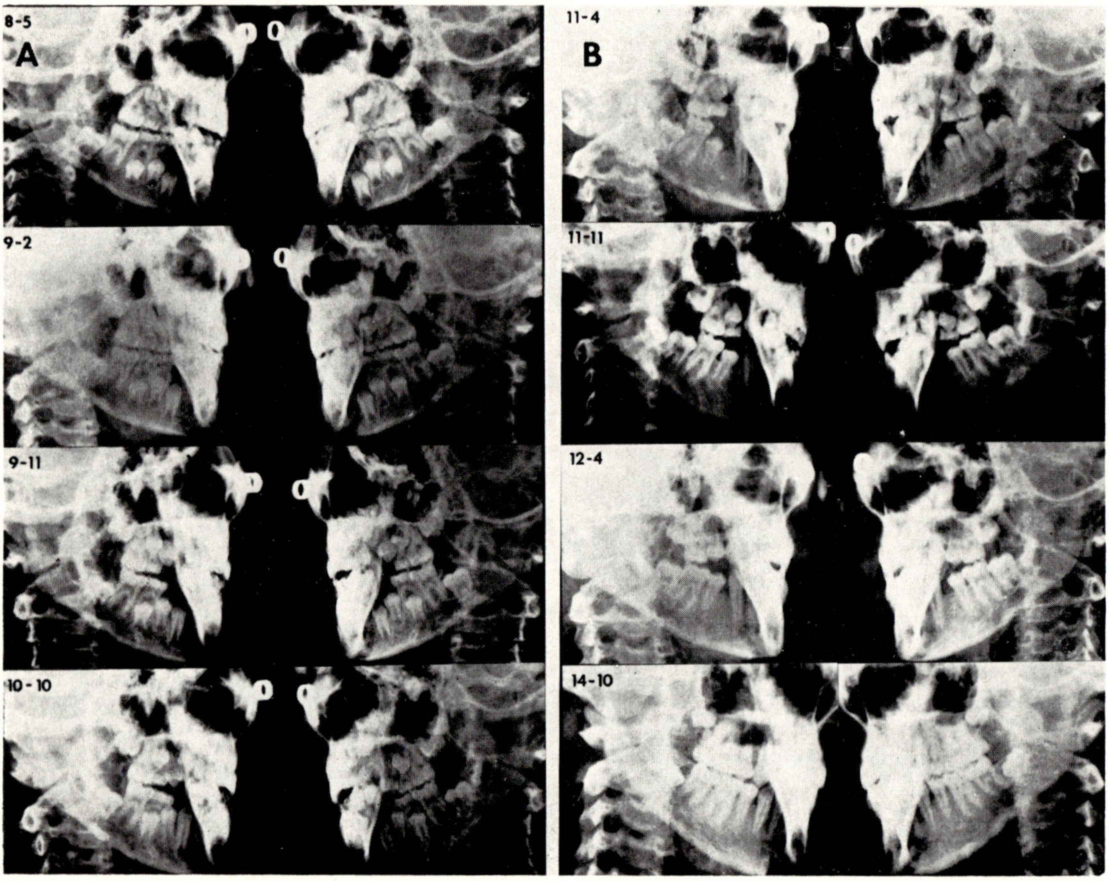

Figure 18-18. Serial oblique roentgencephalometric films utilized to monitor serial extraction from age eight years, five months to age fourteen years, ten months. Note the spontaneous closure of extraction spaces. Orthodontic treatment was essential to correct axial inclinations and level the occlusal plane after age 12–4.

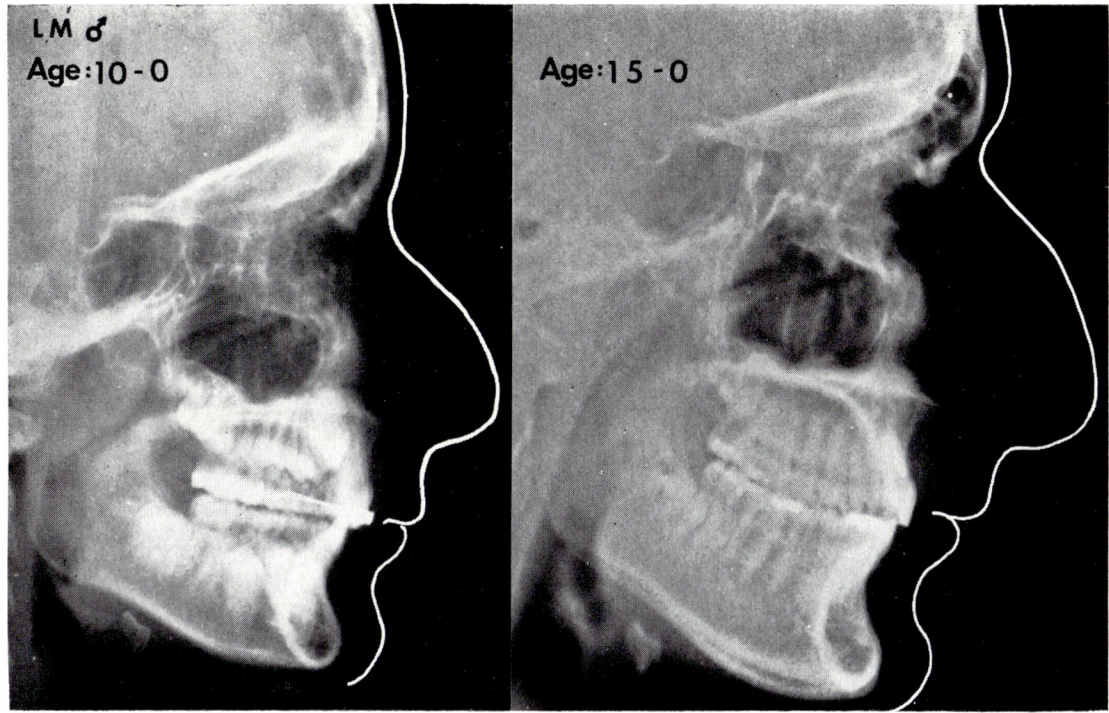

Figure 18-19. Postpubertal growth of the nose. Serial lateral roentgencephalograms demonstrating excessive postpubertal nasal growth and the resultant imbalance in the facial profile. Rhinoplasty to produce a more pleasing profile is indicated in this type of case.

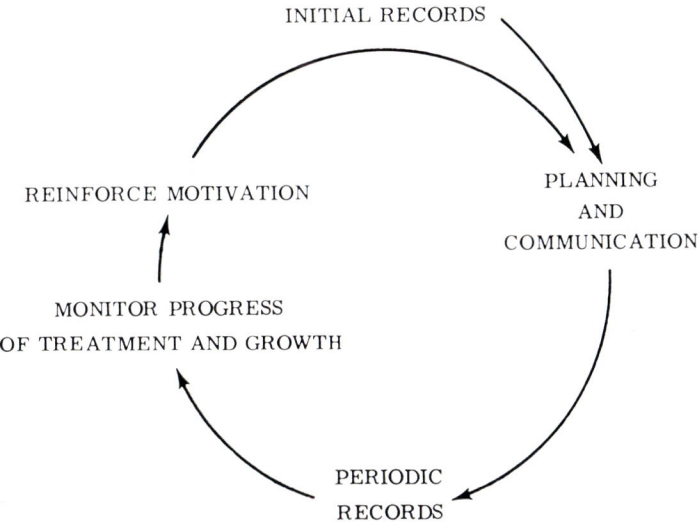

Figure 18-20. A flow chart demonstrating how diagnostic records are employed for treatment planning, counseling, and motivation and to monitor the progress of treatment and growth.

It has not escaped unnoticed that temporomandibular joint crepitus is not an uncommon, though asymptomatic, finding in preschool children.

Another common problem about which there is some controversy has to do with thumbsucking and its effect on the developing dentition. There is no question that prolonged and intense thumbsucking, particularly during the mixed dentition, will result in marked, generally asymmetric, overjet of the maxillary incisors. The controversy is not one of cause-and-effect but has to do with management. The insertion of a palatal crib, in our view, imposes transient and sometimes complicating adaptive muscle habits and speech patterns that require correction at a later time. Alternative methods for correction of this pernicious habit, including patient counseling, should be explored prior to the random prescription of a palatal crib.

PERIAPICAL AND PANORAMIC RADIOGRAPHS

A full series of periapical radiographs are generally supplied by the referring dentist. These are invaluable for the detection of incipient and active carious lesions, for evaluation of the lamina dura and supporting bone and for defining the length and shape of roots.

In recent years, orthodontists have supplanted full-mouth periapical films with the panoramic projection coupled with bite-wing radiographs for the detection of caries. This is particularly true in the young child where a full-mouth series of films are not routinely taken or where such films are difficult to obtain because of discomfort or gagging. The wider area covered by the panoramic radiograph allows the detection of a variety of pathologies which might go undiscovered with the conventional series of periapical films. Such pathologies include cysts, tumors, congenitally missing teeth, supernumerary teeth, impacted teeth and fractures of the condyle (Fig. 18-14).

ROENTGENCEPHALOMETRY

Although roentgencephalometry is generally associated with orthodontic diagnosis and practice, its value transcends its application to orthodontic treatment and is finding increasing and indispensable diagnostic application in maxillofacial surgery, prosthetic and reconstructive dentistry. The technique affords a standardized film, with controlled enlargement and distortion, that allows for reliable measurement. The most common projections employed include lateral, posteroanterior and 45 degree oblique films. Functional analyses can be made by the use of films taken at rest, wide open, sustained phonation of the vowel /u/ or the sibilant /s/ (Figs. 18-15 and 18-16).

The basic evaluation to be made from such radiographs include an estimate of the size and shape of the jaws, their spatial configuration, the position of teeth within the jaws as well as their relationship to the integumental profile. The functional dynamics of jaw movement and labial-lingual musculature can also be assessed from serial films in several postures. In addition, it is possible to prognosticate, within certain limits, ultimate configurations following realization of the full growth potential and maturation of the structures involved. Although a detailed exposition on this subject is beyond the compass of this chapter, it may be useful to make certain general statements.

In his diagnostic considerations, the orthodontist makes use of certain standards of normal development that prevail for boys and girls and which take into account future increments of growth. While such generalizations are useful, the individual must always be considered because chronologic age and developmental age do not always coincide. For example, the child with a precociously erupted permanent dentition may not have achieved his full jaw development, and so a definitive judgment regarding the position of the chin in relation to the facial profile may be premature at an early age (Fig. 18-17).

The utilization of roentgencephalometry as part of a guidance system for self-audit of treatment and growth is indispensable. For example, the use of the lateral and 45 degree oblique projections in a planned program of serial extraction may be used to graphically plot the pattern of craniofacial growth and dental eruption and to determine the most advantageous time for extractions (Fig. 18-18).

The frontal or posteroanterior radiographic projection is generally neglected in orthodontic diagnosis. It is particularly valuable in estimating craniofacial symmetry or, as demonstrated earlier in Figure 18-12, in defining the position of unerupted or impacted canines. The posteroanterior projection can also be employed to define deviations of the nasal septum, asymmetry of the nasal chambers and variations between paired facial structures.

As noted earlier, most children conform to predictive patterns and increments of growth established for the normal child. It is in the case of the unusual child that monitoring with periodic cephalometric films becomes particularly useful. Abnormalities in the growth pattern are important determinants of the type and timing of treatment. For example, the development of an unusual chin point, may affect the predetermined positioning of incisors with respect to the apical base and the integumental profile. By the same token, the development of a large nose during the course of treatment, or subsequent to treatment, will alter facial balance and esthetics. Counseling patient and parents to consider rhinoplasty may be necessary, if the desired esthetic goals are to be achieved (Fig. 18-19).

Aberrant growth changes, whether during active orthodontic treatment or at a later time, can be documented by the orthodontist. The cephalometric film not only provides a method for this monitoring but is also a visual aid that is used in counseling patients and parents (Fig. 18-20).

THE PHOTOGRAPH

The photograph is basic to the diagnostic routine followed in orthodontics. It provides an objective assessment of facial form and a basis for communication between patient and doctor. Of particular concern are the contour of the lips and how they are affected by the position of the teeth. Lip posture may be assessed with the mandible at rest, with the teeth in occlusion or during a swallow. Whether a static or dynamic evaluation, the photograph clearly discloses discrepancies between tooth position and soft tissues and defines abnormal patterns of muscle activity.

Since orthodontic diagnosis and treatment planning are concerned with value judgments regarding aesthetic considerations, it is useful to gain insight into the parental or the patient's self-image. Often by asking the patient, particularly the adult candidate for orthodontic treatment, as to what he sees in his photograph we gain valuable insights concerning self-image and avoid the hazards of imposing one's own value judgments of esthetics on others.

It should be remembered that the patient posing for photographs becomes aware of self-image and postures his lips in a way to minimize, as he thinks best, any dentofacial anomaly that is disturbing to his self-image. These compensatory postures result in discrepancies between what is seen in the radiograph and the photograph and provide an unspoken insight into the patient's self-image.

DENTAL CASTS

Detailed, well-polished, dental casts provide a permanent record of the patient's occlusion. They offer a three-dimensional model which can be examined and measured from a variety of perspectives not possible by direct clinical examination. Such examination includes the simple procedure of counting the teeth in each arch. It is remarkable how frequently it is possible to fail to recognize congenitally missing dental units in an otherwise well-formed arch unless a systematic count is made. Anomalies of dental crowns, cuspal relationships, abnormal wear, gingival recession and erosion are significant findings which may be missed in a routine clinical examination. Finally, dental casts provide an opportunity to estimate or determine arch length requirements by direct measurements of erupted dental units.

AT WHAT AGE SHOULD TREATMENT BEGIN?

If the examination and consultation, as previously outlined, is applied to every child visiting the dentist the following could be expected. First, a variety of pathologies would be detected and treated early. Secondly, orthodontic correction of deciduous crossbite occlusion or the correction of habits may obviate the need for treatment following eruption of the succedaneous teeth. Finally, even if no treatment is instituted, the baseline records—the data base, in the form of casts, photographs or cephalometric radiographs —provide a foundation for the assessment of subsequent growth and development.

When should an adult be referred to an orthodontist? This can be best answered by pointing out that the potential for successful orthodontic treatment is not dependent on chronologic age but on the health of the supporting structures. Orthodontic problems seen in adults are not unlike those observed in children, except they are surrounded by a more complex psyche. Orthodontics for adults can involve full appliance therapy or be limited to the correction of axial inclinations on abutment teeth preliminary to prosthetic restoration.

The armamentaria employed in orthodontic diagnosis can be used as an ancillary service in a variety of prosthetic or restorative procedures. Rest position, free way space and symmetry of mandibular movements are but a few of the many bits of information that can be recorded on film and used in treatment planning. This type of orthodontic diagnostic service is very much like that provided for the physician by the radiologist or laboratory pathologist.

SUMMARY

The rigid data base requirements, consonant with sound orthodontic diagnosis, provide a rational basis for treatment planning and continuous monitoring of dental and craniofacial development. Even more significant is the application of such methodologies and concepts to the wider range of diagnostic problems in general dental practice. Diagnosis of malocclusion is a team enterprise involving the family dentist and orthodontist. It should begin at an early age or as soon as any aberration in tooth development or jaw growth or function is observed. Obtaining a baseline of cephalometric radiographs, dental casts and photographs is a useful device for monitoring a child's growth long before orthodontic treatment is deemed necessary or desirable. By this procedure, the prescription of preventive measures is placed on a rational basis with programmed follow-up.

Orthodontic diagnostic procedures are finding increasing application in the treatment of adults and in cosmetic and reconstructive dental and surgical procedures.

REFERENCES

1. Weed, L. L.: *Medical Records, Medical Education, and Patient Care* (Revised ed.) Chicago, Year Book Medical Publishers, 1970.
2. Solow, B., and Helm, S.: A method for tabulation and statistical evaluation of epidemiological malocclusion data. *Acta Odontol Scand*, 26:63–88, 1968.

Chapter 19

The Role of the Oral Surgeon in Oral Diagnosis and Treatment Planning

STANLEY KENNETT

IN RECENT YEARS, there have been significant changes in the scope of oral surgery. This has been, undoubtedly, due to the advent of antibiotics, advances in anesthesia and a better understanding of oral physiology and anatomy. Not only has it been possible to develop new major oral surgical procedures, but there has been a revival of older techniques, particularly from Europe which were discarded because of problems such as sepsis and difficulties in anesthesia.

Although the general dental practitioner has an appreciation of the scope of oral surgery, he may not be entirely aware of the oral surgeon's role in preprosthetic surgery, in the treatment of facial deformities and in the replantation and transplantation of teeth. It is important for the dentist to have some knowledge of the various procedures which are available. Although he need not know the details of these operative procedures, he should have an intelligent appreciation of the various techniques together with some of their advantages and disadvantages so that he can properly advise his patients.

PREPOSTHETIC SURGERY

"An artificial appliance, no matter how correct it may be in its construction and in the mode of its application, cannot be worn with impunity in a diseased mouth." This statement made by C. A. Harris [1] in 1855 summarizes the aims of oral surgery regarding prosthodontics, since all procedures are aimed at correcting conditions in the oral cavity which make the wearing of dentures unsatisfactory. Before discussing these procedures, however, it is essential to recognize the ideal situation which should exist before denture construction is undertaken.

1. The dental ridges should be of sufficient surface area to provide adequate support. Equally important is that they be smooth and rounded with no undercuts or protuberances.

2. The soft tissue covering the ridges should be healthy and firm.

3. There should be adequate depth of sulci. In this respect, however, it should be noted that normal peripheral tissue elasticity is equally as important.

4. There should be no abnormally high muscle attachments, frena or fibrous bands present which could displace the denture.

5. The mandibular and maxillary ridges should be in normal relationship to each other.

Considering these criteria, it is possible

to discuss the various surgical procedures under several headings: bony abnormalities, soft tissue abnormalities and atrophic dental ridge.

Bony Abnormalities
Sharp and Irregular Ridges

Prophylaxis should be mentioned here at the outset. The construction of satisfactory dentures commences with the extraction of the teeth. Unfortunately, this old adage is often forgotten and is responsible for the great majority of minor prosthetic difficulties.

Atraumatic planned exodontia with trimming of sharp bony spicules and careful suturing will prevent many cases of sharp or uneven dental ridges. In the surgical removal of roots, impacted teeth, cysts, etcetera, every effort must be made to preserve bone, particularly the alveolar crest. This may often be accomplished by a lateral approach—the "buccal window" method in the case of the deeply buried root or impaction (Fig. 19-1). The osteoplastic "flap" is another example of bone and ridge preservation. It may be employed in the removal of the unerupted canine in the palate. In this technique, the bony flap is hinged buccally and following removal of the tooth is replaced, the original contour thus being preserved (Fig. 19-2).

In the diagnosis of abnormal ridges, it is important to differentiate the undercut ridge from the sharp ridge, as the treatment may be quite different. In the latter, all that is usually required is a general recontouring using vulcanite burrs (Fig. 19-3). In the former, however, the aim should be to fill out the undercut areas thus preserving ridge height (Fig. 19-4). This may be accomplished by packing material such as sulphadiazine, oxidized cellulose or bone into the undercut area.

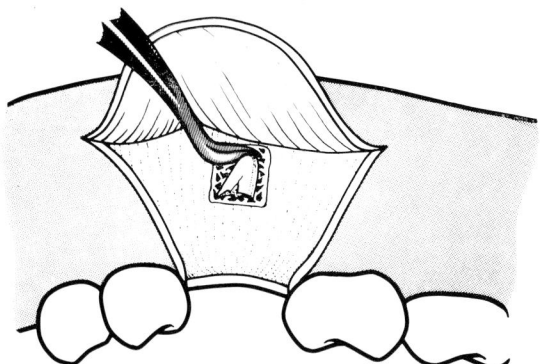

Figure 19-1. The removal of a root via the "buccal window" approach. Note the preservation of the alveolar crest.

MYLOHYOID RIDGE. In cases where sharp or overhanging mylohyoid ridges prevent the correct extension of the lingual flange of the denture, these may be surgically removed. This procedure may be accompanied by repositioning of the posterior portion of the mylohyoid muscle at a lower level if a deeper lingual sulcus is required (Fig. 19-5).

ALVEOLECTOMY. This term is used to denote removal of alveolar bone. When the major portion of the alveolus is removed, the term "radical alveolectomy" is employed. The latter technique popularized in the early 1900's was at first used extensively as it had the advantage of a greatly reduced postextraction healing time and produced what appeared to be an excellent dental ridge. However, since that time it has fallen into disrepute as it was shown that excessive ridge resorption rapidly took place. The technique should now be reserved for cases where there is an abnormal ridge relationship which prevents the correct positioning of the artificial teeth from an esthetic or functional point of view (Fig. 19-6). Careful planning in these cases is essential. Study models must be prepared and trimmed to the desired amount, keeping in mind that bone re-

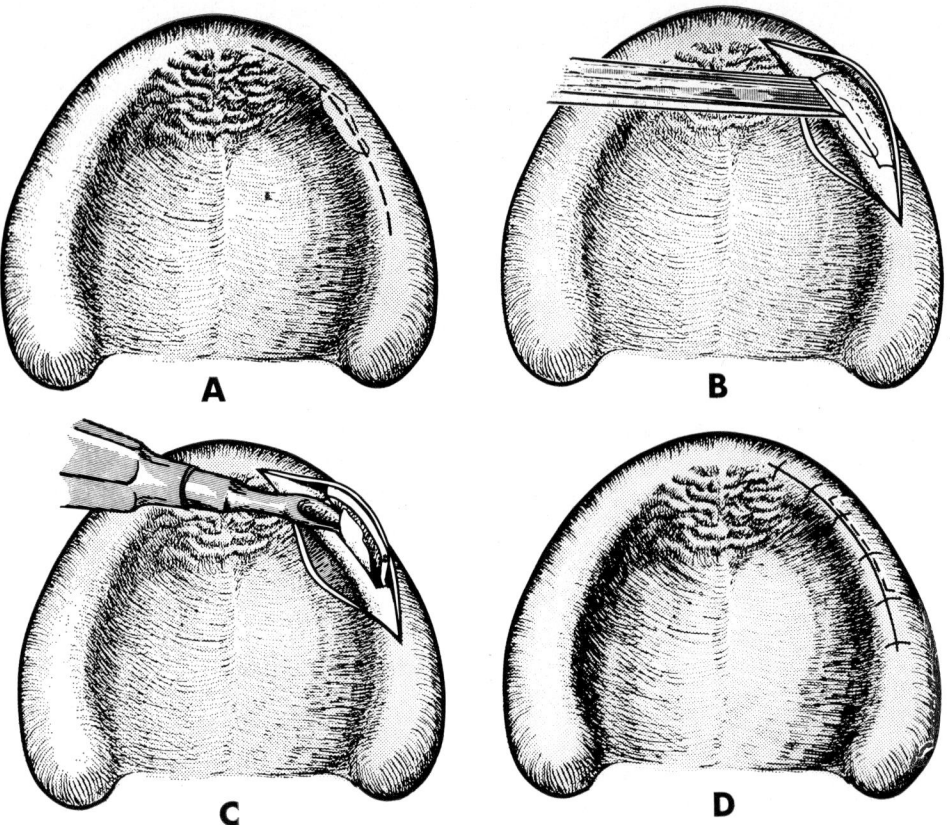

Figure 19-2. The osteoplastic flap technique for the removal of an unerupted canine. (A) Incision. (B) Raising the osteoplastic flap with a chisel. (C) Elevation of the canine. (D) Replacement of osteoplastic flap.

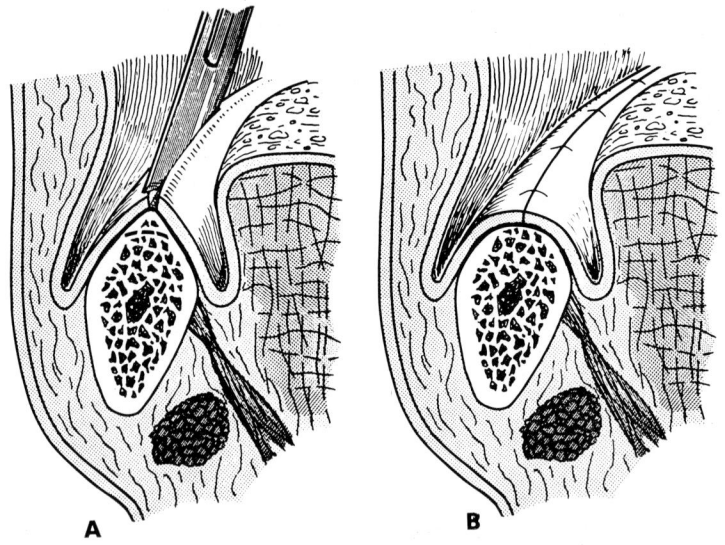

Figure 19-3. Trimming of a sharp mandibular ridge. Cross section through mandible. (A) Area to be trimmed indicated by dotted line. Note position of incision on alveolar crest. (B) Recontoured ridge. Depth of sulcus maintained.

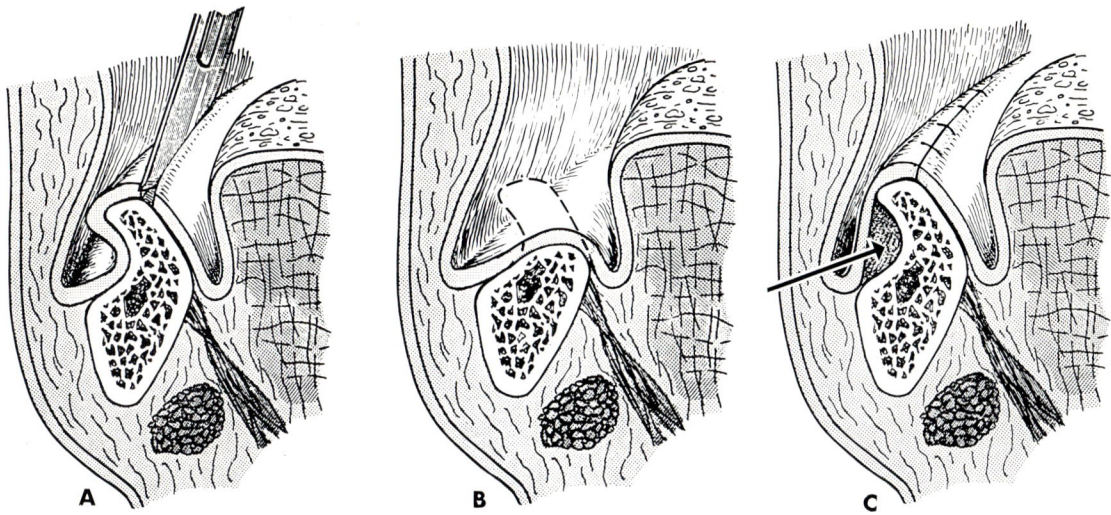

Figure 19-4. Treatment of undercut alveolar ridge. (A) Severely undercut mandibular ridge. (B) Incorrect technique. Removal leading to loss of ridge height and shallow sulci. (C) Correct method. Undercut area packed with bone (see arrow). Ridge height and depth of sulci preserved.

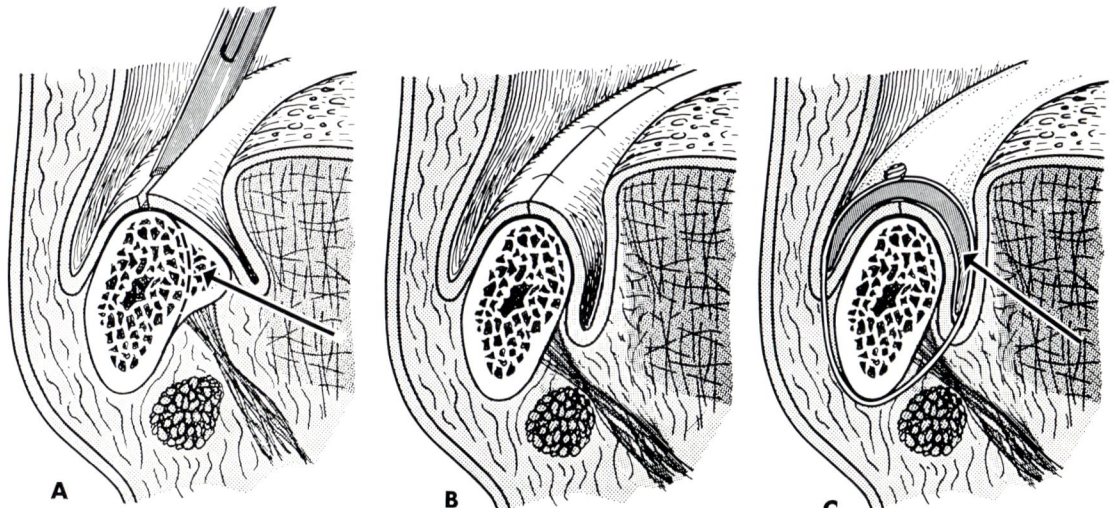

Figure 19-5. Mylohyoid ridge resection and lowering of posterior part of mylohyoid muscle. (A) Undercut mylohyoid ridge (see arrow). (B) Mylohyoid ridge removed and muscle freed. (C) Splint (see arrow) circumferentially wired to mandible. Required to maintain new position of mylohyoid muscle.

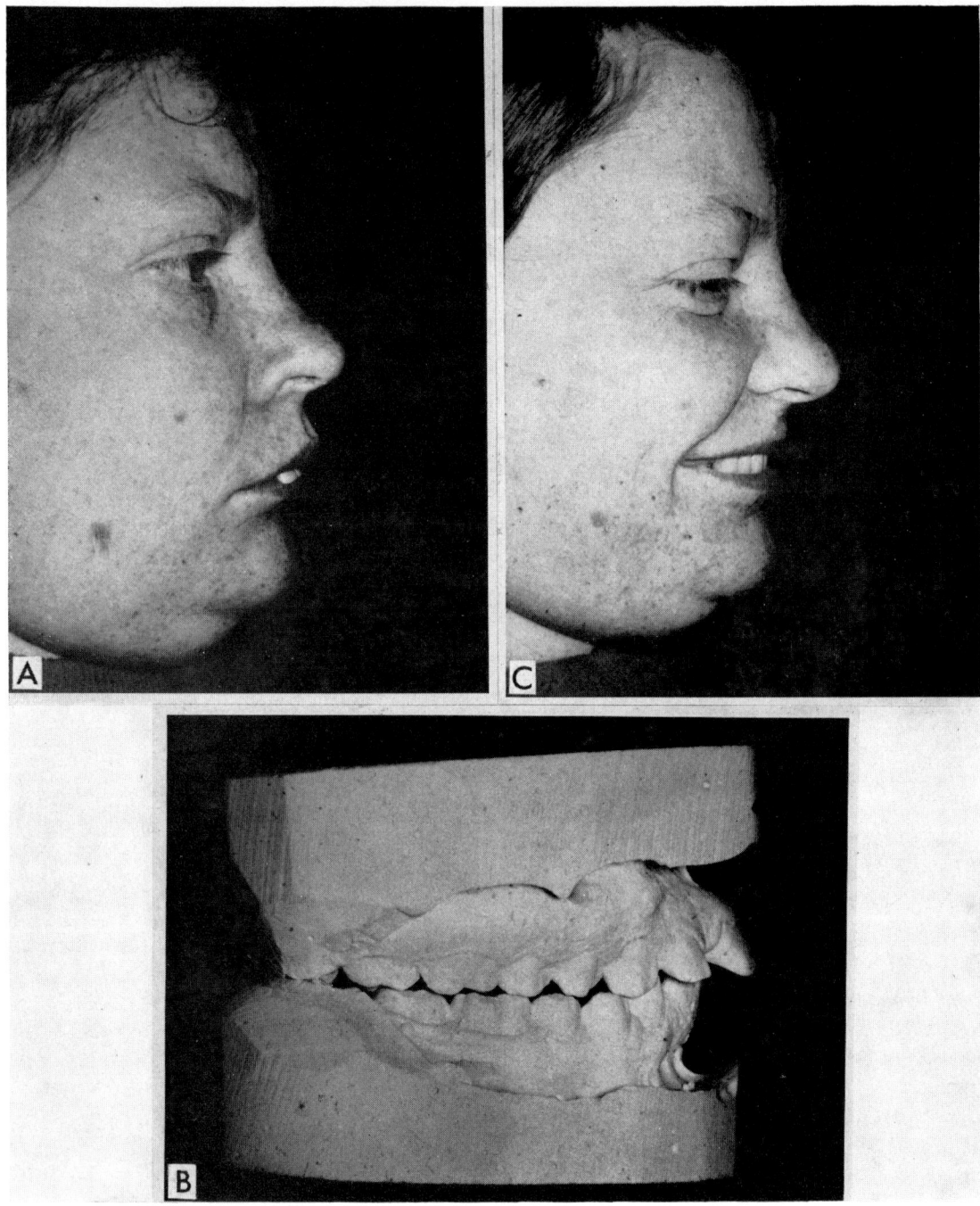

Figure 19-6. Radical alveolectomy. (A) Class II profile. (B) Study models. Note Class II relationship, closed bite with insufficient intermaxillary space for denture construction. (C) Postoperative result after radical alveolectomy and immediate denture insertion.

moval should be kept to a minimum. The use of a clear acrylic template made to the trimmed model is of value in this respect.

Enlarged Maxillary Tuberosities

Great care must be taken in assessing the indications for tuberosity reduction. A disservice may, in fact, be rendered if a large tuberosity is reduced which may have proved useful in the retention of the denture. Similarly, a unilateral undercut tuberosity may be helpful in this respect and does not necessarily require surgical intervention. However, excessive or bilateral undercut areas will interfere with denture insertion. Enlarged tuberosities that encroach on the intermaxillary space must be reduced and recontoured as there may be insufficient space for correct denture extension. The maxillary tuberosities may be enlarged either because of fibrous hypertrophy or bony exostoses. The former is by far more commonly responsible. It is important to distinguish between these two causes clinically since the surgical techniques vary in each case. Radiographs are essential in this respect and these also help in establishing the possible presence of associated pathological features. A not uncommon finding is the presence of an unerupted wisdom tooth which is causing the enlargement. It should be remembered that fibrous dysplasia, Paget's disease of bone and occasionally down-growth of a carcinoma of the maxillary antrum may be responsible (Fig. 19-7). Surgical technique in the case of the fibrous tuberosity entails an elliptical excision of the central wedge of tissue over the tuberosity followed by the undermining of the buccal and palatal

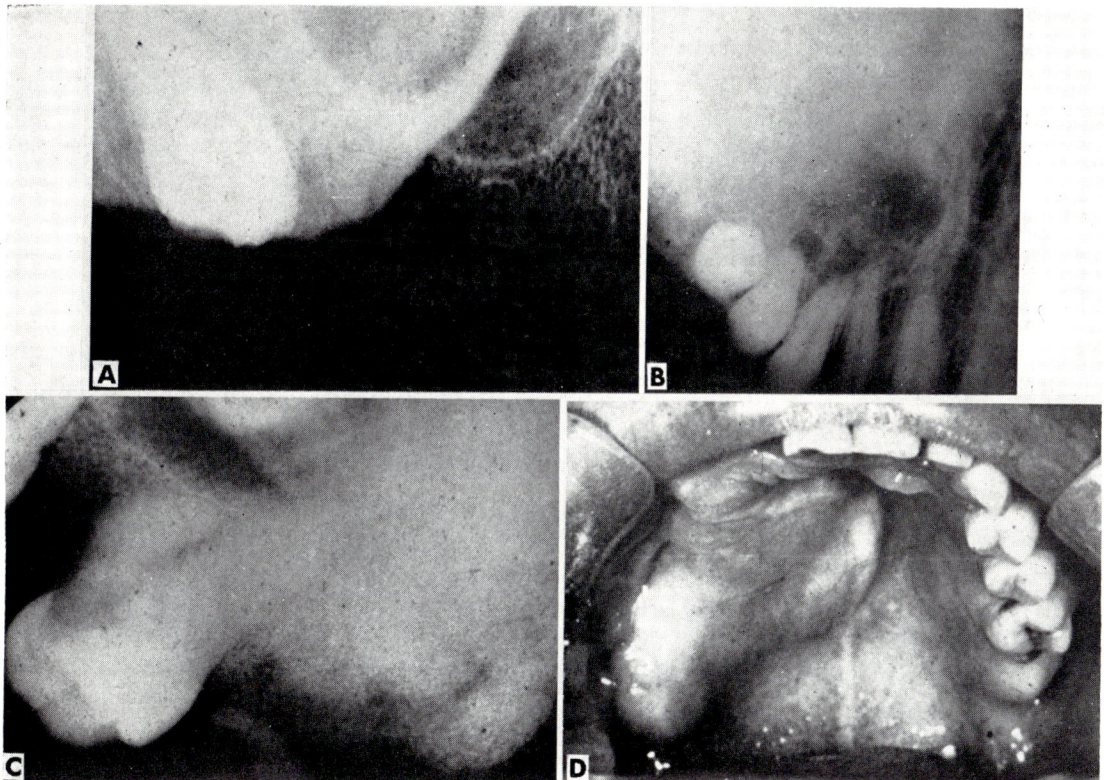

Figure 19-7. Some causes of enlarged maxillary tuberosities. (A) Unerupted wisdom tooth. (B) Paget's disease. (C) Fibrous dysplasia. (D) Carcinoma of maxillary antrum.

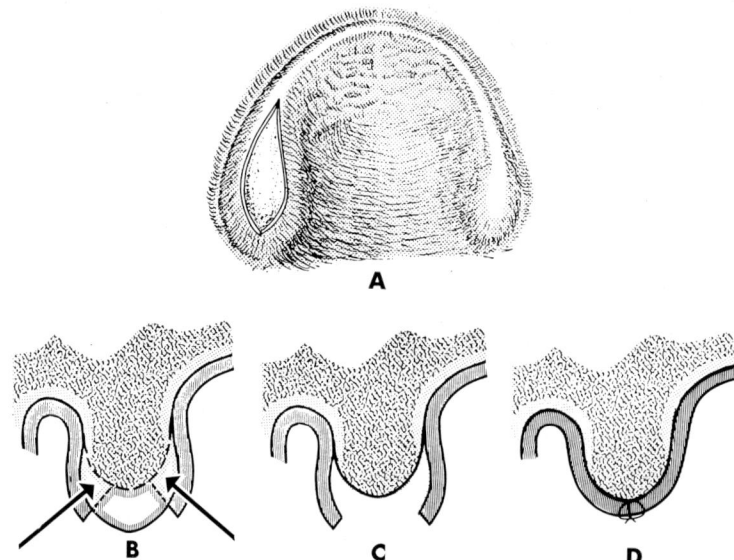

Figure 19-8. Technique of reduction of enlarged maxillary tuberosities. (A) Incision outline. (B) Removal of central wedge and undermining of mucosa (see arrows). (C) Area removed. (D) Mucosa sutured.

mucosa in that area and its closure by suturing (Fig. 19-8). If bony exostoses are involved, a conventional mucoperiosteal flap must be raised in the area and the bone removed with burrs, rongeurs or chisels.

Torus Palatinus

This is an example of an exostosis occurring in the midline of the hard palate. It is probably the result of an overlapping and fusion of the medial surfaces of the palatal processes of the maxilla leading to the formation of a single protuberance. Approximately 20 percent of adults are affected and it is said to be more prevalent among certain races such as the Eskimos.[2] The clinical appearance may vary from a smooth oval swelling in the vault of the palate to a multilobed structure. It consists of dense compact bone with minimal cancellous bone occasionally present in the center. The exostosis shows up as a distinct radiopaque area on occlusal and lateral jaw radiographs.

Surgical removal is indicated in those cases where relief of the denture over that area will result in loss of retention (Fig. 19-9). Pressure ulceration is also extremely common as the mucosa overlying a torus is extremely thin.

Torus Mandibularis

This is another example of an exostosis. It occurs on the lingual aspect of the mandible in the cuspid or bicuspid region and may be unilateral or bilateral. There is con-

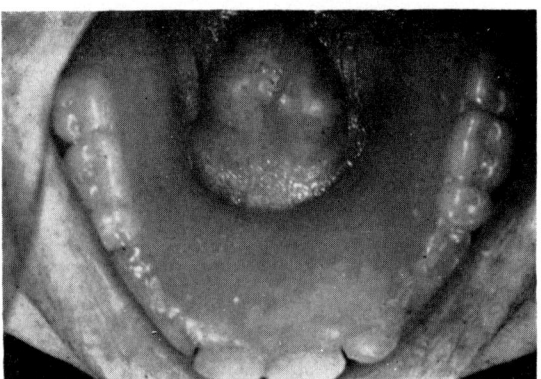

Figure 19-9. Torus palatinus interfering with correct extension of maxillary denture.

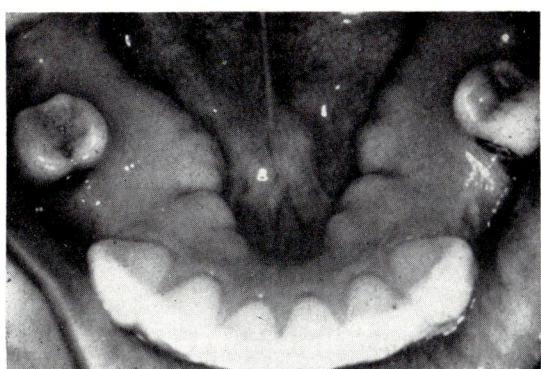

Figure 19-10. Torus mandibularis. Note multilobular nature of the abnormality.

siderable variation in its appearance which may vary from a small globular excrescence to a large multilobed projection occupying a major portion of the floor of the mouth (Fig. 19-10).

Surgical removal, as in torus palatinus, is again only required if interference with a lower denture is likely.

Soft Tissue Abnormalities

Epulis Fissuratum (Denture Hyperplasia)

The prolonged wearing of ill-fitting dentures is often responsible for inflammatory mucosal hyperplasia known as epulis fissuratum and which appears in the oral cavity as redundant folds of mucous membrane. The size is dependent largely upon such factors as patient tolerance, tissue tolerance and the length of time the ill-fitting denture has been present. The appearance may vary from small tags of redundant mucosa attached to the alveolar ridge to extremely complex variegated folds of tissue completely obliterating the sulcus.

Surgical removal is almost invariably indicated together with removal of the cause of irritation which in most instances necessitates either modification or construction of a new denture. Removal is necessary as these redundant folds not only provide an unstable base for dentures but also cause reduction in the depth of the sulci. Furthermore, denture hyperplasia may occasionally be associated with chronic ulceration and frank malignancy (Fig. 19-11). It would be an overstatement to say that the lesion is premalignant, but it is true to say that whenever chronic irritation is of long duration, the possibility of neoplastic change must be considered. In this respect, it becomes imperative that all tissue removed be sent for histopathological examination.

In planning operative procedures several important features must be borne in mind. The denture should be left out for a period of two to three weeks prior to surgery. This will not only cause considerable shrinkage of the hyperplastic tissue but will reduce the inflammatory hyperemia. Both these factors will facilitate surgery. Removal of the redundant tissue is relatively straightforward. However, closure of the resulting defect may present difficulties, a factor which the general practitioner should be aware of. In some instances, primary closure of the wound may be possible, but in others more complex procedures such as secondary epithelializa-

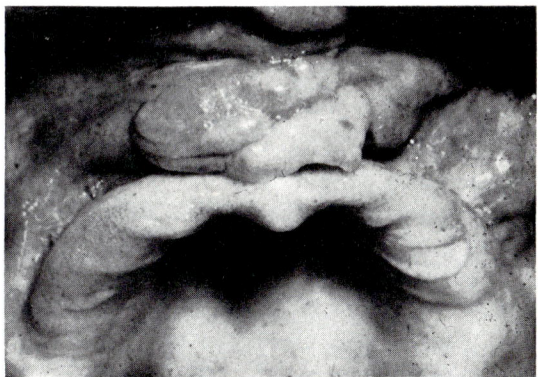

Figure 19-11. Denture hyperplasia in maxillary frenum area which was associated with an early squamous cell carcinoma.

tion vestibuloplasty or split skin grafting (*see* under surgical techniques) may have to be used. If numerous redundant folds are to be removed, each fold should be excised separately; a wide excision which incorporates all the folds in their entirety should not be employed. If the former method is used, the defect will be minimal and closure accomplished with little difficulty often obviating the need for skin grafting procedures.

Another important aspect in planning is the concept that oral mucous membrane postoperatively requires close adaptation to underlying submucosal tissue to prevent hematoma formation, displacement and scarring. This is rarely accomplished by sutures alone and additional support by means of splints may be required. The patient's own dentures adjusted with modeling compound or lined with a zinc oxide eugenol paste may be employed for this purpose.

Abnormal Muscle Attachments, Frena, Scar Bands

These entities are found particularly in the labial and buccal sulci. Except for anatomical structures such as the maxillary labial frenum, the great majority of bands and so-called abnormal muscle attachments are, in fact, due to scar formation following poor exodontic technique. Their removal is often desirable as full utilization of the sulcus is interfered with and displacement of the denture will occur if the prosthesis is not relieved over the band.

Various surgical techniques are available and include diamond-shaped excision of the band with subsequent undermining of

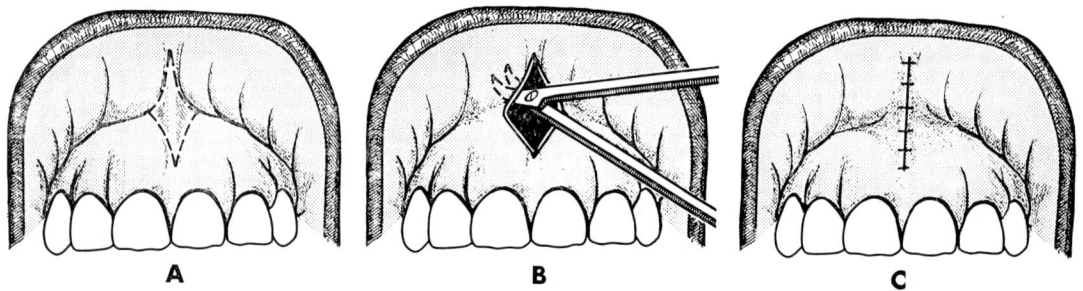

Figure 19-12. Diamond-shaped method of excising a labial maxillary frenum. (A) Outline of incision. (B) Undermining the mucosa. (C) Mucosa sutured.

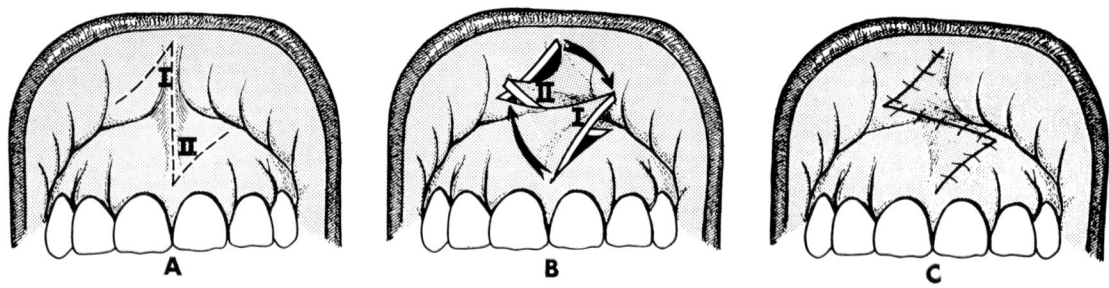

Figure 19-13. "Z" plasty method for treating a maxillary labial frenum. (A) Outline of incision. (B) Transportation of flaps. Note new positions of flap apices I and II. (C) Incisions sutured. Note the new horizontal position of the frenum.

the adjoining oral mucosa in order to close the defect (Fig. 19-12). Certain "plastic" procedures such as the "Z" plasty is a useful alternative in selected cases (Fig. 19-13).

Atrophic Dental Ridge

Despite the advances made in the prosthodontic field, there still remain, particularly in the older age group, a significant number of patients who, because of atrophy of the alveolar ridges and loss of sulci, cannot wear dentures satisfactorily. In the past decade there has been a revival of interest in these cases initiated by the introduction of new techniques, particularly from Europe. Basically, these procedures entail a repositioning of tissues on the bone with the object of extending the depth of the sulcus and increasing the amount of ridge available as a denture bearing area. If there is insufficient bone present, as is often the case in the atrophic mandible or maxilla, these procedures alone would be obviously unsuccessful and it is possible to supplement the dental ridges using materials such as cartilage or bone as free grafts.

Surgical Techniques

Although there are numerous operations advocated to obtain these objectives, only some of the more common techniques will be described.

SUBMUCOSAL VESTIBULOPLASTY. This procedure is applicable in the maxilla where the clinical ridge is inadequate due to muscle or mucosal attachment to the crest of the ridge. Redundant connective tissue between the mucosa and periosteum is removed through a small midline incision by tunneling as far back as the tuberosity area on both sides. The mucosa is then readapted directly to the periosteum, thereby increasing vestibular height (Fig. 19-14). This technique gives excellent results provided certain conditions are ful-

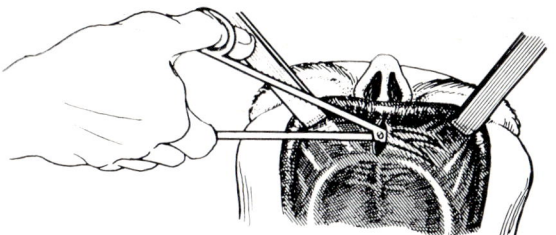

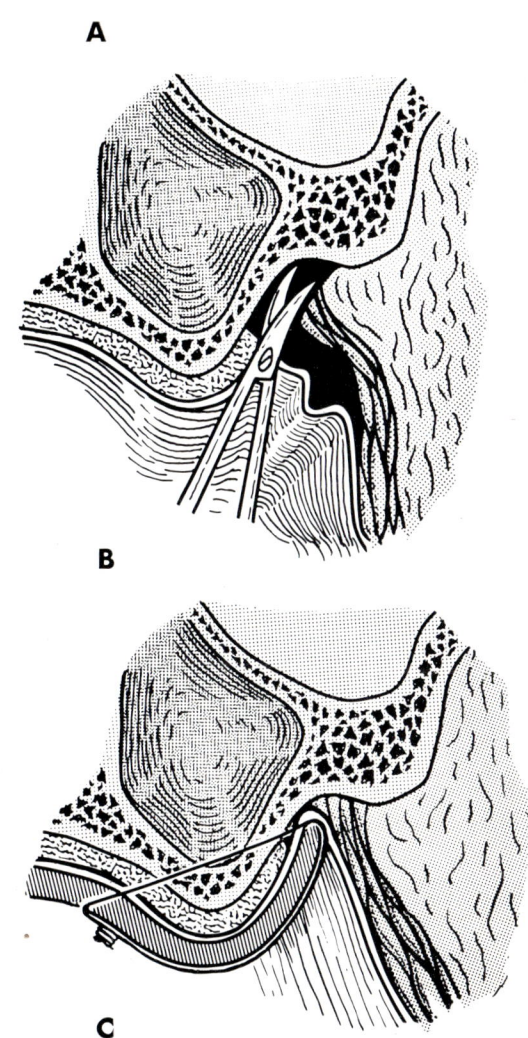

Figure 19-14. Submucosal vestibuloplasty. (A) Midline incision and supraperiosteal dissection. (B) Cross section through maxilla illustrating area where connective tissue (black zone) has been removed. (C) Splint *in situ* retained by peralveolar wire. Note increased depth of sulcus.

filled. The bone must be of sufficient height to support a denture and the mucosa must be absolutely healthy. A simple clinical test described by Obwegeser[3] is the placing of a mouth mirror into the labial sulcus displacing the vestibule as far as it prosthetically required and observing if the lip is elevated and drawn inwards. If this occurs, there is insufficient mucosa for this technique to be effective. It also is not advisable to carry this out in the mandible since being a somewhat blind procedure, damage to the mental nerve is likely.

SECONDARY EPITHELIALIZATION VESTIBULOPLASTY. This procedure is applicable to both jaws and consists of elevating a mucosal flap. Supraperiosteal dissection is then carried out as far, superiorly or inferiorly, as is permitted by anatomical factors. This results in a release of tissues laterally away from the alveolus and a new increased sulcus depth is obtained by suturing the free edge of the mucosal flap as high up as possible to the periosteum in the maxilla and as low down as possible in the mandible. The periosteum overlying the bone which has thus been exposed is left uncovered and allowed to epithelialize over, hence the name of the procedure.

The main principle which this technique is based upon is that raw areas on bony surfaces cannot contract. However, there is some tendency postoperatively for the tissues to return to their previous attachment and as much as 50 percent of the new sulcus may be lost. In view of this, it becomes important in these cases for overcorrection to be obtained in the first instance.

SKIN GRAFTING. This procedure is similar to secondary epithelialization vestibuloplasty but differs in that the mucosa after dissection is not sutured to the periosteum and the raw area is not allowed to epithelialize over. Instead the raw surface is covered by a split thickness skin graft usually taken from the inner aspect of the thigh. The graft is retained by a denture lined with modeling compound. The denture, in turn, is attached to the mandible or maxilla by circumferential or peralveolar wires and retained for ten days (Fig. 19-15).

MUCOSAL GRAFTS. The use of skin in the oral cavity has the disadvantage that a second distant operation site is involved. Furthermore, as skin is relatively inelastic, the peripheral seal between the denture and the grafted area is not as good as normal mucosa. For these reasons, techniques have been recently evolved where free mucosal grafts instead of skin are used. The mucosa may be obtained from the cheek by means of a fine dermatome or palatal mucosa may be used. Initial results with these techniques have been extremely promising, but as yet it is too early to assess the long-term results.

TUBEROPLASTY. A not infrequent finding is the loss or atrophy of the maxillary tuberosity. This may be due to excessive resorption or damage occurring during the extraction of the maxillary molar teeth. As this area is vital in obtaining a peripheral seal in denture construction, the procedure of tuberoplasty has been devised. The operation entails the raising of a mucosal flap distal to the tuberosity and the cutting of the attachments of the medial pterygoid and tensor palati muscles to the tuberosity, thus providing access to the fissure between the tuberosity and the pterygoid plate. A chisel is then used to separate these structures, thereby gaining additional depth distal to the tuberosity. The free mucosa is then sutured to the periosteum as high up as possible. The raw defect created is allowed to granulate over or may be covered with a skin graft. The early results of this procedure are extremely encouraging although some regression of tis-

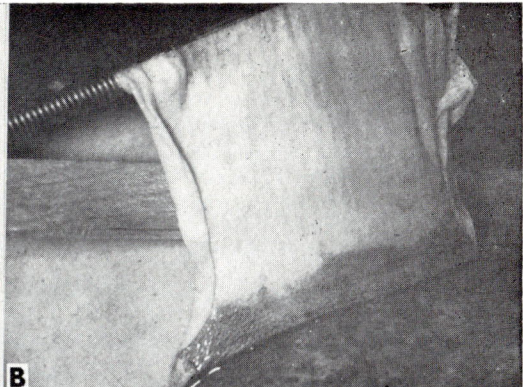

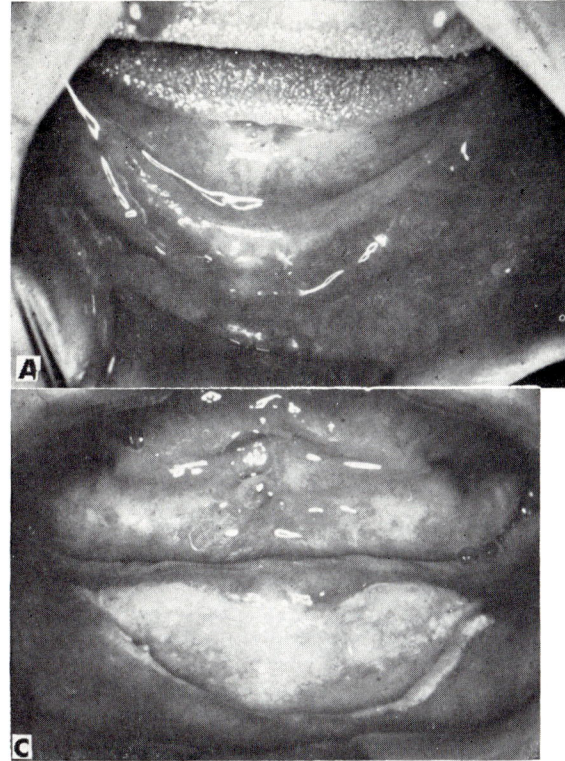

Figure 19-15. Epithelial inlay. (A) Mandibular ridge with shallow labial sulcus. (B) Split skin graft from inner aspect of thigh. (C) Epithelial inlay three months postoperatively. Note new depth of labial sulcus.

sues and loss of depth postoperatively does occur.

LOWERING OF THE FLOOR OF THE MOUTH. In patients where there has been loss of sulci, but there is sufficient mandible present, it is possible by lowering the entire floor of the mouth to make more bone available to serve as a dental ridge.

The technique involves two mucosal incisions, one slightly buccal and the other slightly lingual to the alveolar crest and extending from the retromolar fossa of one side to the retromolar fossa of the opposite side. The mylohyoid muscle is then detached from its insertion together with the superior portion of the genioglossus. On the buccal aspect a supraperiosteal dissection is carried out as far laterally and inferiorly as is required. Great care is taken to avoid injuring the mental nerves. A series of sutures connecting the free margins of both buccal and lingual mucosa are passed under the mandible and tied so that the flaps are drawn down towards the inferior border of the mandible (Fig. 19-16). Impressions are taken utilizing a preprepared stent which is then used to carry a skin graft to the buccal aspect of the exposed mandible. The stent and graft are retained *in situ* for approximately ten days by means of circumferential wires or nylon sutures. After this time a definitive denture is constructed. The technique gives excellent results, but it must be remembered that it is a major oral surgical procedure and as such should be reserved only for cases which are exceptionally difficult from the prosthetic point of view.

RIDGE GRAFTING. As mentioned previously in those cases where bone resorption is so advanced that maximum ridge exposure by any of the vestibuloplasty techniques discussed would be insufficient for denture retention, various ridge grafting

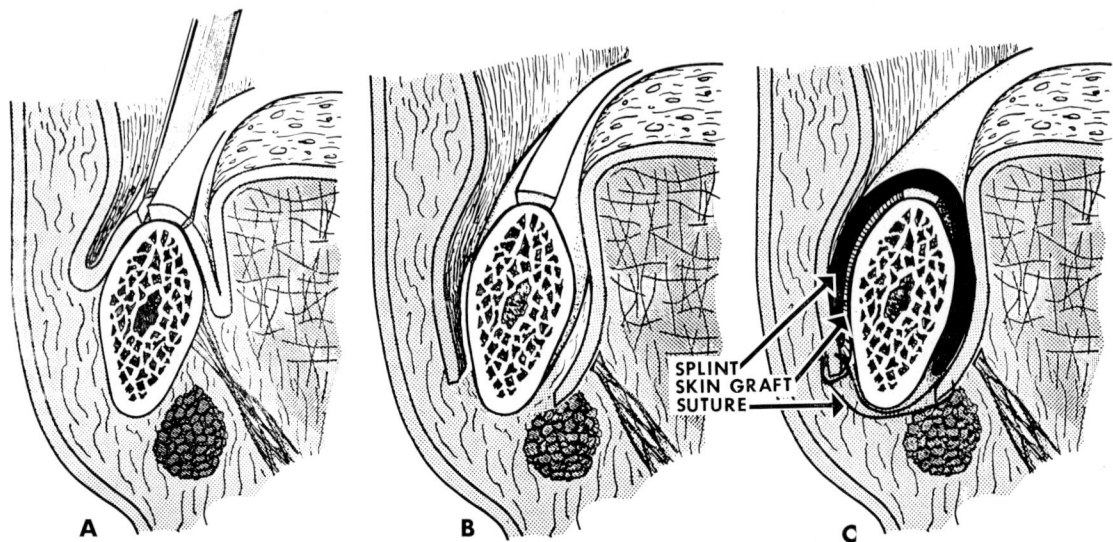

Figure 19-16. Lowering of floor of mouth (Obwegeser technique). Cross sections through mandible. (A) Buccal and lingual incisions. (B) Dissection involving detachment of mylohyoid muscle on lingual and buccal supraperiosteal dissection. (C) Buccal and lingual mucosal flaps sutured under lower border of mandible. Note skin graft on buccal aspect and splint in place.

procedures may be used. Numerous types of materials have been tried in this respect including allelografts such as acrylic, silicone, stainless steel and homografts of cadaver bone. All these, however, are foreign bodies and are rejected by the tissues in a great number of cases. By far the most success has been achieved when autogenous bone grafts utilizing iliac crest or rib have been employed. The bone is contoured to fit the shape of the existing alveolar ridge and inserted subperiosteally. Stabilization is achieved by means of direct wiring. Good tissue coverage of the graft is essential and this necessitates considerable undermining of the mucosa with subsequent further loss of sulci. In view of this feature a further vestibuloplasty procedure must be performed at a later date before denture construction may be undertaken.

Summary

From the foregoing, the scope of oral surgery in the preparation of the mouths for dentures may be divided into minor and major procedures. The former would include most of the conditions discussed in the first two sections, and these techniques should be used routinely and without hesitation in the relevant situation. When the patient has an atrophic jaw, major procedures are required to remedy this defect and many of these have not been widely accepted on this continent. This fact must be taken into account in the treatment planning and weighed carefully against the difficulties which the patient is experiencing prosthetically. This may be summarized in the following manner.

Mandible

1. *Atrophy more marked in posterior region.* Mylohyoid ridge resection with lowering of the mylohyoid muscle in the posterior region may overcome this problem by increasing the depth of the lingual flanges thus giving added lateral stability.

2. *Atrophy associated with anterior*

region and marked mentalis muscle activity. Skin grafting vestibuloplasty is the method of choice in dealing with this problem. The mentalis muscle may be detached and repositioned at the same time.

3. *General atrophy and loss of sulci, but sufficient mandible present.* This is the ideal case for a "lowering of the floor of the mouth" (Obwegeser) procedure. The severity of the operation must be explained to the patient.

4. *Atrophy, loss of sulci and insufficient bone present.* There is no really satisfactory method for dealing with this problem. However, if the patient is determined to wear dentures and all other methods have failed, the use of an iliac autogenous bone graft to the ridge followed by lowering of the mouth or vestibuloplasty would give the best chance of success. It must be emphasized that this procedure is still experimental and the long-term results have not been assessed, particularly in respect to the further resorption of the graft.

Maxilla

1. *Loss of sulcus.* Secondary epithelialization vestibuloplasty is probably the treatment of choice. It may be eventually replaced, however, by mucous membrane grafting when this technique is simplified. The use of skin is contraindicated in the maxilla as the peripheral seal is not as adequate because of the inelastic qualities of skin when compared with mucous membrane.

2. *Submucosal vestibuloplasty.* This technique has a limited place in the treatment of the atrophic maxillary ridge since the conditions necessary for its satisfactory use are rarely present.

3. *Loss of tuberosities.* Tuberoplasty should be carried out in these cases. It is a more minor procedure than bone grafting the tuberosity and despite some regression of the sulcus created, retention of the denture is considerably improved.

4. *Extreme maxillary atrophy.* As in the mandible, bone grafting may have to be carried out in severe cases if all other methods have proved unsatisfactory.

FACIAL DEFORMITIES

In the management of facial deformities, the oral surgeon is concerned mainly with the treatment of those acquired and developmental conditions of the jaws associated with excessive degrees of malocclusion. The single most important reason for the correction of these deformities is an esthetic one, for it is well known that a patient's personality is dependent to a large extent on facial appearance. The entire mental outlook may be changed by successful surgery.

It should be mentioned at the outset that possibly in no other branch of dentistry is the close cooperation of the various clinical disciplines so essential. Orthodontics plays an integral role in this respect and surgical correction should not be undertaken without prior consultation.

Conversely, it must be realized that the scope of successful orthodontic therapy is mainly limited to dento-alveolar abnormalities and that where there is marked basal bone discrepancy, orthodontic treatment can only alter facial growth pattern to a limited extent. The scope of surgical correction, however, is not limited solely to these cases. In many instances, orthodontic treatment may be unavailable or unacceptable to the patient for such reasons as financial or the length of time appliances have to be worn. Furthermore, the older patient is more difficult to treat orthodontically even for dento-alveolar abnormalities.

From the above considerations, it is possible to classify the more common facial deformities which are amenable to surgical correction: (a) prognathism—mandibular and maxillary; (b) micrognathic—mandibular and maxillary; (c) apertognathia; (d) mandibular asymmetry; (e) chin correction; and (f) orthodontic surgery (dento-alveolar surgery).

Diagnosis and Treatment Planning

In establishing a diagnosis and formulating a treatment plan the following are important: (a) clinical assessment, (b) cephalometry and (c) study models.

Clinical Assessment

In all facial deformities, it is essential to arrive at the correct diagnosis and treatment plan, not only at the local "jaw level" but after considering the patient as a whole. A patient with mandibular prognathism may, in fact, be suffering from acromegaly and obviously surgical treatment in such a case will result in relapse. Similarly, surgery prior to the cessation of skeletal growth will result in failure since stability of the corrected facial skeleton is the most important criterion of success. Thus surgery before the late teens is unwise in most cases. Psychological considerations must be taken into account and far better results are obtained if the patient requests surgery for esthetic reasons rather than the practitioner insisting on surgery with a view to increasing masticatory efficiency. Clinical assessment must include a thorough examination of the teeth and their periodontal status. A complete radiographic survey is essential in this respect. It is futile to subject a patient to major jaw surgery if the prognosis of the teeth is poor and a comparable result could be achieved by means of prosthodontics.

Any existing abnormal patterns of behavior must be noted. Habits such as thumb and lip sucking or tongue thrust, if not corrected, will result in relapse following surgery.

Cephalometry

This branch of radiography has now become an essential and integral part of preoperative planning. Its importance lies in the fact that in many cases it is not possible to decide in which jaw the abnormality lies. Thus at first sight a case of prominence of the lower jaw may not be due to mandibular prognathism but, in fact, to under-

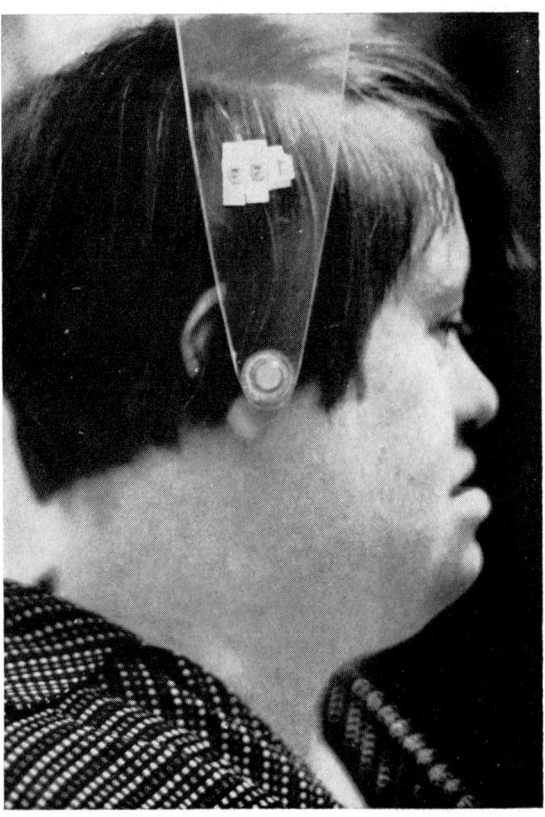

Figure 19-17. Pseudomandibular prognathism.

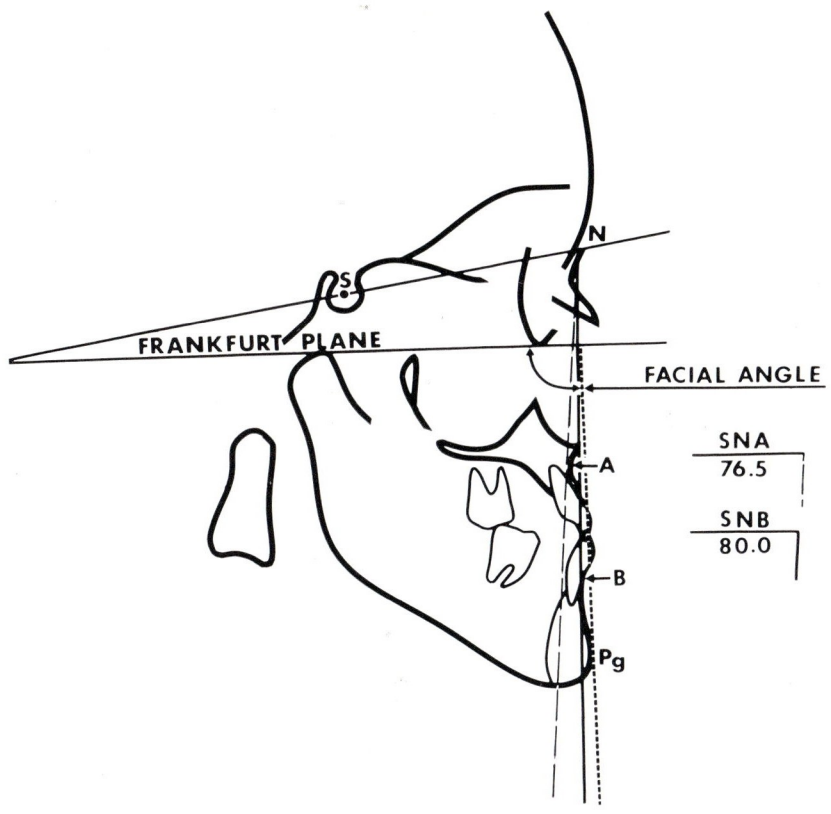

Figure 19-18. Cephalometry of patient in Figure 19-17. Note the low SNA reading, indicating deficient growth of maxilla. (Normal SNA = 82° SNB = 80°)

development of the maxilla (Fig. 19-17 and 19-18).

Study Models

Duplicate study models in artificial stone are a prerequisite in preoperative planning. They are required to serve as a permanent record to assess the improvement attained by surgical correction. Their major use, however, is in the planning of the type of surgical procedure that is most suitable for a particular case. Occlusal discrepancies that will occur after surgery may be forecast by positioning the models in the new postoperative position (Fig. 19-19). These may require occlusal equilibration or in the more excessive cases, orthodontic treatment may be necessary.

Mandibular Prognathism

This abnormality is extremely unsightly and in addition function may be severely disrupted. The incisor teeth cannot be approximated and thus incision is impossible. The gonial angle is markedly obtuse and correction of this is an integral part of treatment. In many cases there is a strong hereditary tendency. Various surgical techniques have been described for the treatment of this abnormality which is usually outside the scope of orthodontic therapy alone. Basically, these can be divided into those where surgery is carried out in the body of the mandible (ostectomy—excision of bone) and those through the ascending ramus (osteotomy—surgical cutting of bone).

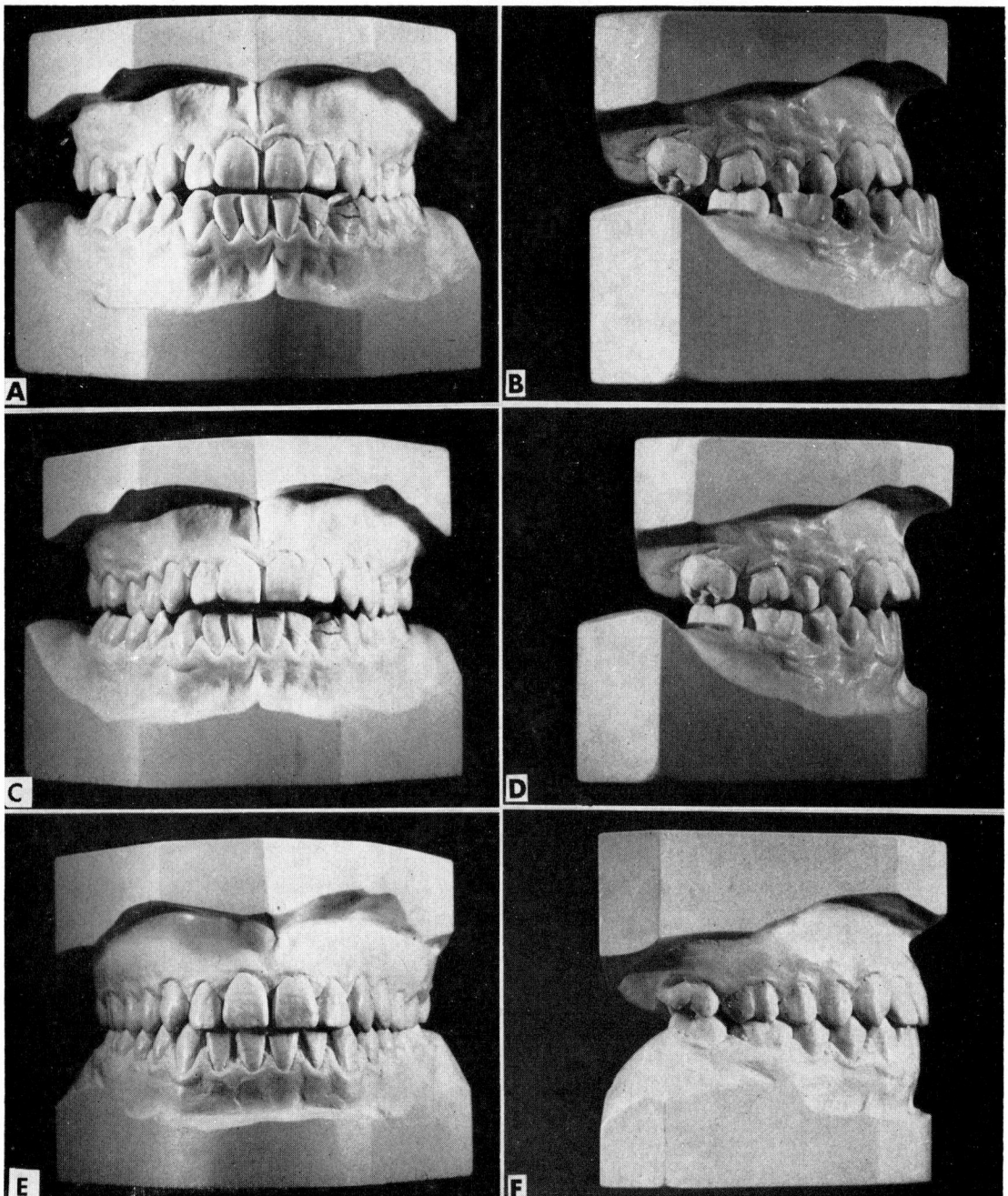

Figure 19-19. Study models in a case of mandibular prognathism. (A) and (B) Initial occlusion demonstrating class III relationship and anterior open bite. (C) and (D) Optimum occlusion possible with surgery alone. (E) and (F) Occlusion achieved with combined orthodontic-surgical management.

Body Ostectomy

This operation which may be performed either intraorally or extraorally consists of the bilateral removal of a measured piece of bone usually in the bicuspid area. The anterior segment is then set back establishing a correct incisal relationship (Fig. 19-20). Obviously if there are teeth present in the segment of bone to be removed, these must be extracted prior to operation.

Although this operation still has its advocates, it has lost favor in recent years due to certain inherent disadvantages.

1. Although the mandible is prognathic, there is rarely marked disparity between the mandibular and maxillary arches and hence removal of bone leads to a relatively small mandibular arch.

2. Extraction of mandibular teeth is always necessary, which not only reduces masticatory efficiency but necessitates the construction of a partial denture or bridge work postoperatively.

3. There is a greater incidence of operative morbidity; nonunion is more frequent and damage to the inferior alveolar nerve almost invariable.

4. Cosmetically, the results are only satisfactory in minor abnormalities since there is often a bunching up of tissues in the bicuspid area causing the so-called "Chipmunk" appearance. Furthermore, the gonial angle remains obtuse as it cannot be corrected by this method.

Operations Through the Rami

The most commonly used procedures consist of the subcondylar (subsigmoid) osteotomy and the sagittal splitting procedure of Obwegeser.

Subsigmoid Osteotomy

This is usually performed through an extraoral approach. It involves stripping off the pterygomasseteric sling from its attach-

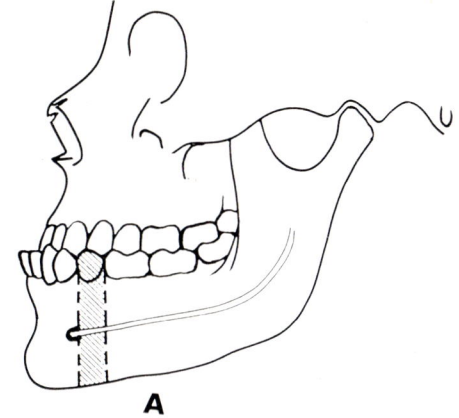
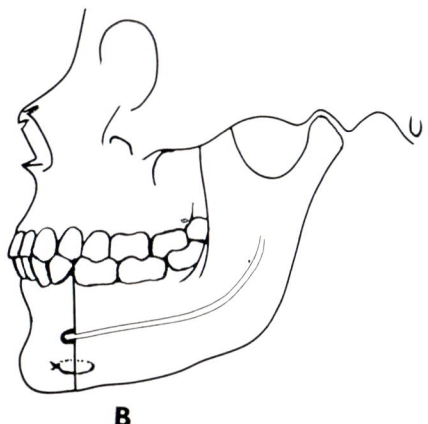

Figure 19-20. Body ostectomy. (A) Mandibular prognathism. Removal of premolar and section of body (shaded area). (B) Anterior segment set back and wired in place.

ment to the ramus and sectioning the ramus as shown in Figure 19-21. The entire body of the mandible is then repositioned in the correct relationship to the maxilla. Variations in the line of cut may be employed but they do not essentially alter the operation.

Sagittal Split (Obwegeser)

This is an entirely intraoral procedure. By using certain cuts, the ramus of the mandible is split in the sagittal plane (Fig. 19-22). The body of the mandible is again repositioned as an entire unit.

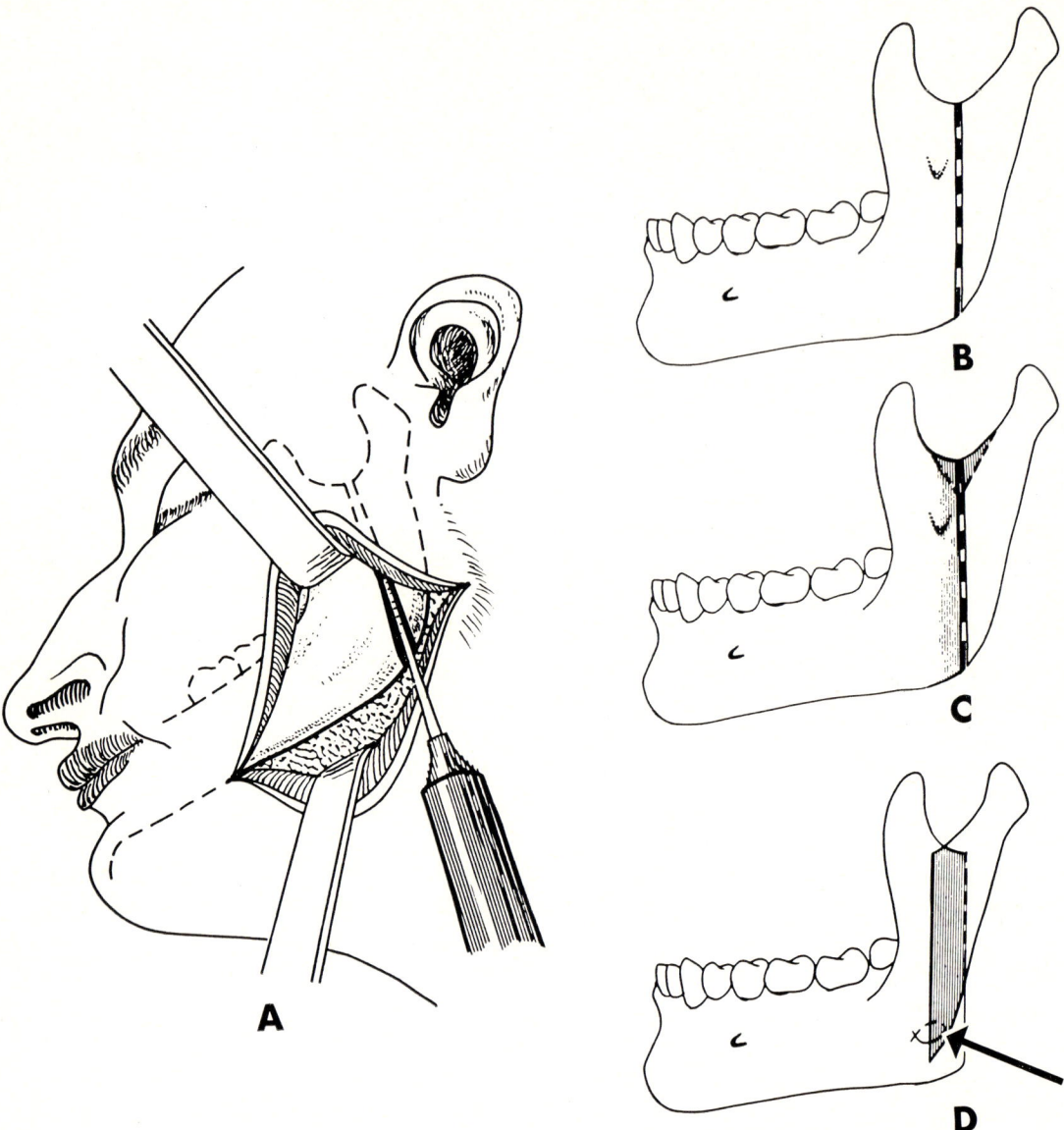

Figure 19-21. Subsigmoid (subcondylar) osteotomy. (A) Extraoral approach to ramus. Vertical osteotomy illustrated. (B) Line of cut in vertical osteotomy. (C) V-shaped wedge removed from sigmoid notch area, decortication of proximal (shaded area) ensures good apposition. (D) Distal fragment overlapped. Intraosseous wire (arrow) for fixation.

Advantages and Disadvantages

Both these techniques have significant advantages and explain the trend toward ramus surgery. Backward movement of the entire body of the mandible moves back all the attachments of the tongue and floor of the mouth as a unit thus preventing relapse due to tongue pressure. Cosmetically, the results are excellent as the gonial angle can be modified and there is no bunching up of tissues. The morbidity

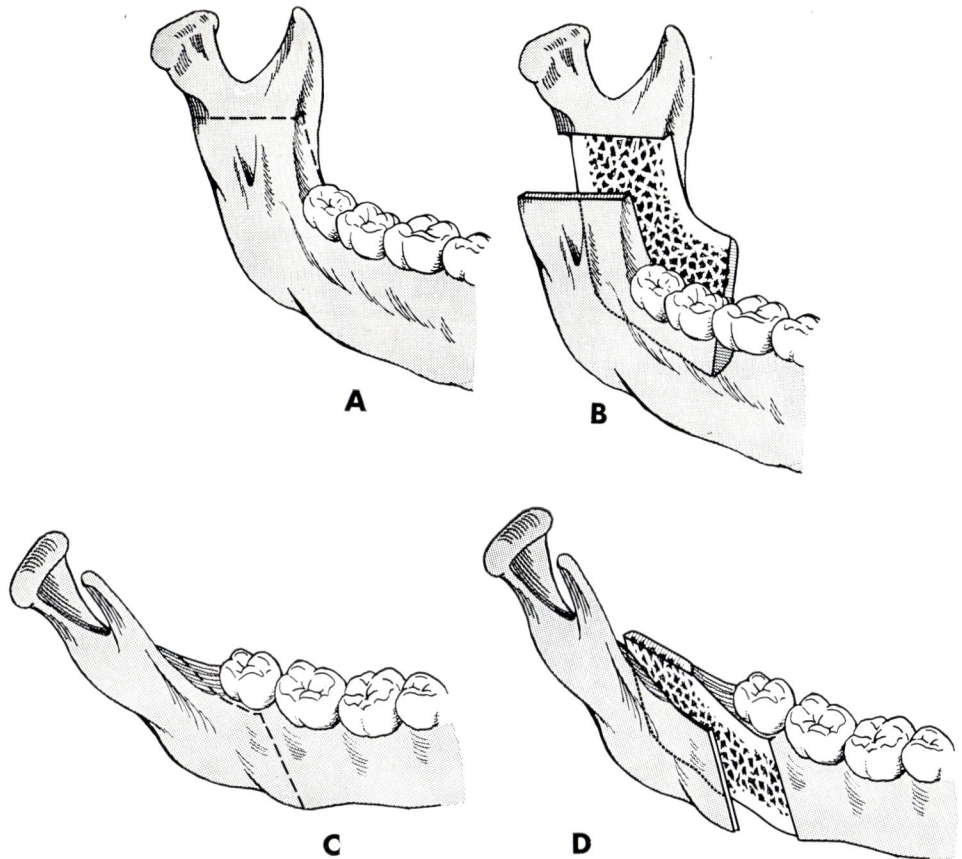

Figure 19-22. Sagittal split osteotomy (Obwegeser). (A) Outline of lingual cut (lingual view of mandible). (B) Buccal and retromolar cuts (lingual view of mandible). (C) and (D) Proximal and distal fragment of mandible after split carried out (buccal view of mandible).

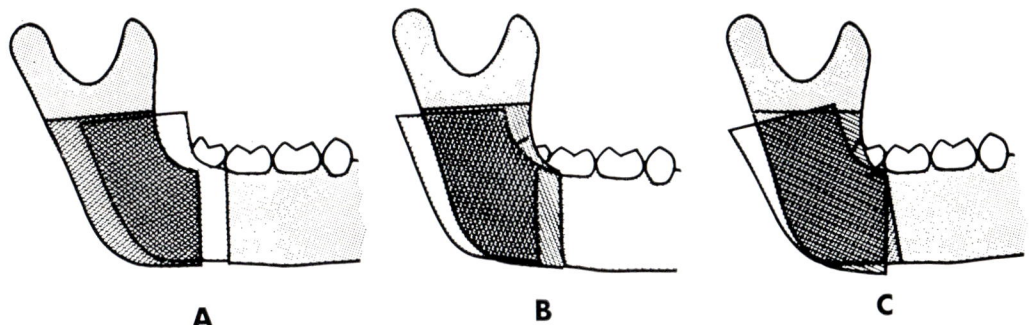

Figure 19-23. Versatility of sagittal split osteotomy (Obwegeser). (A) Mandible advanced for micrognathia. (B) Mandible retruded for prognathism. (C) Mandible rotated upwards in anterior open-bite case. (Note good bony contact in all positions).

is far less, non union is excessively rare and damage to the inferior alveolar nerve less likely in the case of the subcondylar approach.

The Obwegeser sagittal split procedure has the advantage that it is performed intraorally and hence a facial scar is not created. It is also an extremely versatile procedure which is suitable for cases with apertognathia (open bite) or micrognathic deformities (Fig. 19-23). However, it must be stated that it is a technique which is extremely difficult, requiring a great amount of skill and experience. Furthermore, in inexperienced hands, it carries a high morbidity. Complications, such as severe hemorrhage, damage to the inferior alveolar nerve, severe postoperative edema necessitating tracheostomy have all been reported.

The subcondylar osteotomy on the other hand, although producing almost universally acceptable results, has a far less degree of morbidity. The technique is simple, visualization of the operative site is excellent and damage to the inferior alveolar nerve is completely avoidable. The only objection that can be raised is the production of facial scars. However, these can be kept to a minimum if limited to 3 cm and placed correctly in a skin crease (Fig. 19-24).

In summary, it may be stated that with few exceptions, operations on the ramus are preferable for mandibular prognathism and in most instances the subcondylar

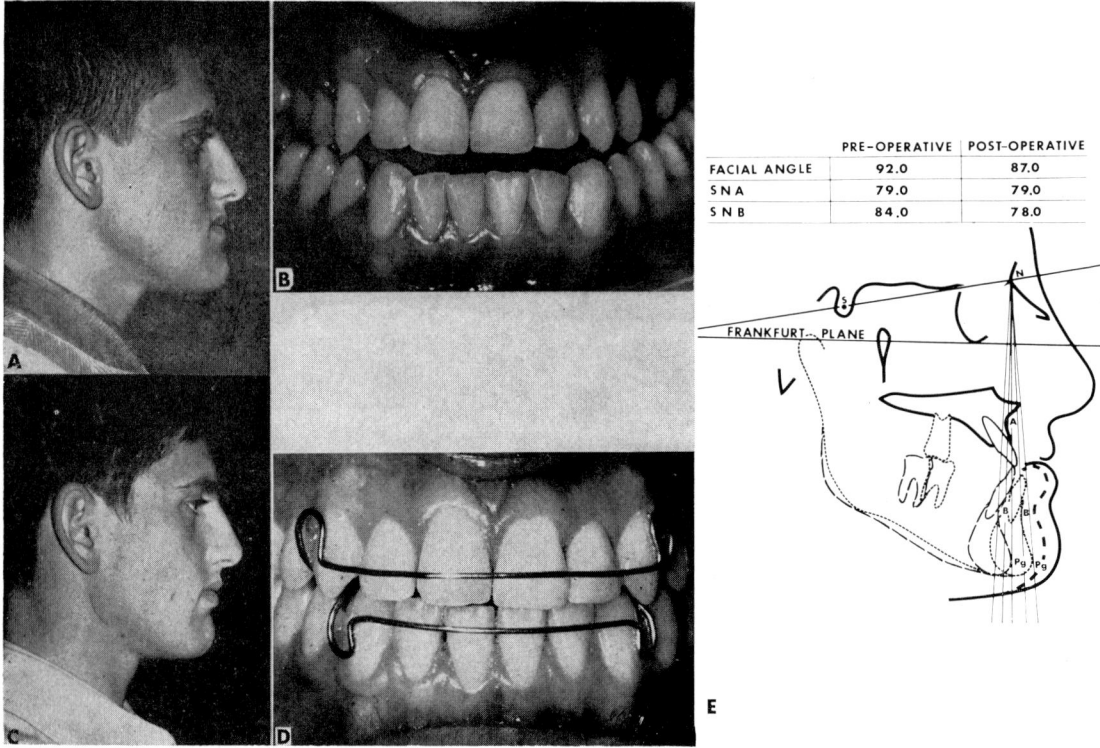

Figure 19-24. Mandibular prognathism and apertognathia treated by subcondylar osteotomy. (A) and (B) Preoperative profile and occlusion. (C) Profile six weeks postoperatively. Note the size and position of scar. (D) Postoperative occlusion with orthodontic retaining appliances. (E) Cephalometric analysis of case.

osteotomy is the operation of choice. In those patients where it is imperative that no facial scars be created, the Obwegeser sagittal split osteotomy should be employed.

Maxillary Prognathism

This common facial abnormality not only is often unacceptable to the patient on esthetic grounds, but there is often accompanying soft tissue trauma due to the abnormal incisor relationship. Thus in the class II, division I case with proclined upper incisors, the palatal gingival margin is traumatized and stripped by the lower incisors causing alveolar resorption and early loss of teeth. Similarly with the class II, division II, the retroclined maxillary incisors may traumatize the labial mandibular mucosa.

Orthodontic treatment alone in many of these cases cannot correct these abnormalities to the required degree since there is a limit to the amount of apical torque and movement of the incisors that is possible or desirable.

Surgical correction for these types of malocclusions is now well established and is being performed more frequently. It is interesting to note that the procedure carried out today varies little from Wassmund's operation [4] which he first carried out in 1935. It involves firstly the extraction of both maxillary first premolars. This is followed by palatal and buccal ostectomy through the extraction sites to the level of the floor of the nose. The anterior maxillary segment is then mobilized by a horizontal osteotomy above the apices of the teeth and joining the vertical cuts. This segment may then be pushed back into the correct predetermined position. A midline split between the central incisors may or may not be required to achieve the desired result (Fig. 19-25).

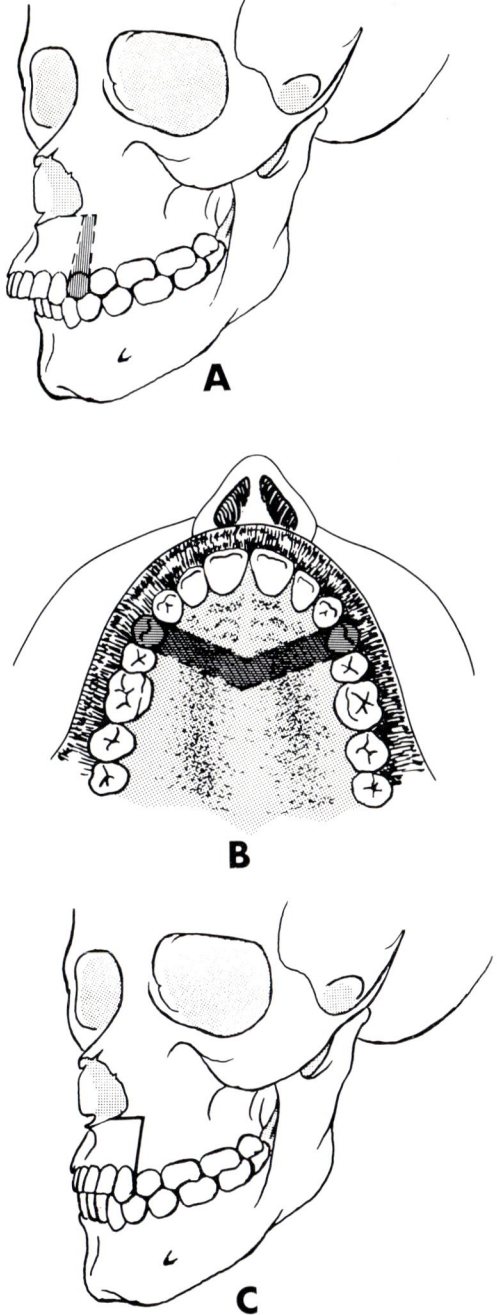

Figure 19-25. Premaxillary ostectomy (Wassmund procedure). (A) Extraction of 1st premolar and line of buccal cuts. (B) Palatal view of bone removal (shaded area). (C) Premaxilla set back into class I relationship.

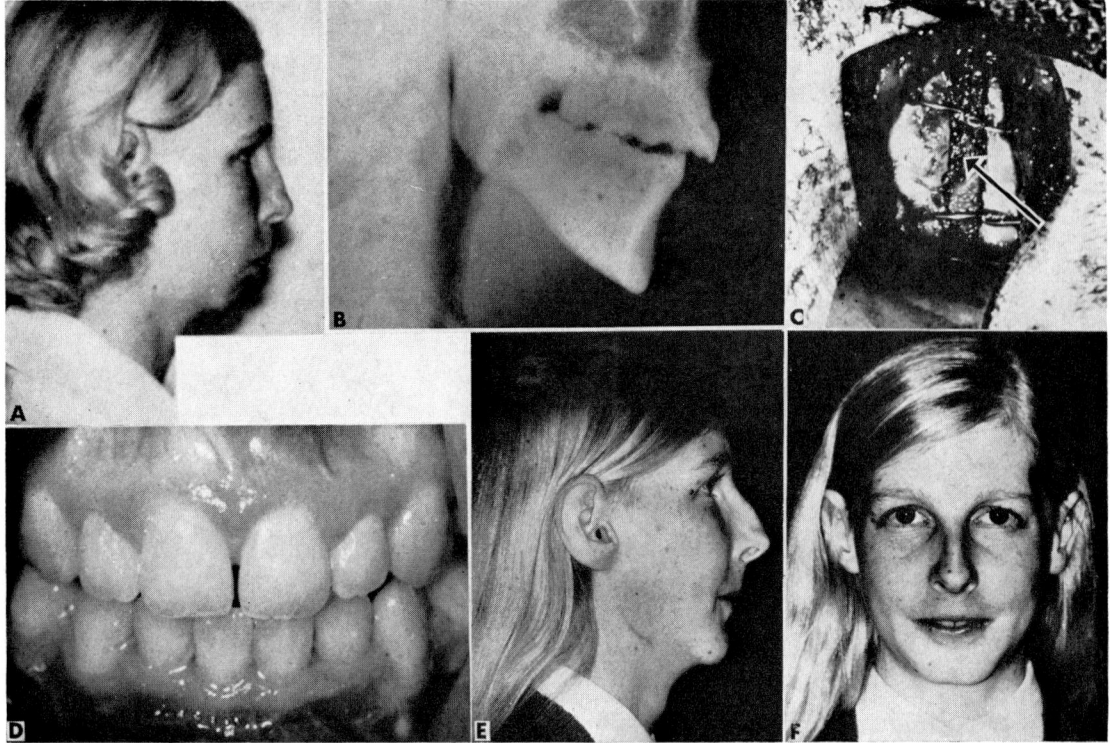

Figure 19-26. Mandibular micrognathia treated by subcondylar osteotomy and bone graft. (A) and (B) Preoperative profile and radiograph of patient. (C) Photograph taken at operation. Note the bone graft inlaid in the ascending ramus (arrow). (D) Postoperative occlusion. (E) and (F) six weeks postoperatively.

Mandibular Micrognathia

True micrognathia or "bird face" deformity presents a formidable problem as far as surgical correction is concerned. Although, as in mandibular prognathism, numerous techniques have been used particularly through the body of the mandible, again current opinion favors procedures through the ramus. In this respect, it is agreed that the Obwegeser sagittal split osteotomy is the operation of choice. When carried out for micrognathia, the body of the mandible is slid forward into the desired position instead of backward as in mandibular prognathism.

Occasions arise, however, when the ramus is too thin for a splitting procedure to be carried out. In these cases, subcondylar osteotomy via an external approach combined with bone grafting may be used (Fig. 19-26). Recently a modification employing "C" sliding osteotomy[5] (Fig. 19-27) has been shown to achieve good results without the necessity for bone grafting.

Maxillary Retrognathism

Of all the facial deformities, maxillary retrognathism offers the greatest challenge to management. The majority of cases in the past have been treated by surgery in the mandible to reduce the mandibular pseudoprognathism. However, the results of this therapy often leave the patient with a rather "flat" profile which is esthetically unacceptable. Recently, techniques have been developed whereby the entire maxilla may be mobilized and brought forward to the desired acceptable position. This procedure referred to as horizontal maxillary osteotomy consists of creating a horizontal fracture above the apices of the teeth so that the alveolar portion is loose. The maxilla is then immobilized until union in the new position has been achieved. It has been found that relapse, although evident in a number of cases, may be greatly reduced if cancellous bone chips taken from the iliac crest are packed into the space created behind the maxilla after its mobilization (Fig. 19-28).

Apertognathia (Open Bite)

In this condition there is a lack of occlusal contact anteriorly which extends distally to a varying degree. It may arise as a result of skeletal factors or structural or functional soft tissue abnormalities. In many cases, both skeletal and soft tissue factors are involved. Soft tissue causes such as abnormal swallowing, tongue thrusting and lip sucking are responsible for the high incidence of relapse following both orthodontic and surgical correction.

In the skeletal type of open bite, surgical correction becomes the treatment of choice. There are basically two procedures which may be employed. When the open bite extends to the first molar, the mandible should be divided in the ramus in order to rotate the body of the mandible upward. In this type, the sagittal split procedure offers the best results (Fig. 19-23, C). An inverted L osteotomy may be employed, but this may necessitate a bone graft (Fig. 19-29). Where the open bite is confined to the anterior region only, the Kole procedure gives excellent results.[6] In this technique, the anterior lower segment of teeth and bone is elevated to correct the open bite and the defect created filled with bone obtained from the lower border of the mandible (Fig. 19-30).

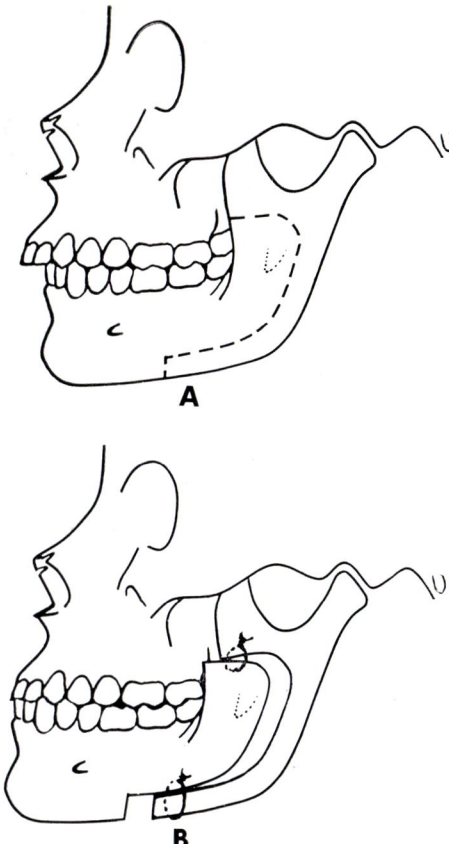

Figure 19-27. Mandibular micrognathia. "C" sliding osteotomy. (A) Outline of cuts. (B) Mandible advanced. Note good bony contact obviating need for bone graft.

Tongue Reduction

If the tongue is large, it has been shown that the postoperative relapse of the open bite may occur.[7] In these cases, tongue reduction should be undertaken prophylactically although some surgeons prefer to carry this out later at the slightest sign of a relapse.

Mandibular Asymmetry

This is usually due to either unilateral hyperplasia or unilateral hypoplasia. The most common variety of the former is a lateral deviation of the mandible to the normal side with an increased amount of

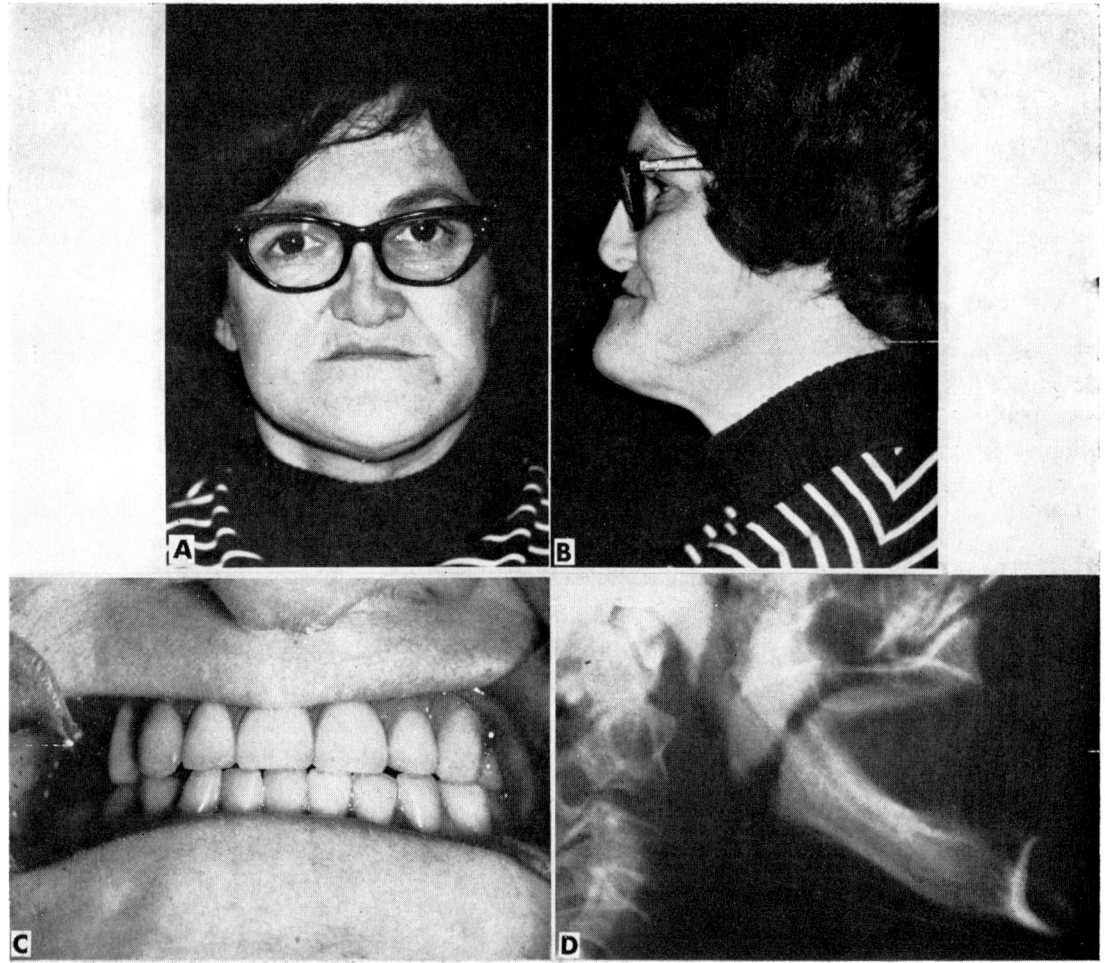

Figure 19-28. Maxillary retrognathia as a result of trauma. Treated by total maxillary osteotomy. *Preoperative:* (A) and (B) Severe retrusion of maxilla and pseudoprognathism. (C) Occlusion with dentures in place. (D) Lateral jaw radiograph. *Postoperative:* (E) and (F) Postoperative appearance at six weeks. (G) Occlusion with new dentures. (H) Lateral jaw radiograph. Note the new position of maxilla. Bone graft shown by arrow.

prognathism. In the latter, a shortening of the mandible is produced with deviation to the affected side and the chin is more posterior than normal retrognathia.

Surgical correction is required in the majority of instances where the deformity is gross. The operative procedures used in surgical correction are modifications of the techniques already described and careful planning becomes imperative in their choice.

Chin Correction (Genioplasty)

An extremely useful adjunct in the surgical management of facial deformities, particularly of the prognathic or micrognathic variety, is the technique of genioplasty. These procedures may be performed via an intraoral approach—the so-called degloving procedure (Fig. 19-31). Once access has been obtained to the chin, it may be advanced forward in the case of

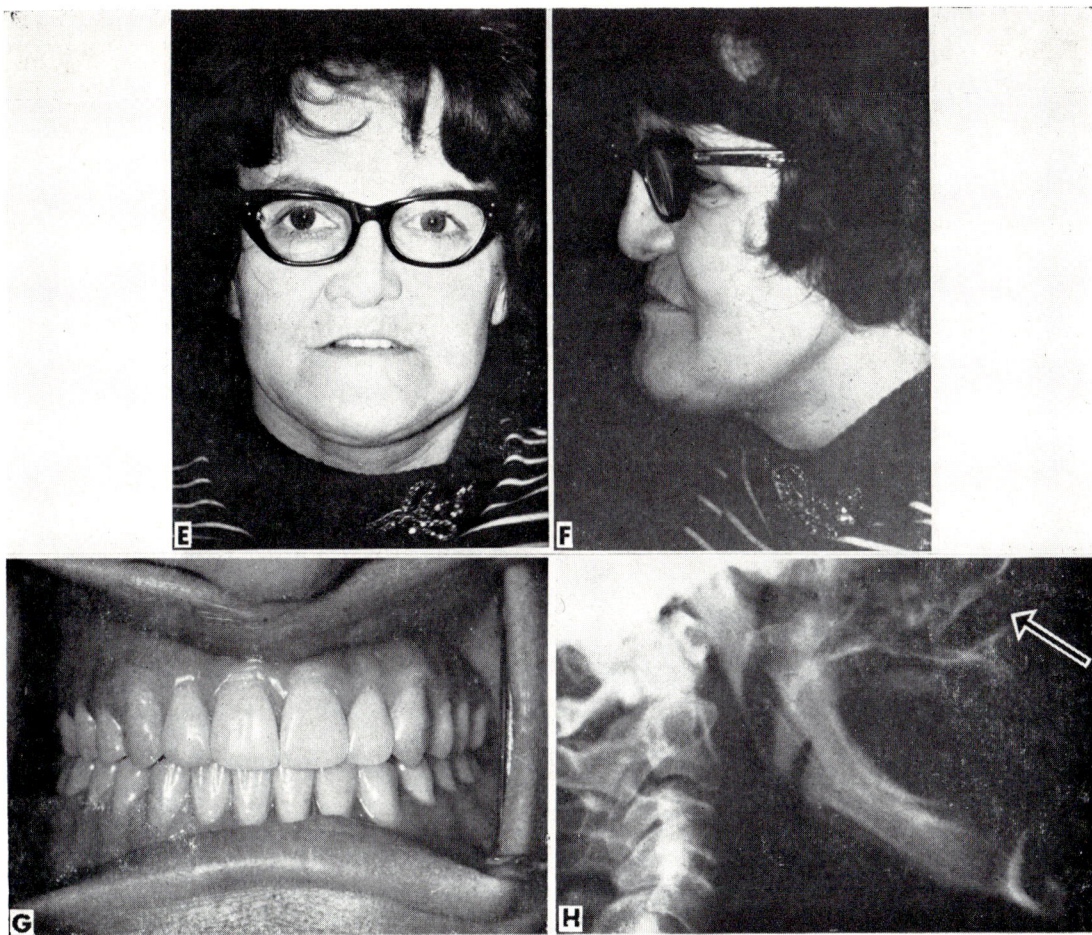

micrognathia or reduced in the prognathic mandible. A further variation in the micrognathic case is the insertion of a bone graft or alleloplastic graft such as silicone to improve the contour.

Orthodontic Surgery (Dento-alveolar Surgery)

This term has been coined to describe techniques whereby in the treatment of dental malocclusions, a segment of teeth and investing alveolar bone is detached surgically and repositioned en bloc, without complete section of the jaw. These techniques were first described by Cohn-Stock in 1921[8] and numerous modifications have since been developed. In the past few years, there has been a tremendous revival of interest in these methods and they are now used routinely in many centers. The surgical principles involved may be illustrated by considering several types of malocclusion where orthodontic surgery is used.

Mandibular Prognathism

In cases where, although the teeth are in a class III relationship, the chin point is

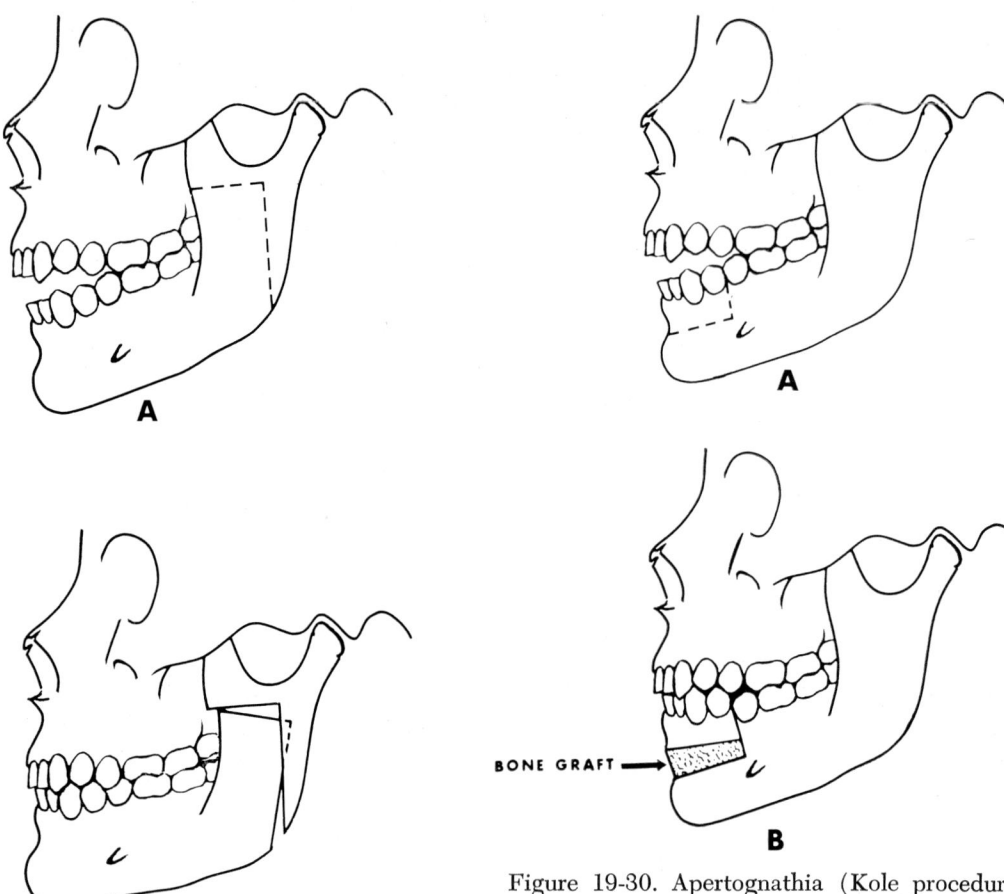

Figure 19-29. Apertognathia (open bite). Reverse "L" osteotomy. (A) Outline of cut. (B) Mandible rotated upwards. Note poor bony apposition.

Figure 19-30. Apertognathia (Kole procedure). (A) Outline of cut. (B) Anterior segment lifted to correct open bite. Note position of bone graft to fill in defect.

correct, it is possible to set back the lower anterior teeth in a normal relationship without completely dividing the mandible (Fig. 19-32). The blood supply of the anterior teeth moved is maintained through the lingual tissues.

Closed Bite

In cases where there is a severe overbite present as in Angle class II, division I cases, a portion of bone may be removed from the apical area of the lower anterior teeth and these may then be lowered to obtain a normal occlusal contour to the lower occlusal plane (Fig. 19-33).

Maxillary Protrusion

The surgical technique used to set back the anterior maxillary teeth has already been discussed (Fig. 19-25) and is another illustration of orthodontic surgery.

Corticotomy

The term "corticotomy" is also used in orthodontic surgery and is a method of facilitating rapid tooth movement by means of orthodontic appliances. In this technique, complete separation of the alveolar process is not required, but cuts are made through the cortical plates so that the segment of bone to be moved is held in place solely by cancellous bone. It

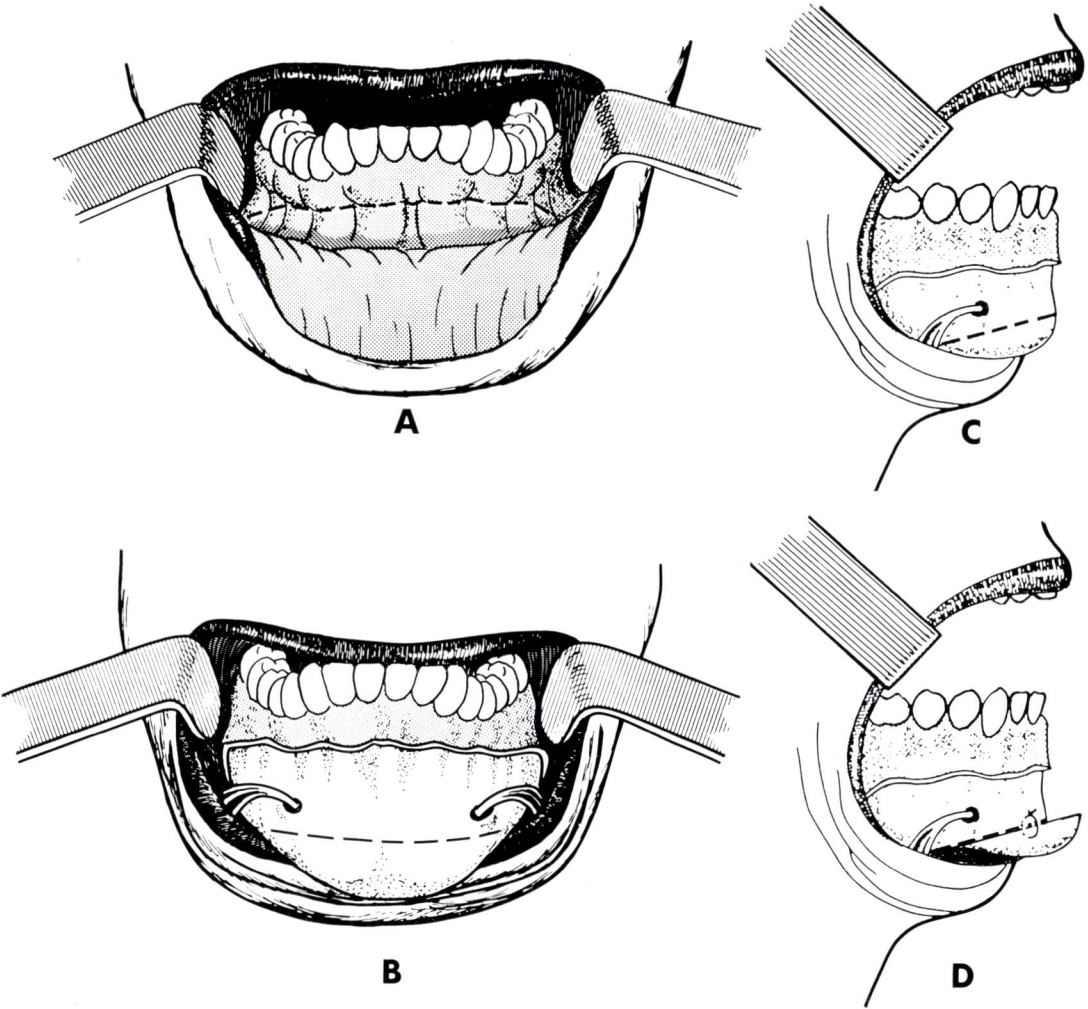

Figure 19-31. Genioplasty—intraoral degloving procedure technique. (A) Intraoral view showing line of incision. (B) and (C) Reflection of mucoperiosteal flap. Note the preservation of the mental nerves. (D) Sliding genioplasty carried out. Note new forward position of chin.

is thus possible to produce rapid orthodontic movement of the demarcated alveolar segment whilst maintaining adequate blood supply and innervation to the teeth and bone involved.

Complications and Risks in Surgical Corrections

Although it is essential for the practitioner to be familiar with the risks involved before referring his patient for surgical correction of a malocclusion, experience has shown that in fact, the risks and complications employing modern surgical techniques correctly are surprisingly low. These can be discussed under several headings.

Nonunion and Malunion

Both these complications are rare and usually result from either inadequate fixation or poor planning in selecting the

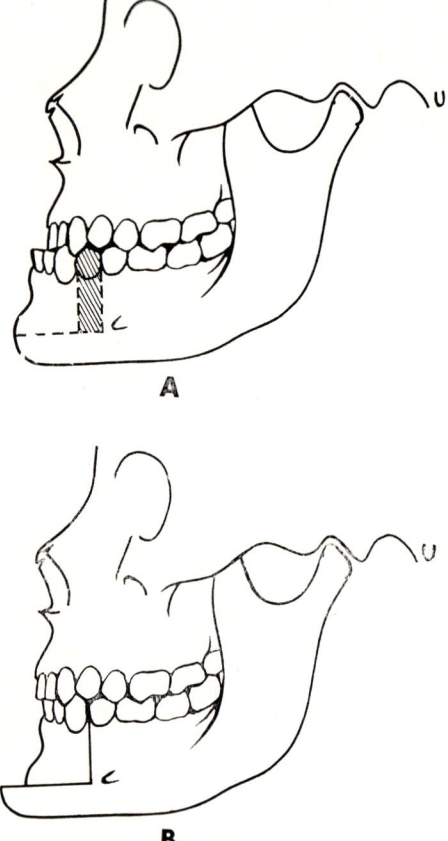

Figure 19-32. Mandibular prognathism. "Orthodontic surgery." (A) Outline of cuts. Segment of bone removed in premolar area (shaded). (B) Anterior segment set back. Note that mandible is intact and chin position not altered.

countered. The teeth undergo a temporary period of up to three to six months whereby they do not respond to pulp testing, but during that time they are still vital from the vascular standpoint. After this period, it has been found that response to pulp testing returns.

Relapse

Similar factors operate in both surgical and orthodontic cases of relapse. If the original stimulus which was responsible for the malocclusion is still in evidence postoperatively, such as thumb sucking and tongue thrust, or growth has not been completed, then relapse will follow in-

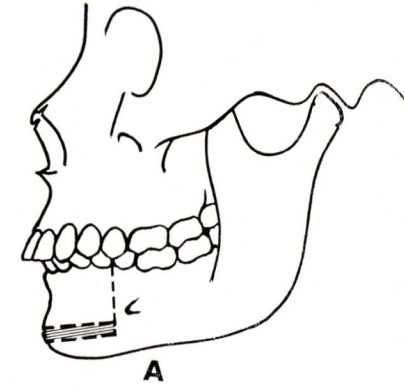

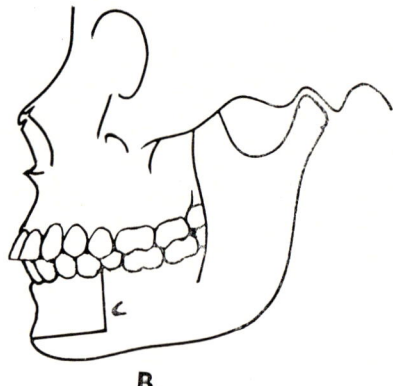

Figure 19-33. Closed bite—subapical ostectomy. (A) Line of cut with segment of bone removed subapically (shaded area). (B) Anterior segment lowered into new occlusion.

wrong operative procedure. Techniques described in the ramus of the mandible have a particularly low incidence in this respect.

Devitalization of Teeth

This hazard has mainly applied to orthodontic surgery and has been largely theoretical. Logically, one could assume that because the alveolar bone is cut subapically and hence the apical blood supply of the teeth interfered with, that devitalization would occur invariably. However, this, in fact, is not the case and is rarely en-

dependent of which modality is used. However, it has been shown that surgical correction offers the most stable result, particularly if the technique used enables muscles to be repositioned.

Sensory Nerve Loss

This is a definite risk but can be minimized by careful surgical technique and choice of operation. As mentioned previously, operations through the ramus, particularly the subcondylar osteotomy which is the most frequent operation performed, have a low incidence of damage to the inferior alveolar nerve since the cuts are distal to the lingula. In the case of dentoalveolar procedures if the mental nerve is carefully dissected out for some distance into the tissues and protected with a retractor whilst the cuts anterior to it are made, only minor temporary mental anesthesia will result.

Summary

In summary, it is fair to say that a whole new era in the treatment of facial deformities has been opened up.

Surgical correction is not advocated as a replacement of orthodontic therapy, but as an adjunct particularly in those cases where the malocclusion is of such severity that successful treatment by appliances alone is not possible or, as in the case of adults, would have to be unacceptably prolonged. Careful orthodontic planning must precede the surgical procedure and in many instances actual active orthodontic therapy must be carried out, prior to surgery, in order to obtain a balanced postoperative occlusion.

REPLANTATION AND TRANSPLANTATION OF TEETH

Although these procedures have been known and practiced since ancient times, they have, on the whole, gained few advocates. This is due to the fact that despite numerous reports in the literature, the success rate has been difficult to assess and at the present time little agreement exists whether or not these procedures should be recognized as acceptable therapy. If a fair appraisal of this subject is to be obtained, however, each technique must be evaluated independently in the light of current knowledge and comparison with standard procedures in each case. Before discussing the value of the various techniques involved, it is essential to understand precisely the terminology employed.

Replantation: Refers to the replacement of a tooth in its own alveolar socket following its removal either surgically or as a result of trauma.

Autogenous transplantation: The transferral of a tooth from one site to another in the same individual.

Homogenous transplantation: The transplantation of a tooth from one individual to another of the same species.

Heterogenous transplantation: The transplantation of a tooth from one species to another.

Homogenous Tooth Transplantation

Several problems are evident in the appraisal of this procedure. Since transplanting teeth from one person to another is involved, the immunological phenomenon must be considered. There is now ample evidence that teeth possess antigenic properties which contribute to their rejection. So far, there is no method available which overcomes this problem. Furthermore, it becomes extremely difficult to have a donor tooth immediately available when it is required. Attempts have been made to overcome this problem by the setting up of "tooth banks" and by various storage techniques.[9] These have included refrigeration, dehydration, storage in saline and antibiotic solutions. However, it has not been possible to preserve the pulp by any known method, and therefore, further root development, which is an important factor in successful transplantation, has not been possible. The end-result of the great majority of attempts, therefore, has been ankylosis of the tooth with progressive resorption of the root usually during the first six months. Similar results have been reported where the donor tooth has been root filled prior to transplantation.

It would seem, therefore, despite some claims of limited success that unless the immunological and storage problem is overcome homogenous tooth transplantation is doomed to failure and its present status should be considered as purely experimental.

Autogenous Tooth Transplantation

Far more success has been achieved in the transplantation of teeth from one site to another in the same individual than in homogenous transplants. For the most part, however, it has been confined to the transplantation of the unerupted third mandibular molar with incompletely developed roots into the extraction site of the first molar (Fig. 19-34) and the repositioning of the unerupted maxillary canine in the adult.

Careful patient selection and meticulous

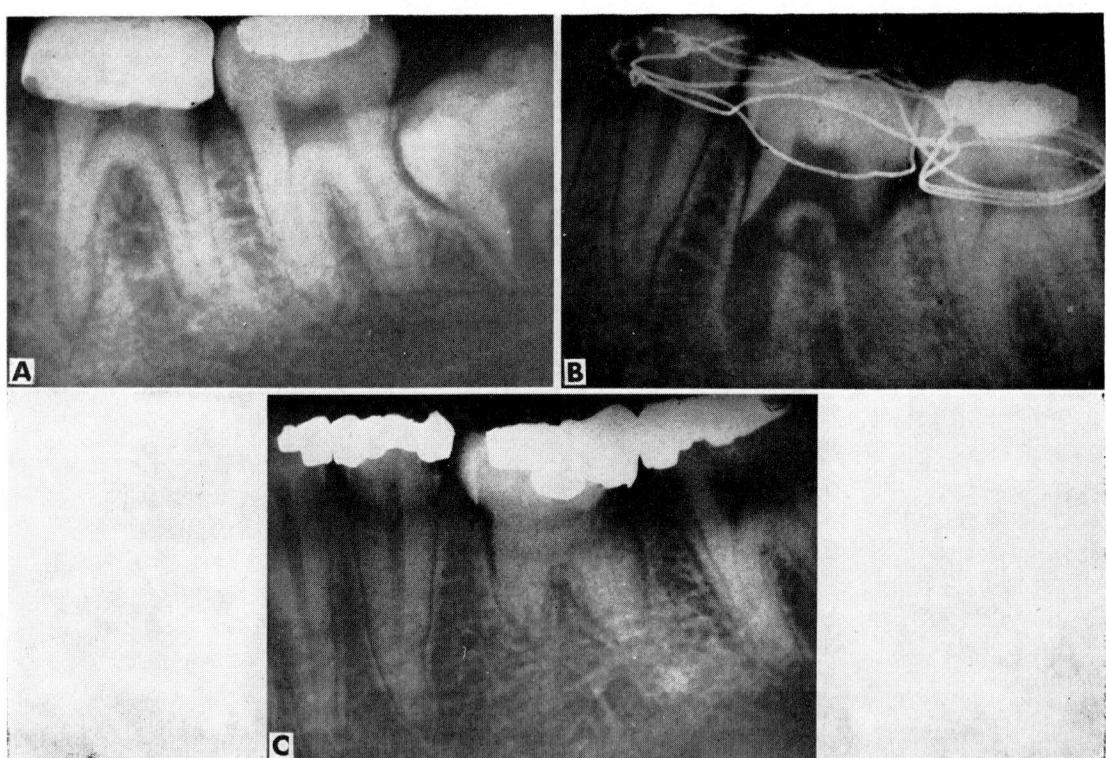

Figure 19-34. Autogenous transplant of mandibular third molar. (A) Carious first permanent mandibular molar with periapical involvement. Note stage of development of third molar. (B) Immediate postoperative radiograph. Third molar wired in place in extraction site. (C) Five years postoperatively. Note the root formation and periodontal membrane.

surgical technique is imperative. The general oral health of the patient must be excellent and no acute periapical or paradontal disease should be present in the recipient site. The ideal situation in the case of the third molar is that it should have 3 to 5 mm of root developed at the time of transplantation. Surgical technique must be such that the soft tissue of the root sac is not damaged and adequate immobilization obtained. The overall success rate judging from the reports in the literature is in the order of 50 percent.[10] The criteria for success vary, but usually consist of retention of the tooth for a period of five years with normal root development, the absence of ankylosis and root resorption.

In the transplantation of the impacted maxillary canine a different situation is in evidence. These cases involve a fully developed root and reattachment of the periodontal ligament must occur for success to be achieved. Successful retention of the tooth has been claimed for varying lengths of time although root resorption eventually occurs in the great majority of cases.

Replantation

In the great majority of cases, this procedure has been carried out when anterior teeth have been avulsed as a result of facial trauma. Accidents occurring during such procedures as tonsillectomy or laryngoscopy account for a small percentage of cases. Recently another indication has been added, and that is, in endodontic therapy where, because of problems encountered such as blockage of root canals, perforation or unfavorable inaccessible root canals, the tooth is extracted, endodontically treated and immediately replanted. The success rate, according to different investigation, was found to vary from 20 to 50 percent when taken over a five-year period.[11] A consistent finding present in all the series reported was that those teeth which had been replanted after being out of the socket for over thirty minutes had the worst prognosis and usually showed marked resorption within the first few months. The consensus of opinion in these cases is that the teeth should be endodontically treated before replantation. Where the tooth has only been out of its socket for a few minutes, minimum handling and no root canal treatment is advocated. As in transplantation, adequate splintage is essential.

Summary

1. Unless a breakthrough is achieved in the problem of immunity, rejection mechanisms and tooth storage, it is probably fair to say that homogenous or heterogenous tooth transplantation has no place in dental therapy.

2. In considering the autogenous transplantation of the unerupted third molar into the first molar socket, it can be stated that there is probably a limited place for this procedure in the carefully selected patient. It must be remembered, however, that a far more satisfactory and reliable technique is orthodontic closure of the space created by the extraction of the first molar and allowing the third molar to erupt normally.

3. Similarly in the case of the impacted cuspid when it is not possible to bring the tooth into the dental arch by orthodontic means, the treatment of choice is to surgically remove the cuspid and close the space between the lateral and first premolar. The first premolar may then be fashioned by careful grinding to simulate a cuspid. An indication for repositioning exists, however, in those cases where orthodontic treatment is not available. If the patient is young, it may not be possible to construct a fixed bridge for fear of

pulpal injury, and rather than a partial denture be worn, the transplanted canine may act as a space maintainer in the interim period.

4. Of all the procedures discussed in this section, replantation has the most accepted place in dental treatment. It should be attempted in all cases of avulsion of teeth, particularly in young individuals where the alveolus has not been too grossly disrupted or the root fractured. In cases where a considerable time has elapsed between avulsion and treatment, endodontic therapy should be performed prior to replantation. Even if resorption takes place several years later, the tooth has served as an excellent space maintainer, making the attempt worthwhile.

REFERENCES

1. Harris, C. A.: *The Principles and Practice of Dental Surgery*, 6th ed. Philadelphia, Lindsay & Blakiston, 1855, p. 609.
2. Thoma, K. H.: *Oral Pathology*, 6th ed. St. Louis, Mosby, 1970, p. 45.
3. Obwegeser, H. L.: Surgical preparation of the maxilla for prosthesis. *J Oral Surg*, 22:127, 1964.
4. Wassmund, M.: *Lehrbuch der Praktischen Chirurgie des Mundes und der Kiefer*. Leipzig, Meuser, 1935, vol. I, p. 289.
5. Kruger, G. O.: *Textbook of Oral Surgery*, 3rd ed. St. Louis, Mosby, 1968, p. 497.
6. Kole, H.: Surgical operations on alveolar ridge to correct occlusal obnormalities. *Oral Surg*, 12:277, March, 1959; 12:413, April, 1959; 12:515, May, 1959.
7. Egyedi, P.: Reduction of tongue size in the surgical correction of jaw deformity. *Br J Oral Surg*, 3:13, 1965.
8. Cohn-Stock, G.: Die Chirurgische Immediatregulierung der Kiefer, speziell die Chirurgische Behandlung der Prognathie. *Vjschz Zahnheilk*, 37:320, 1921.
9. Jonck, L. M.: An investigation into certain aspects of transplantation and reimplantation of teeth in man. *Br J Oral Surg*, 4:137, 1966.
10. Apfel, H.: Autoplasty of enucleated prefunctional third molars. *J Oral Surg*, 8:289, 1950.
11. Grossman, L. I.: Intentional replantation of teeth. *JADA*, 72:1111, 1966.

Selected Reading

1. Barton, P. R., and Rayne, J.: The role of alveolar surgery in the treatment of malocclusion. *Br Dent J*, 126:11, 1969.
2. Hayward, J. R.: Surgical correction of malocclusion. *Dent Clin North Am*, 13:607, 1969.
3. Hinds, E. C.: Diagnosis and selection of surgical procedures in management of open bite. *J Oral Surg*, 27:939, 1969.
4. Kruger, G. O.: *Textbook of Oral Surgery*, 3rd ed. St. Louis, Mosby, 1968, Chs. 7 and 23.
5. MacIntosh, R. B., and Obwegeser, H. L.: Preprosthetic surgery: A scheme for its effective employment. *J Oral Surg*, 25:397, 1967.
6. MacIntosh, R. B. Orthodontic surgery: Comments on diagnostic modalities. *J Oral Surg*, 28:249, 1970.
7. Natiella, J. R., Armitage, J. E., and Greene, G. W.: The replantation and transplantation of teeth: A review. *Oral Surg*, 29:397, 1970.
8. Thoma, K. H.: *Oral Surgery*, 5th ed. St. Louis, Mosby, 1969, Chs. 20 and 53.

Chapter 20

Diagnosis and Treatment Planning for the Child

ALLEN W. ANDERSON AND DONALD E. ORE

T HE DIAGNOSIS and planning of dental treatment for the child differs from that in the adult to the extent that the child is a dynamic individual who is continually changing. He is growing and maturing physically, mentally and emotionally. The facial complex undergoes rapid change from birth through puberty unlike any other part of the growing child. The practitioner must constantly keep this in mind when treating the child patient.

The parents are an integral part of the diagnosis and treatment of the dental problems observed in children. They take part in the diagnosis by providing information regarding prenatal, natal and postnatal events and episodes as well as the current medical and dental history of the child. The instructions and some demanding aspects of the treatment (diet, home care and appliance care) are additionally carried out by the parents. Thus, in developing a treatment plan from the diagnosis, a triad consisting of the patient, the doctor and the parent is necessary for the correct diagnosis and treatment plan.

FORMULATION OF THE TREATMENT PLAN

The child is usually brought to the dental office for reasons of (a) pain; (b) advice concerning a developmental problem, such as retained primary teeth; (c) a required school examination; or (d) routine oral examination.

The mechanics of the formulation of a treatment plan for the child does not vary appreciably from that for an adult. There are several broad categories of treatment that a child may require. A checklist may be developed to ensure a thorough diagnosis and complete treatment. The following is the usual sequence in carrying out an orderly treatment plan.

Emergency Treatment

A child usually presents for emergency treatment because of pain. Pain may be caused by dental caries, infection or trauma. Whatever the cause of the pain, treatment must be immediately instituted to ensure its alleviation. A swift and thorough diagnosis is required; information and data not pertinent to the emergency treatment may be gathered at the next visit when an adequate amount of time should be set aside. This tends to reduce the immediate patient and parent anxieties.

Pain from dental caries may be of two types depending on whether there is dentinal or pulpal involvement. Dentinal pain is characterized as a sharp, lancinating type of pain usually occurring when sweets are eaten or when the dentin is exposed to nonphysiologic stimuli. Pulpal pain is characterized as a dull, throbbing type of pain occurring spontaneously or when the patient is lying down. It is important to distinguish between these two types of pain since treatment for each is complete different. Removing the caries and placing a sedative dressing of zinc oxide and eugenol (ZOE) will relieve pain due to dentinal involvement. Some form of pulp therapy is indicated for pulpal pain (*see* pulp therapy).

Traumatic Injuries

All traumatic injuries to the mouth or teeth of the child patient should be seen by the dentist as soon as possible following the episode. The immediate clinical examination should include a thorough radiographic survey.

The clinical examination *must* include, aside from a history of the injury, any history of unconsciousness, dysphasia or prolonged vertigo. The pupillary reflexes should be evaluated, and any signs of diplopia (double vision) should be ruled out. Any facial asymmetry should be noted and all the facial bones should be palpated and tested for mobility to rule out fractures.

Fractured, intruded, displaced or avulsed teeth should be individually accounted for. A missing primary tooth should be related to the exfoliation time or mobility of the contralateral tooth. If a missing tooth cannot be accounted for, a chest x-ray should be considered to rule out aspiration; this is paramount in the younger patient and infant.

THE CROWN FRACTURE. This is the most common injury seen in the dental office. Treatment of crown fractures is important to (a) maintain arch length and integrity, (b) maintain a healthy periodontium, (c) preserve pulpal vitality, (d) maintain esthetics and (e) prevent psychological effects.

The *class I fracture* which involves little or no dentin usually requires nothing more than smoothing the rough edges of the fractured crown (Fig. 20-1). In addition, the parent should be cautioned about the possible complications of pulpal degeneration and necrosis which require further treatment. Periodic follow-up at regular recall visits is recommended.

The *class II fracture* which involves considerable dentin but not the pulp requires more definitive treatment since the fracture is usually very near the pulp (Fig. 20-1). Either ZOE or calcium hydroxide

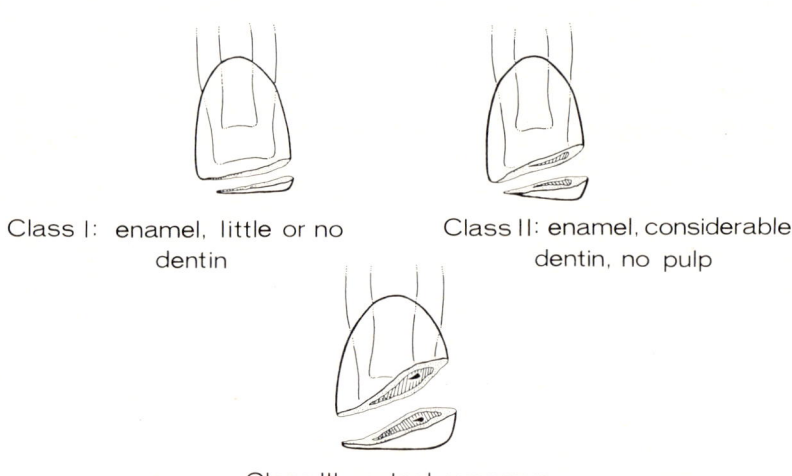

Class I: enamel, little or no dentin

Class II: enamel, considerable dentin, no pulp

Class III: pulpal exposure

Figure 20-1. The Ellis classification of crown fractures.

should be placed over the exposed dentin. Since the treatment is to aid the recovery of the pulp, ZOE is the material which will sedate the pulp and promote pulpal healing. Calcium hydroxide with its high pH and irritating properties may not allow the hyperemia and mild inflammatory response to subside quickly. The medicament should be protected with either a stainless steel band or crown (Fig. 20-2). A stainless steel band or open face crown will allow for pulp testing at a later time.

Pulp testing at the time of injury is very unreliable and serves no useful purpose. A pulp which has sustained a severe injury may give a false negative response. It is also possible that the various pulp tests may add nothing but insult to injury (see diagnostic aids).

The medicament should be left in place for at least two months when the tooth should be evaluated clinically and radiographically to determine the progress of healing. If healing has progressed satisfactorily, a transitional restoration (see restorative treatment) or perhaps a permanent restoration may be placed. Again, the parent should be cautioned about possible complications.

The *class III fracture* involves the pulp (Fig. 20-1). The first consideration in treating these teeth is to attempt to determine the type of final restoration. It is very embarrassing to perform a successful pulpotomy only to find that endodontic treatment is needed because a post type of crown is required to restore the tooth.

If the exposed pulp is treated within a few hours of the accident and the exposure is minimal, less than 1 mm, a direct pulp capping with calcium hydroxide may be performed. If the exposure is seen after twenty-four hours or is larger than 1 mm, a calcium hydroxide pulpotomy is the treatment of choice. When the exposure has been present for longer than seventy-two hours and there is complete root formation, endodontic treatment is indicated. If an open apex is present and the exposure has been present for more than seventy-

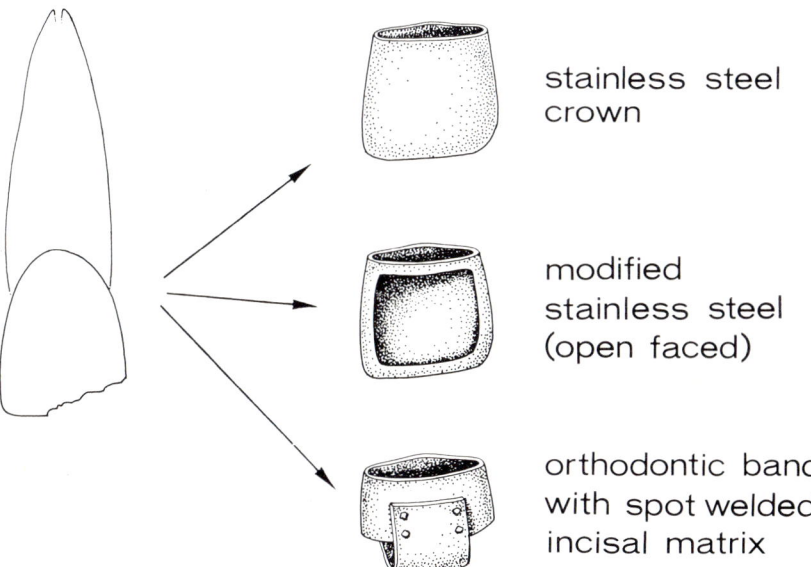

Figure 20-2. Three methods used for emergency coverage of a crown fracture to protect the medicament applied to the dentin or pulp and temporarily restore function.

two hours and the pulp is not necrotic, a pulpotomy should be attempted with calcium hydroxide with the hope that continued root formation will continue. When the pulp is necrotic, Frank's technic (see pulp therapy) should be employed.

The pulp treatment should be protected for two months with either a band or a stainless steel crown (Fig. 20-2). When the pulp treatment appears to have been successful, a transitional restoration may be placed.

ROOT FRACTURES. These are more likely in the adult than in the child because the alveolar bone in the child is more plastic than in the adult. Root fractures may occur in the apical one-third, middle one-third, or cervical one-third with the middle one-third the most common.[1] When trauma to the anterior teeth has occurred and a crown fracture is not evident, a root fracture is a distinct possibility. Rarely will there be a root fracture and a crown fracture in the same tooth because the blow is dissipated at the fracture site—either the crown or the root (Fig. 20-3). The more apical the fracture, the better the prognosis for healing. The pulp retains its vitality in a large number of root fracture cases.[1] In children, vertical fractures of the tooth involving extensive parts of the root are infrequent and these teeth should be extracted.

In cases of root fracture, the two fragments should be brought into apposition and splinted. The type of splint to be used is at the discretion of the dentist. The splint should not interfere with the occlusion and should remain in place for at least two months. As healing progresses, resorption in varying degrees usually takes place at the fracture site near the cementum.

DISPLACEMENT. These usually occur in the young child when the bone is still in a relative plastic state and root formation is incomplete. The prognosis is good but complications may arise depending on the displacement and developmental stage of the tooth. Usually there are no crown or root fractures associated with displacements.

Labial or lingual displacements and extruded teeth should be repositioned and splinted. Sometimes, however, blood and edema fluid may interfere with the repositioning of an individual tooth or an entire segment. When the tooth is repositioned, the dentist can feel the tooth move into its original position since the bone is compressed around the displaced tooth. The tooth should be followed at monthly intervals and the splint should remain in place for approximately two weeks. The relatively short period of time of splinting is to help reduce the possibility of ankylosis. Other complications are pulp necrosis, internal and external resorption, and discoloration.

Intruded teeth should not be reposi-

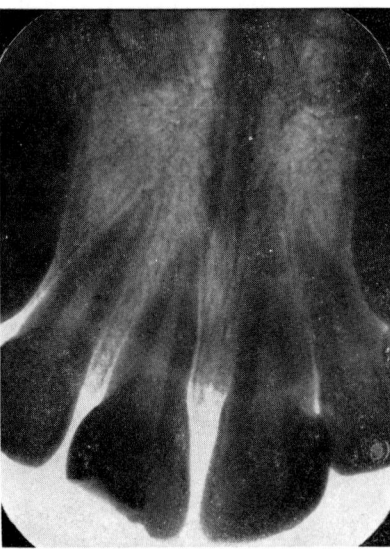

Figure 20-3. Radiograph of two central incisors showing a crown fracture of one central and a root fracture in the other. Note the intact crown in the tooth with the root fracture. Root fracture and crown fracture rarely occur in the same tooth.

tioned but allowed to reerupt into their original position. They should be followed at monthly intervals to determine if eruption is occurring. Complications are similar to those mentioned above.

AVULSED TEETH. Avulsed teeth should be replanted although the prognosis is very poor. These teeth usually undergo external resorption until exfoliation.[2] The best chance of success is with teeth where there is incomplete root formation.[3] The extraoral period also is of significance and thirty minutes elapsed time appears to be critical.[4] The method and temperature of storage does not appear to be an influencing factor.[5] The cases which seem to be the most successful are those in which the patient has performed the replantation.

The suggested technic is as follows:

1. Anesthetize and radiograph the area.
2. Clean the tooth gently in a 2% NaF solution. Avoid disturbing the periodontal ligament. The fluoride solution inhibits the external resorption.[6]
3. Remove the blood clot with suction and establish bleeding. Do not scrape the surfaces of the alveolus.
4. Replant the tooth with gentle finger pressure.
5. Splint the tooth with a fast-setting acrylic applied with a paintbrush or some other suitable splinting material. Maintain the splint for approximately two weeks for reasons cited above. Bands, arch bars or wire should not be used to splint replanted teeth as they usually produce orthodontic forces which may accelerate resorption of the root.
6. Radiograph the area and follow with radiographs at biweekly intervals for two months. Follow at monthly intervals for six months and then semiannually.
7. Check with the physician regarding a tetanus booster and administer an antibiotic (not tetracycline prior to age eight because of the danger of tooth discoloration).
8. If at any time there are clinical signs of pulpal degeneration, institute endodontic treatment. In teeth with open apices, the pulp will become necrotic in approximately 50 percent of cases; while in the mature teeth, pulpal necrosis will occur in 90 percent of the cases.[3]

Although replantation is not very successful, the procedure is warranted by the service the tooth will perform in providing space maintenance during the development of the occlusion, speech development and esthetics. The procedure, however, is not recommended in the primary dentition because the teeth are usually mature necessitating endodontic therapy, splinting is difficult, and patient cooperation is usually minimal in this age group. In addition, the resorption potential of the primary teeth appears to be higher than the permanent teeth and the primary tooth will usually be replaced by a permanent tooth within a relatively short period of time.

When and if the replanted tooth is lost, either a space maintainer or a fixed bridge may be placed.

Routine Oral Examination

A thorough oral and facial examination and the collection of diagnostic aids and records can usually be accomplished by the second nonemergency visit.

Diagnostic Aids

Many diagnostic aids may be employed to make or confirm a diagnosis. The most commonly used aids in pedodontics are (a) radiographs (intraoral and extraoral), (b) study models, (c) caries activity tests and (d) pulpal vitality tests.

INTRAORAL RADIOGRAPHS. Bite-wing radiographs are essential for the detection of

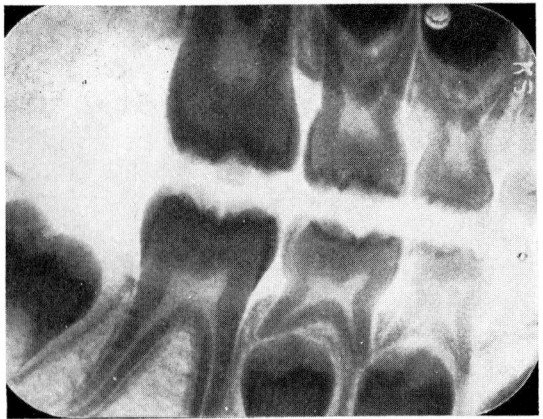 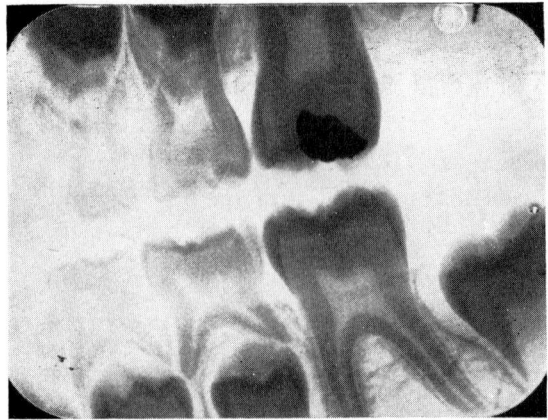

Figure 20-4. Bite-wing radiographs. Interproximal contact areas must be clearly visible for accurate diagnosis. Note the large radiolucent area beneath the mesiobuccal cusp of the maxillary second primary molar. This is observed in many of these particular teeth and should not be confused with caries.

incipient interproximal caries (Fig. 20-4). Full-mouth surveys are necessary for the early detection of dental anomalies in number and form and the assessment of the progress of dental development.

Generally, it is consistent with good practice to obtain anterior periapicals and posterior bite-wings at about age three as a caries detecting measure.

At about age five a full-mouth survey should be taken. This survey will show the development and position of most of the permanent dentition as well as the integrity of the developing teeth.

It is not always necessary to take a full-mouth survey at one sitting unless it is required in special instances such as developmental disturbances. Radiographs of different individual teeth or groups of teeth may be taken at intervals over a period of years. Thus, if a patient begins routine dental care at age three, a complete survey could be accomplished by age five. A complete full-mouth survey can readily be accomplished at one sitting with patients above the age of five. Anterior teeth, because of their vulnerability to injury at early ages, should be one of the first groups of teeth to be radiographed. The posterior quadrants may be radiographed at subsequent recall visits.

EXTRAORAL RADIOGRAPHS. These include the cephalometric headplate, the panoramic radiograph, lateral jaw views of the mandible, special views of the head, for example Water's, and the wrist plate. The cephalometric headplate is utilized for the diagnosis of orthodontic problems and growth analysis. The panoramic radiograph may be used in lieu of a full-mouth intraoral survey but must be supplemented with bite-wing radiographs for caries detection and occasionally intraorals of selected teeth, for example, a tooth suspected of having periapical pathology. The wrist plate is used to determine the skeletal age of the patient versus the chronologic age.[7] Both intraoral and extraoral radiographs may be used to determine dental age versus chronologic age. If the dental age does not coincide within limits with the chronologic age, an endocrine disturbance or familial tendency for delayed dental development may be suspected.

STUDY MODELS. Study models are necessary for the diagnosis of malocclusions and potential malocclusions. They can be used as an aid in the presentation of the treatment plan to parents by helping the parents visualize the dental problems of their child. Additionally, they are of importance from a forensic standpoint.

CARIES ACTIVITY TESTS. Many caries activity tests have been introduced to the dental profession. The most widely used tests are the Snyder test and the *Lactobacillus* count. Sims[8] prepared a definitive article on their interpretation and use. He emphasized their use in preventive dentistry; that is, determining the effectiveness of home-care procedures—diet and plaque control. The Snyder test may be easily and efficiently used in the dental office rather than the *Lactobacillus* count.

Caries activity testing is of value in determining the acid-producing potential of the oral flora by measuring the quantity of an acid-producing microorganism, *Lactobacillus acidophilus* (see Ch. 9).

A rampant caries patient will have a high degree of caries activity as measured by the tests. Similarly, a patient on a caries control program will have a minimal degree of activity.

The tests are valuable in differentiating between active and arrested caries, the completion of caries control and the effectiveness of a recall program.

PULPAL VITALITY TESTS. Although no pulpal vitality test can accurately determine the status of the pulp, they can provide an indication of pulpal status when used in conjunction with radiographs, the history of the tooth, mobility and tenderness to percussion. Electric pulp testing is not completely reliable and diagnosis of pulpal status should not be based solely on this test. The electric current may pass over the enamel surface to the periodontal ligament and give a false positive response. On the other hand, the pulp may be in a state of shock after trauma and consequently a normal pulp may not respond to the stimulation and give a false negative.

Thermal testing with heat and cold are somewhat more reliable than electric pulp testing, but again these tests can not be considered conclusive. A tooth with a small pulp chamber may not elicit a response to thermal tests because of the thickness of the enamel and dentin. In addition, a fearful child may not give a true response because of the control testing on adjacent teeth and the reaction he is expecting. Fear of further pain may cause the child to elicit false positive responses. Two to four weeks after the injury, pulp tests may be conducted with more reliability and should be continued at periodic recall visits. The nerve elements in the pulp may require considerable time to recover from a blow to the tooth. Consequently, absence of a response to pulpal vitality tests does not indicate endodontic treatment in the absence of pronounced clinical symptoms.

Soft Tissue Abnormalities

The soft tissues in children must be examined very closely as in adults.

The mucosa along the alveolar process and the attached gingivae should be examined carefully when deep carious lesions in the teeth are present. A fistulous tract

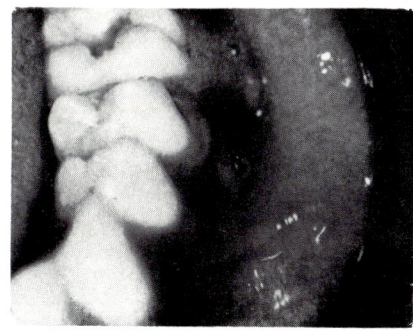

Figure 20-5. Chronic dento-alveolar abscesses of the second premolar and first permanent molar with fistulous tracts below the attached gingivae.

(parulis) may be noted which indicates a chronic dento-alveolar abscess (Fig. 20-5). The drainage of an abscess may also occur via the periodontal ligament and the gingival sulcus.

Occasionally an eruption hematoma is present just prior to the eruption of a tooth (Fig. 20-6). It appears as a blue or purple elevation on the alveolar ridge similar in appearance to a contusion or "bruise." No treatment is necessary since it will disappear with the eruption of the tooth. This must be differentiated from a "tattoo" caused by a heavy metal or foreign body.

The frena, especially the maxillary and mandibular labial frena, may have an abnormal attachment or shape (Fig. 20-7). The maxillary labial frenum may cause a speech problem or, more frequently, spaced central incisors (*see* elective oral surgery). The mandibular frenum may cause a stripping of the gingivae around the anterior teeth (Fig. 20-8). This will result in the destruction of the periodontal tissues of these teeth. Treatment should not be delayed as may be the case for the maxillary frenum.

In ankyloglossia the lingual frenum is attached near to or at the tip of the tongue and may restrict tongue movement. If the speech is normal and abnormal spacing in the mandibular anterior segment is not apparent, frenectomy is not indicated.

RECURRENT APHTHAE AND TRAUMATIC LESIONS. The gingivae and mucosa of children may be involved by recurrent aphthous ulcers which are usually found near the buccal frena or in the mucobuccal fold (Fig. 20-9). This is *not* a viral lesion. Currently it is believed that an "L" form of bacteria may be the causative factor.[9] Often a child brushes his teeth harshly prior to a dental visit and occasionally will abrade the gingivae. After a few days this

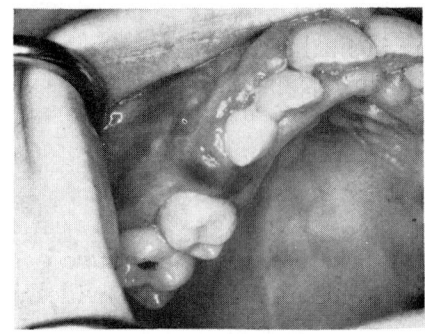
Figure 20-6. Eruption hematoma in the area of the first premolar. It is more commonly associated with the maxillary second primary molar and first permanent molars.

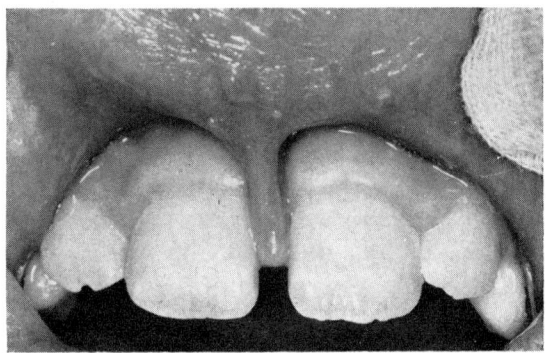
Figure 20-7. Abnormal labial frenum with a thick fibrous band of tissue extending lingually. This case will require surgery. (Courtesy of Dr. Gerald B. Winter.)

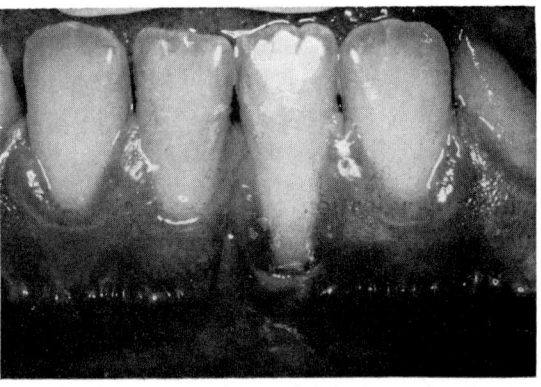
Figure 20-8. Gingival stripping around the left central incisor which is attributable to the mandibular frenum. Periodontal surgery is necessary to prevent further destruction of tissue in the area. (Courtesy of Dr. Gerald B. Winter.)

may resemble an aphthous lesion (page 102).

ACUTE HERPETIC GINGIVOSTOMATITIS. In this condition numerous ulcers occur throughout the oral cavity including the gingivae (Fig. 20-10). Gingival involvement is useful in differentiating this condition from erythema multiforme in which the gingivae are rarely involved. Acute herpetic gingivostomatitis is found in the younger age groups, usually under the age of six. Treatment should be palliative (Dyclone® and perhaps an antihistamine). Secondary infection and dehydration are possible complications (page 101).

STREPTOCOCCAL GINGIVITIS. Acute beta hemolytic streptococcal gingivitis can only be diagnosed by culturing the organism (Fig. 20-11). This disease must be quickly diagnosed and antibiotic therapy instituted in order to prevent the possible development of rheumatic fever or acute glomerulonephritis.

GINGIVAL DISTURBANCES FOLLOWING RUBELLA VACCINATION. Recently the German measles vaccine (rubella) has been implicated in the development of gingival disturbances in a few children. In some instances the disturbance is a gingival recession on the buccal surface and mobility of the mandibular first primary molar although other teeth may be affected. A radiograph of the area appears normal. This lesion appears about six weeks to three months after vaccination and will heal without treatment in about six to eight weeks. Sensitivity is usually present when the root surfaces are exposed.

DILANTIN HYPERPLASIA. Dilantin hyperplasia occurs in most of those epileptic children taking the drug. In many instances the hyperplasia is so extensive that a gingivectomy must be performed (Fig. 20-12). A gradual increase in the tissue is usually noted after the surgery but use of the electrosurgery appears to retard this increase in tissue.

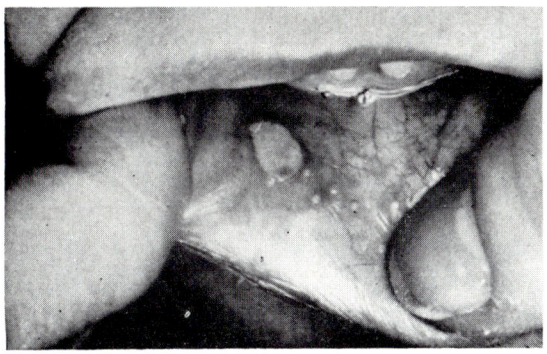

Figure 20-9. Recurrent aphthous ulcer on labial mucosa. This lesion must be differentiated from acute herpetic gingivostomatitis. (Courtesy of Dr. Gerald B. Winter.)

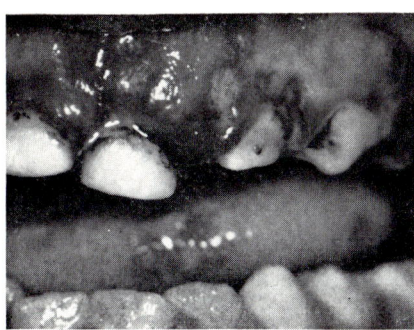

Figure 20-10. Acute herpetic gingivostomatitis. Note the vesicle near the lateral incisor and associated gingival hemorrhage.

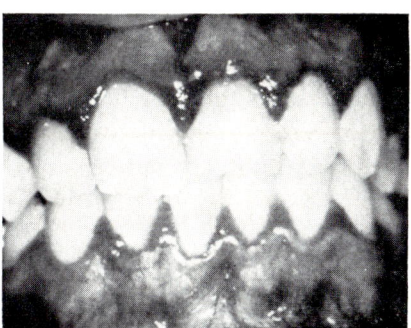

Figure 20-11. Acute beta hemolytic streptococcal gingivitis. Although this appears similar to "filth" gingivitis, the fever and malaise dictate that a culture be obtained.

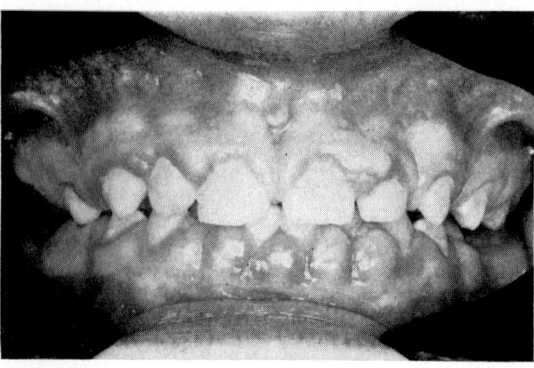

Figure 20-12. Dilantin hyperplasia of the gingival tissues. Gingivectomy is necessary and will probably need to be repeated at some future time if the patient remains on Dilantin. (Courtesy of Dr. Gerald B. Winter.)

Dental Abnormalities

STAINS AND PIGMENTATIONS. A stain is a discoloration which can be removed by scaling or prophylaxis whereas a pigmentation is a discoloration incorporated in the tooth structure which cannot be removed. Normal primary teeth are usually whiter than the normal permanent teeth which tend to be grayish-yellow in color.

The most common stain is green stain which is difficult to remove. Orange stain is much easier to remove. Both stains are associated with poor oral hygiene and are caused by chromogenic bacteria. Black stain is usually found on the lingual and/or labial surfaces of the teeth and is very tenacious. A thorough scaling and prophylaxis is required. When children are taking iron supplements, a brownish stain appears on the teeth and is easily removed. Stannous fluoride will produce a brownish stain in areas of decalcification but not on sound tooth structure.

Erythroblastosis fetalis produces a characteristic blue-green color in the enamel and dentin (and is usually associated with hypoplasia). A history of rhesus incompatibility will substantiate the diagnosis.

Tetracycline will discolor the forming enamel and dentin a brownish-yellow to gray. The discoloration is dose related but duration of administration may also have an effect. Most of the drug is deposited in the dentin.[10] The diagnosis can be confirmed with ultraviolet light since recently erupted teeth will fluoresce. Care should be taken to cover the child's eyes to prevent retinitis from exposure to ultraviolet. Long-term exposure to light produces a change in color from yellow to brown. The hypoplasia sometimes seen in these teeth has been associated with illness rather than the drug.

Porphyria will stain teeth a wine color (purplish-brown). Both the primary and permanent teeth may be affected. This is a generalized pigmentation and should not be confused with internal resorption which produces a similar color.

HEREDITARY DEFECTS. Dentinogenesis imperfecta and amelogenesis imperfecta are hereditary defects of the teeth, each affecting one of the hard tissues of the crown and are readily discernible.

Dentinogenesis imperfecta is characterized by the (a) grayish-brown opalescent color of the teeth, (b) marked abrasion of the teeth and (c) marked narrowing or obliteration of the pulp chamber (Fig. 20-13 A & B). The condition may be associated with osteogenesis imperfecta. Treatment usually consists of restoring the teeth with stainless steel crowns and restoring vertical dimension.

Amelogenesis imperfecta affects the enamel and may be of two main types hypoplastic or hypocalcified. In the hypoplastic type, the enamel is hard but matrix formation is defective. In the hypocalcification type, the matrix formation is normal but calcification is inadequate. Several types of amelogenesis imperfecta have been demonstrated within the two main types (Figs. 20-14; 20-15, A and B; 20-16, A and B). The teeth affected with amelogenesis may be stained and the foods in the diet are believed to be responsible. Radiographically, the dentin and pulp chamber appear normal while the enamel appears

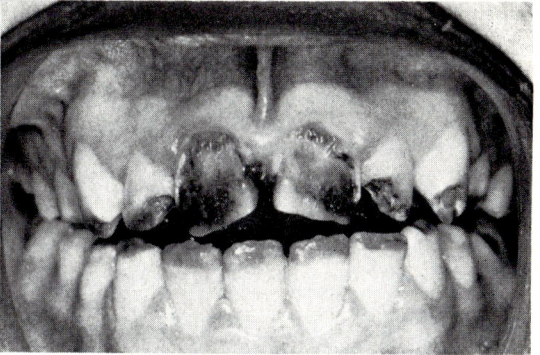

Figure 20-14. Amelogenesis imperfecta of the generalized hypocalcification type. There are areas of more normally calcified enamel near the cervical margins. (Courtesy of Dr. Gerald B. Winter.)

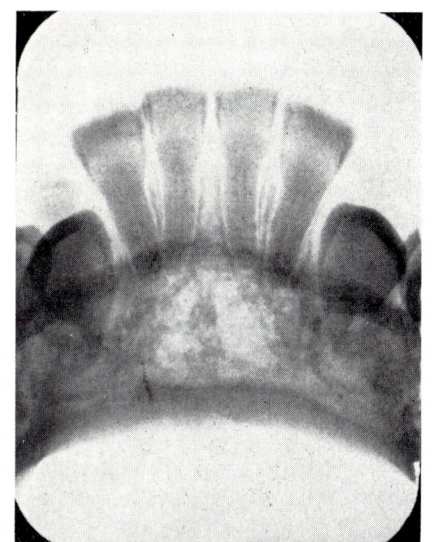

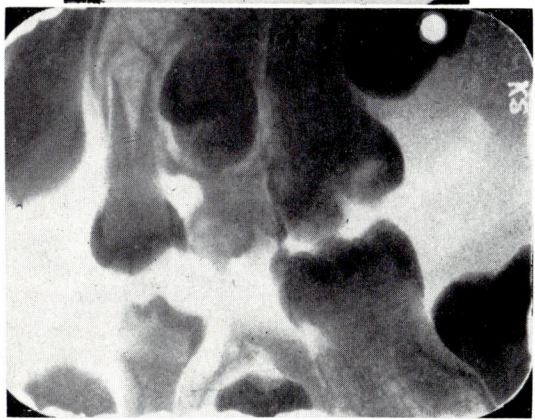

Figure 20-13. (A) Mandibular anterior periapical radiograph in dentinogenesis imperfecta. The pulp chambers and root canals are virtually absent. Enamel and dentin are easily distinguished. Note the "tulip-shape" of the mandibular incisor teeth. (B) Posterior bite-wing radiograph in dentinogenesis imperfecta depicting obliteration of pulp chambers even before root formation is complete.

as a thin layer or may be absent. Treatment is essentially the same as for dentinogenesis imperfecta.

DEFECTS RESULTING FROM LOCAL CAUSES AND SYSTEMIC DISEASE. Any systemic or local disturbance severe enough to affect matrix formation and calcification will produce hypoplasia of the enamel (Fig. 20-17). Usually high fevers will cause hypoplasia in all teeth developing at that time. The age at which the systemic disturbance occurred can be determined by noting the amount or level of the tooth which is hypoplastic. This is known as tooth ring analysis.[11] Trauma and chronic infection may also produce a localized hypoplasia which is frequently found only on one surface. This may appear as an isolated white spot especially in the anterior region.

CONGENITAL ABSENCE OF TEETH. Congenital absence of teeth occurs in 5 percent of all patients and is frequently diagnosed initially in the child patient. The premolars and maxillary lateral incisors are the teeth most frequently absent (Fig. 20-18, A, B and C).[12] Every effort should be made to retain the primary tooth predecessors. If

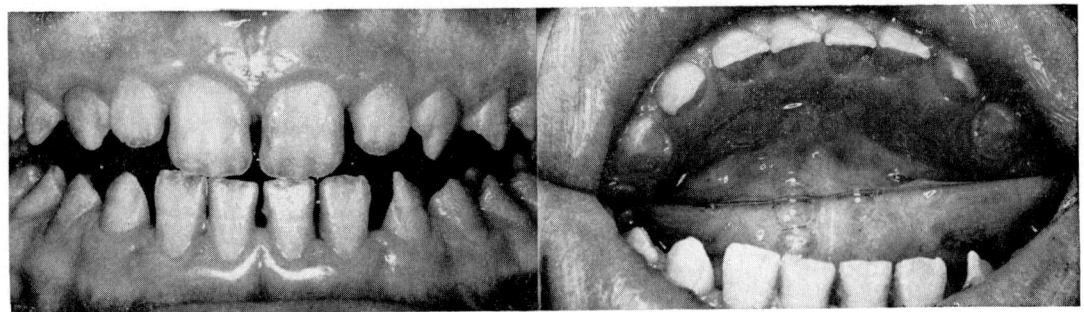

Figure 20-15. (A) Amelogenesis imperfecta with generalized enamel hypoplasia (thin type). Spacing between the teeth is due to the very thin enamel layer. Very fine pitting and wrinkling of the enamel is present on some teeth, for example, maxillary lateral incisors. (B) Incisal view of above which also shows the thin layer of enamel. (Courtesy of Dr. Gerald B. Winter.)

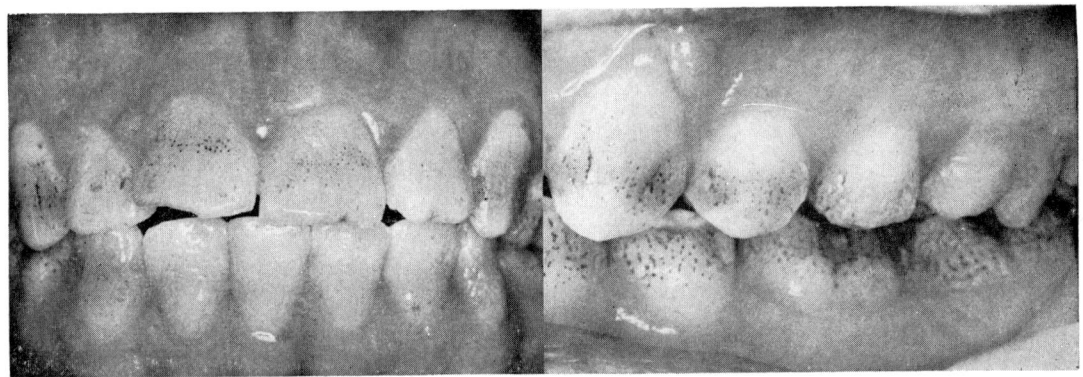

Figure 20-16. (A) Amelogenesis imperfecta with generalized enamel hypoplasia (random pitting type). Anterior view of teeth with stained pits in the enamel surface. (B) Posterior teeth of same case. (Courtesy of Dr. Gerald B. Winter.)

arch length is needed to provide space for proper alignment of the remaining permanent teeth, the primary teeth may be restored with stainless steel crowns of a narrower mesiodistal dimension and appropriate contour. It is difficult to retain the primary lateral incisors and careful consideration must be given to the orthodontic problems. A decision must be reached whether the space should be maintained or regained for the construction of a fixed bridge, or the canines must be recontoured to some extent toward the appearance of lateral incisors.

ANKYLOSED TEETH. These are easily diagnosed and require careful observation. They are often called "submerged teeth" but this is a misnomer (Fig. 20-19). The tooth has become attached to the alveolar process by a bony union. This prevents the tooth from moving occlusally as the alveolar process continues to grow. Therefore, the condition results from growth of the alveolar process up and around and the tooth and not from a submerging of the tooth.

The primary molars are the teeth which become ankylosed most frequently, although after trauma an anterior tooth may become ankylosed. The amount of deviation from the occlusal plane will depend on the age at which the ankylosis occurs.

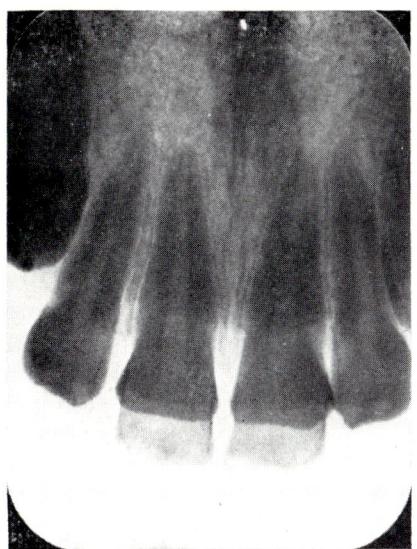

Figure 20-17. Chronic enamel hypoplasia (birth to twelve months) of incisors as seen on the radiograph. Disturbance of enamel formation produced the radiolucent areas in the incisal half of the crown. Clinically, the affected area appears yellowish-brown.

Ankylosis may result in a loss of arch length by allowing the permanent molars to tip mesially since normal contact is lost. Eruption of the succedaneous tooth is usually prevented or abnormal since only rarely does the erupting tooth resorb the bony union with the tooth. Consequently, ankylosed teeth are usually extracted. A general rule of thumb is to have the tooth extracted by an oral surgeon when only one-half of the crown is visible. A space maintainer may need to be placed to hold the proper arch length prior to extraction and after the extraction.

Essential Oral Surgery

After the clinical and radiographic examination, the dentist must determine which teeth are restorable. Those that are not restorable should be extracted—either by the dentist himself or an oral surgeon.

In the young or fearful child, referral to an oral surgeon for extraction under general anesthesia or nitrous oxide analgesia plus local anesthesia may be helpful to the dentist. The child will tend not to associate the dentist with potential unpleasant experiences and thus gain confidence in the dentist sooner. Many children are referred to pedodontists as "management problems" because an extraction was performed either at or soon after the initial visit.

Of course the dentist may find it necessary to extract a tooth as an emergency or first appointment treatment. In the young or fearful child, the dentist should expect to spend the next few visits with the child performing fear-removing treatments, for example, toothbrushing instructions, prophylaxis, etcetera, to allow the child to gain confidence in the dentist and dentistry, especially if the local anesthesia and extraction were painful. The "tell, show, and do" technic as each new instrument or procedure is produced will allay many of the patient's fears of the unknown.

Pulp Therapy

Those teeth which are or may be pulpally involved must be treated as soon as possible. Pulp treatment may be in the form of indirect pulp capping, direct pulp capping, pulpotomy or pulpectomy. It is understood that pulp therapy is performed with a rubber dam in place.

Indirect Pulp Capping

This is a technic which may be used in selected teeth with potential carious exposures (Fig. 20-20). Selection of the teeth is based on the clinical judgment that the pulpal pathology is reversible. The technic is to remove all necrotic and infected carious dentin and as much decalcified (affected) dentin as possible without causing a pulp exposure during the excavation (Figs. 20-21 and 20-22). It is suggested that a large (#4–6) round bur be used rather than a spoon excavator since the spoon

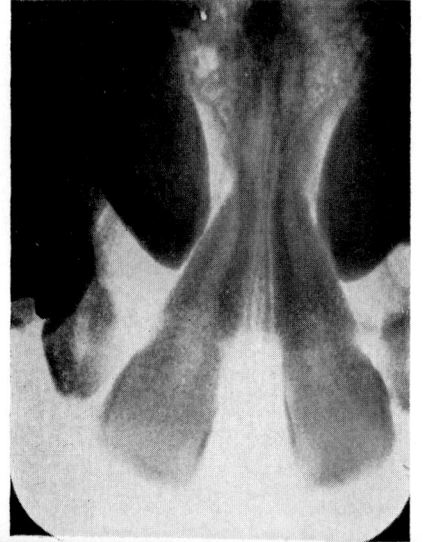

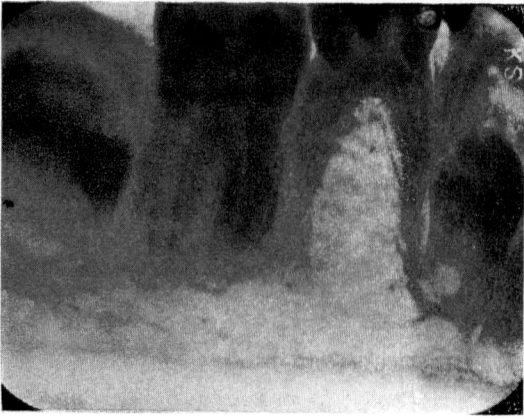

Figure 20-18. (Top, left) Periapical radiograph depicting congenital absence of maxillary permanent lateral incisors and typical eruption pattern of permanent canines. (Top, right) and (Left) Periapical radiographs showing the congenital absence of second premolars and the need for adequate radiographs to diagnose the condition.

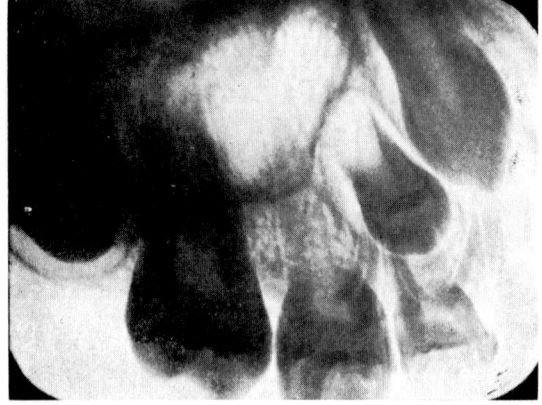

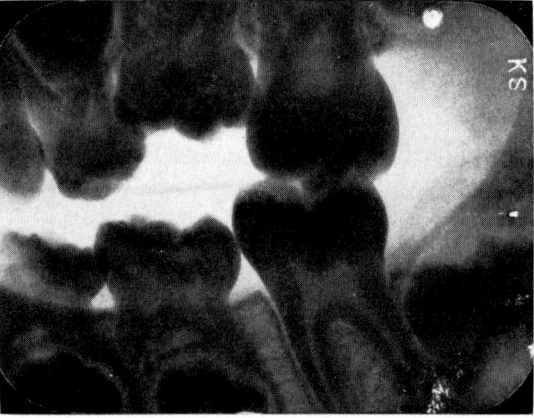

Figure 20-19. Bite-wing radiograph depicting ankylosed teeth (mandibular first and second primary molars and maxillary second primary molar). The teeth are not level with the occlusal plane.

excavator tends to peel large pieces of decalcified dentin from the cavity resulting in numerous exposures. After the initial excavation, the floor of the cavity is sealed with a thick layer of ZOE (Fig. 20-22). The sealing of the cavity is most important since this prevents a reinfection of the tooth structure and renders any remaining bacteria harmless as long as the lesion remains sealed. Since decalcification precedes bacterial invasion of the tubules, only a few bacteria will remain if the excavation is carried out carefully.[13]

It is suggested that ZOE is the medicament of choice for indirect pulp capping because it will sedate the pulp and allow pulpal healing and the ultimate formation of sclerotic and reparative dentin (Figs. 20-21 and 20-22). In addition, it is a good sealant. Calcium hydroxide has been advocated as a medicament because of its capacity to stimulate reparative dentin formation and its supposed remineralization

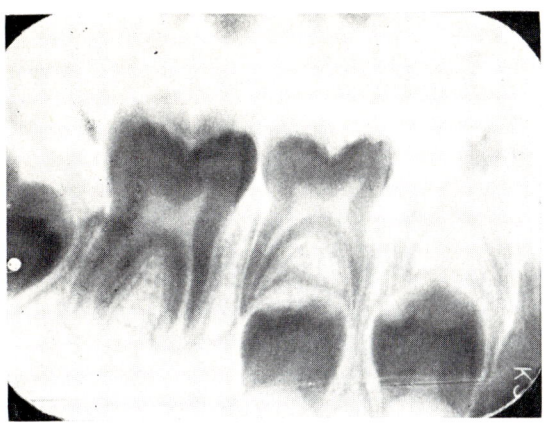

Figure 20-20. Periapical radiograph showing a large carious lesion in the mandibular first primary molar. This is a good candidate for indirect pulp capping. Note the thin radiopaque line on the roof of the pulp chamber (sclerotic dentin) and the absence of visible periapical pathology. The tooth will require a stainless steel crown restoration.

properties. However, the high pH (over pH 11) may cause the already inflamed pulp (from toxic bacterial products) to proceed into an irreversible state necessitating a pulpotomy or pulpectomy.

The ZOE should remain in the cavity for at least six weeks since this is the optimal time needed for adequate reparative dentin formation. If the cavity is sealed for longer periods of time (three to four months), the decalcified (affected) dentin may become remineralized. In those teeth where the ZOE may be easily dislodged, a band around the tooth will be most helpful, and of course, the ZOE may be covered with zinc phosphate or carboxylate cements.

Although it is not necessary always to reenter the cavity by removing the ZOE to inspect the nature of the dentin, it is suggested that this be done in those teeth which initially had a questionable prognosis for indirect pulp capping. The first few teeth for which the dentist attempts indirect pulp capping should also be reentered to familiarize himself with its results and to refine his technic. It should be pointed out that this procedure works equally well for both the primary and permanent teeth.

Direct Pulp Capping

At the present time, the medicament of choice for direct pulp capping is calcium hydroxide and therefore the procedure is best limited to young permanent teeth. With the high degree of success with formocresol for primary teeth, a five-minute vital pulpotomy should be performed in those primary teeth which might be candidates for direct pulp capping.

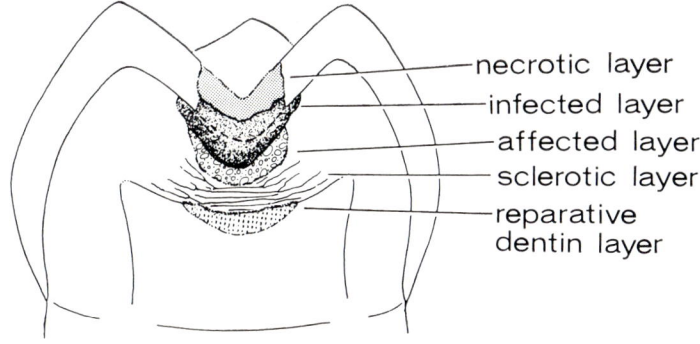

Figure 20-21. Schematic drawing of a carious lesion and the defense mechanisms (sclerosis and reparative dentin) against advancement and pulp exposure. The anatomy of the lesion and its defense are fundamental to case selection for indirect pulp capping.

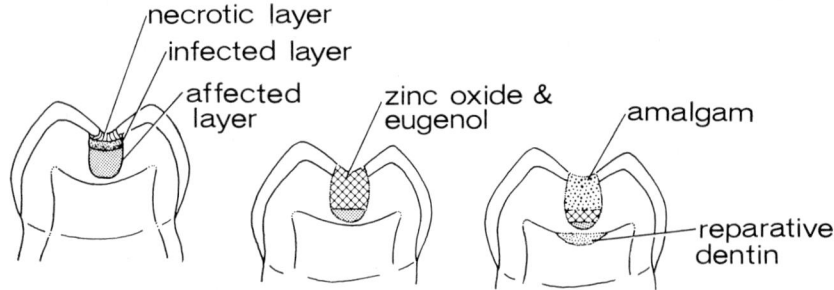

Figure 20-22. Schematic drawing illustrating the steps and response to indirect pulp capping. Remove infected and *some* affected dentin. Place ZOE for at least six weeks, then final restoration.

Pulpotomy

The *vital* pulpotomy is a very useful technic for the primary and younger permanent teeth which have carious exposures and bacterial infection of the coronal pulp. The technic is the same for both types of teeth with the exception of the medicament that is placed in contact with the pulpal stumps at the orifices of the root canals (Fig. 20-23).

For the young (open apices) permanent teeth with healthy pulp tissue in the root canals, calcium hydroxide is the medicament of choice, although research is being conducted on the use of formocresol in these teeth.

For the primary teeth, formocresol is the medicament of choice. Two methods of application may be used:

1. Five minutes. A cotton pellet *saturated* with formocresol is applied to the amputation site for five minutes followed by sealing the pulp chamber with ZOE. This technic is used when clinical judgment indicates that infection has not progressed beyond the amputation site.

2. Seven days. A cotton pellet *slightly moistened* with formocresol is sealed in the pulp chamber for seven days. At the next visit, the pellet is removed and the chamber is sealed with ZOE. This technic is used when clinical judgment indicates infection has progressed beyond the amputation site.

The *nonvital* pulpotomy is useful in those primary teeth which are obviously infected and necrotic and especially in the second primary molar prior to the eruption of the first permanent molar. The technic is similar to the seven-day vital pulpotomy procedure. The pulp chamber is debrided and dried and then the slightly moistened cotton pellet of formocresol is placed in the chamber for seven days. The second visit procedure is the same as for the seven-day vital pulpotomy.

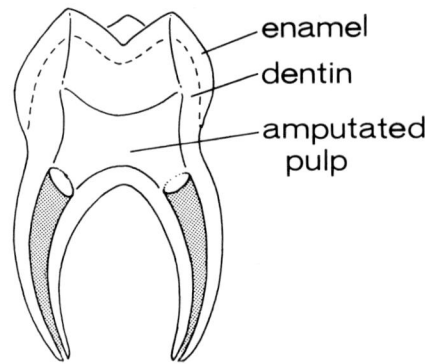

Figure 20-23. Schematic drawing of pulp amputation in a molar tooth. Proper amputation is easiest when the entire roof of the chamber is removed. Pulpal elements should not extend beyond the orifices of the canals into the chamber.

Case selection is important for this technic. Where there is atypical or abnormal resorption areas on the roots of the tooth, it is best to extract the tooth. This type of resorption is usually found on those teeth which have had longstanding dentoalveolar abscesses with the loss of extensive amounts of alveolar bone. However, primary teeth with fistulous tracts, mobility and some loss of interradicular bone can be treated successfully with this technic in most instances. The advantage of using this technic rather than routinely extracting these teeth is that a properly restored primary tooth is an ideal space maintainer.

Pulpectomy

Routine endodontic therapy should be performed on all pulpally involved, mature (closed apices) permanent teeth since the success rate is very high (96 to 98 percent). In those young permanent teeth with necrotic or severely infected pulps, induction of root end closure should be performed. The technic developed by Frank [14] can be performed on anterior teeth as well as posterior. The technic is to clean and fill the canal with calcium hydroxide and camphorated paramonochlorophenol until a good apical seal can be obtained using routine endodontic technics. Although pulpectomy has been advocated for primary teeth, the reasonably good success rate of the nonvital pulpotomy technic indicates that this difficult and time-consuming procedure may not always be necessary.

Caries Control

Diet Analysis

Sucrose is the prime substrate for cariogenic bacteria.[15] The elimination of sucrose in the diet is extremely difficult but it can be eliminated between meals. A diet history (Fig. 20-24) which is analyzed (Fig. 20-25) for the frequency of intake and the form of sucrose (non-retentive versus retentive) and the total nutrition can be an excellent teaching aid toward carrying out a preventive program. It must be emphasized that the frequency of ingestion of sucrose is more important than the amount. The diet analysis must also explain to the parents the interrelationships of the tooth, the substrate and bacteria and that dental caries do not develop because of "soft teeth."

Home-Care Instructions

Although toothbrushing alone cannot completely prevent dental caries and gingival problems, it is an essential adjunct to the prevention of dental disease and maintenance of oral health. Until the age of eight, the parent must aid the child in toothbrushing because the child does not have the dexterity to perform a thorough cleansing of the teeth. Some method of disclosing the location of plaque on the teeth should be used to ensure thorough toothbrushing. Many disclosing agents may be used but the most common is a food dye—erythrosin.

The disclosing tablet or solution may be used prior to toothbrushing for determining the extent of plaque or after toothbrushing to determine the effectiveness of the toothbrushing technic. Almost any toothbrushing method may be used as long as the patient can use it effectively. However, for children the horizontal or "scrub brush" technic appears to work best.[16] The electric toothbrush will perform a more thorough cleansing of the teeth if used in a conscientious manner. It is considered by most children as a novelty for some time and gets good use, but after several weeks the novelty value diminishes and the

Time	Food	7th Day Quantity	Prepared

FOOD INTAKE DIARY

Patient's name_____

Our dental examination of your child's oral health condition has revealed that your child has excessive dental decay. By this we mean that the decay rate in his mouth has become so active that all of the teeth are in danger of being completely destroyed. In order to prevent this your cooperation is necessary.

Far more is known about dental decay today than was known a few years ago. Therefore, we now understand how it can be controlled better. One of the most important factors that affects the dental decay rate is the diet. Therefore, we must obtain an accurate and complete dietary history of your child's eating habits. You will be instructed in how to prepare this diet diary.

Instructions:

1. A complete record of *everything* eaten for seven consecutive days is necessary.
2. Record every type of food consumed, solid or liquid, at mealtime, between meals, at the soda fountain, while watching TV, etc. Record also candies, life savers or lozenges, gum, cough syrups or drops.
3. For each meal, list the food preparation (fried, broiled, etc.) and amount (1 tsp. or 1 Tbl, 1 cup, 1 4-oz. glass, number of pieces.)
4. For fruits and vegetables record whether raw, fresh, frozen, canned or juice.
5. Record amount of sugar or sugar products and cream or milk added to cereal, beverages or other foods.
6. Record foods in order in which they are eaten.
7. Particular information on snacks is most important. Do not leave out the smallest detail.
8. Keep this record in an easy to reach place in order to keep current. It is extremely difficult to be accurate in retrospect.

* Figure 20-24. Front page (right-Food Intake Diary) and back page (left) of a diet history booklet. The booklet consists of two 8½″ by 11″ sheets of paper mimeographed on both sides of the two sheets of paper. The printed sheets are folded to produce a four-page booklet. All the remaining pages are similar to the back page, as illustrated, so that the parent can record the diet for a seven day period in the booklet. When the diet history has been completed by the parent it is returned to the dentist for analysis by the dentist or his auxiliary personnel using the analysis form illustrated below (Figure 20-25). The diet history becomes a part of the patient's record.

electric toothbrush gets about as much use as the manual toothbrush.

The dentifrice is also important in a home-care program. The dentifrice should at least be one that contains an *active* fluoride ion and is a therapeutic rather than a cosmetic dentifrice. Fluoride toothpastes may contain NaF or SnF_2. It is recommended that a SnF_2 toothpaste is the toothpaste of choice for reasons to be stated below.

Fluoride Treatment

The topical fluoride treatment should be a routine office procedure for both the child and the adult. Presently two systems

* The diet history and diet analysis forms were modified (after Nizel, A. E.: Nutrition in Preventive Dentistry, Science and Practice. Philadelphia, Saunders, 1972) by Dr. J. A. Gallios and Dr. D. E. Ore.

Recommendations

R_x

Suggested snack foods for people with excessive decay.

FRUITS: Raw: apple, fresh apricots, melons (watermelon, cantaloupe), cherries, grapefruit, grapes, oranges, peaches, pears, pineapple, tangerines, fresh fruit juices (unsweetened).
VEGETABLES: Raw: cabbage, cauliflower, carrots, celery, cucumbers, lettuce and other salad greens, radishes, tomatoes, turnips. Tomato juice.
MILK: Unsweetened.
CHEESE: All kinds—cheddar, cottage or cream.
NUTS: All kinds.
COMBINATIONS: Apple slices with cheddar cheese; cream cheese balls rolled in chopped nuts; celery stuffed with cottage cheese and chives; baloney slices spread with cream cheese and cut in wedges; shrimp on toothpicks with tomato cocktail sauce made without sugar; deviled eggs; pear halves spread with cream cheese and sprinkled with chopped nuts.

* Figure 20-25A.

* The diet history and diet analysis forms were modified (after Nizel, A. E.: Nutrition in Preventive Dentistry, Science and Practice. Philadelphia, Saunders, 1972) by Dr. J. A. Gallios and Dr. D. E. Ore.

THE DECAY PROCESS

What causes dental decay?
"Too much candy?" "Not brushing the teeth?" "Soft teeth?" All of these answers are partly true and partly untrue. They reflect a superficial understanding of the causes of dental decay, causes that were not understood even by dental scientists until recently. Dental decay is a disease of the teeth, caused, like many other diseases, by germs (bacteria). These germs exist in the mouth. They digest food that is placed in the mouth. When these germs digest this food they produce acid. This acid collects on the teeth in those areas that are difficult to clean (grooves, between the teeth, gumlines), and destroys the hard tooth structure. This destruction of enamel and dentin if allowed to continue may cause death of the pulp or nerve of the tooth. This may lead to pain, infection, abscess formation or other serious complications.

These bacteria make acid readily from carbohydrates (sugars or sweets). These bacteria work with amazing speed. In tests, it was shown that it takes only about 90 seconds to produce enough acid to cause tooth damage. This destructive process continues for a minimum of about 30 minutes. (Far longer when sticky or retentive sugars are used). This period of time we call an "acid attack."

How can dental decay be controlled?
1. Toothbrushing—*at the proper times* has been shown to be helpful. The teeth should be brushed *after* each eating to remove sticky foods from the teeth and to shorten the duration of the acid attack. Brushing in the morning and at bedtime is not as effective as brushing after eating.
2. Selection of nonretentive foods and avoidance of refined carbohydrates (sugars) is extremely important. If the food remains in the mouth a long time (cookies, caramels, candies) one could expect a devastating acid attack of long duration (longer than 30 minutes). If one utilized "detergent" food (fresh fruits, fresh vegetables, nuts, olives, etc.) the acid does not remain in the mouth so long.
3. The *frequency* of eating carbohydrates is especially important. Those who eat frequently (nibble) have far more "attacks" and much more decay than those who eat three nutritious meals a day and do not snack. This is why it is so important to reduce *between-meal snacks*.

SWEETS INTAKE ANALYSIS

SWEETS	WITH MEALS	BETWEEN MEALS	
NON-RETENTIVE			TOTAL MINIMUM EXPOSURES
RETENTIVE			MINIMUM HOURS OF ACID ACTIVITY

COMMENTS: _____

FIGURE 20.25B SWEET INTAKE ANALYSIS

NUTRITIONAL ANALYSIS

FOOD GROUPS	1ST DAY	2ND DAY	3RD DAY	4TH DAY	5TH DAY	AVG. PER DAY	RECOMMENDED BY U.S. GOVERNMENT			DIFF.
							CHILD	ADOL.	ADULT	
MILK Cheese Cream Butter							3-4 SERV.	4 OR MORE	2 SERV.	
MEAT							2 OR MORE			
VEGETABLE FRUIT Deep Color and Citrus							4 OR MORE			
BREAD CEREAL Enriched Whole Grain Cooked Cereal							4 OR MORE			

COMMENTS: _____

FIGURE 20.25C. NUTRITIONAL ANALYSIS

are in use—the stannous fluoride system and the acidulated fluoride phosphate system. Both have been proven effective in significantly reducing dental caries. Although the acidulated fluorophosphate system will incorporate more fluoride into the enamel and give a slightly higher reduction in dental caries, the stannous fluoride system appears to be the more versatile and therapeutic. The stannous ion is taken into decalcified enamel and dentin and thus partially remineralizes a lesion, which is unique to the SnF_2 complex. This will result in incipient lesions becoming arrested or marked reduction in their rate of progress. For this reason, stannous fluoride is presently the system of choice since many incipient or "white spot" lesions are undetectable.

Since the protection offered by the fluoride ion in various systems is additive, the dentist should use a topical fluoride appli-

Figure 20-25A. The diet analysis form (A,B,C) is a one page 8½″ by 11″ sheet of paper mimeographed on both sides and folded. The data collected in the diet history is analyzed and the results placed on the form. The form is given to the parent for use at home as a dietary guide for the patient. It is suggested that the parents be present when the analysis is performed.

The front page of the form (right-The Decay Process) provides a summary of the carious process and its control. The dentist or auxiliary personnel can use this as an outline in discussing the role of diet in prevention.

The back page of the form (left-Recommendations) is filled out after the sucrose analysis (Figure 20-25B) and the nutritional analysis (Figure 20-25C) have been completed. Recommendations can be enumerated and could include phrases such as "Increase daily meat servings," "Decrease daily bread cereal servings," or "Substitute fresh fruit for snacks." A listing of suggested substitute foods to replace cariogenic snacks is presented below the recommendations.

Figure 20-25B. The sweets intake analysis is completed by analyzing the diet history for those foods which contain sucrose. The sucrose content of the diet is analyzed for the form of the sugar (non-retentive or soluble versus retentive) as well as when the sugar was eaten (with meals or between meals). When sucrose appears in the diet history it is recorded in the proper square with a "chit mark." This is a good task for the parent. After the entire diet history is analyzed, the "marks" are totaled from all squares to determine the total minimum exposures (far right) or "acid attacks." This is the minimum number of exposures because it is likely that there may be some sucrose ingestion which has not been recorded.

The minimum number of hours of acid activity is determined by allocating thirty minutes for each non-retentive (soluble) sugar-form ingested and one hour for each retentive sugar-form. This will approximate the hours of acid production to which the plaque covered areas of the teeth have been subjected.

Figure 20-25C. The nutritional analysis is performed by recording each food listed in the diet history in the appropriate square according to the type of food. There will be some foods eaten (colas) which will not be recorded since they have no nutritional value. Only five of the seven days listed in the diet history is used for this analysis. "Chit marks" are made and then averaged to determine the average daily servings of the four food groups. This is compared with the U. S. Government recommendations. The difference is recorded as the number of daily servings above or below the Federal recommendations. Usually the child will be minus one in the milk group, minus one in the meat group, minus two in the fruit-vegetable group, and plus three in the bread-cereal group. The individual diet is then discussed with the parent(s) and recommendations are made as explained above.

cation in those areas where the communal water supply is fluoridated. This will result in added protection to that provided by the fluoridated water. When fluoridated water, topical fluoride applications and a fluoride dentifrice is used, a reduction of approximately 70 percent in DMF may be expected.[17]

Restorative Treatment

Most of the diagnosis and treatment planning for the pedodontic patient will center around the restorative procedures. Many restorative materials are used in pedodontics, for example, silver amalgam, stainless steel bands and crowns, gold and silver inlays, gold foil, composite and acrylic materials, and occasionally silicate cement. In some restorative procedures, these materials may be used in combination.

Silver amalgam is still the material of choice for restoration of posterior teeth, although silver or gold slice preparation inlays may be used. Currently, composite materials are being suggested for posterior teeth [18] but further research and improvement is necessary before composite materials may be used routinely. Powdered gold foil may be used as efficiently as silver amalgam is class I cavities in the first permanent molars, premolars and lingual surfaces of anterior teeth.

The stainless steel band and crown are used frequently in restoring both primary and permanent teeth. Some of the indications for stainless steel crowns are (a) extensive caries in primary or permanent teeth and after pulpotomy or pulpectomy, (b) hypoplastic teeth or teeth with hereditary anomalies and (c) fractured teeth.

The stainless steel band can be used effectively in restoring primary canines and incisors.

Restoration of the fractured incisor presents a challenge to the dentist. After the emergency treatment and when the pulp has had an opportunity for recovery, a transitional restoration (a restoration between emergency treatment and the final restoration) can be placed. The type of transitional restoration will be determined by the extent of the fracture. Examples are

1. Wire reinforced composite or acrylic.
2. Open-face stainless steel crown and composite or acrylic.
3. Pin-ledge inlay and composite or acrylic.
4. Transitional crown—acrylic crown placed over a minimal preparation. The preparation is extended about ½ mm central to the dentino-enamel junction.
5. Acid-etch acrylic restoration.

Transitional restorations are necessary for (a) restoring function, (b) restoring esthetics to some degree, (c) maintaining space and (d) protecting the pulp. In general, most transitional restorations will be replaced at a later age (twelve to sixteen) with some type of jacket crown. However, if the transitional restoration is satisfactory from the standpoint of the purposes enumerated above, there is no need to replace it.

As already indicated, hypoplastic teeth may be restored with stainless steel crowns. Although stainless steel crowns are used primarily for the posterior teeth, they may be used in the anterior region also. The anterior stainless steel crown may be made more esthetic by cutting out the labial surface and covering the hypoplastic area with acrylic or composite material. Recently, a new technic for the restoration of hypoplastic and fractured incisors has been proposed.[19] This is the acid-etch technic. The defective enamel is partially decalcified with 50% phosphoric acid and the etched enamel provides retention for an acrylic build-up of the defective area. The procedure avoids much tooth preparation and the use of stainless steel materials.

Elective Oral Surgery

Elective oral surgery is best delayed until it is necessary to accomplish another phase of the treatment plan. Delaying elective oral surgery will give the patient time to gain confidence in the dentist. In general, elective oral surgery will be performed after the restorative treatment is completed and prior to any orthodontic treatment. Ankylosed teeth may be removed prior to restorative treatment since restorations are sometimes fractured during the removal of the ankylosed teeth.

The maxillary labial frenum presents a problem in diagnosis and treatment planning and is a controversial area of treatment. Spaced central incisors are normal during the mixed dentition period although the frenum may exaggerate this spacing. The anatomy of the frenum must be evaluated before a decision to perform a frenectomy is made. In addition, the wedging action during the eruption of the permanent canines must be considered since pressure atrophy of the frenum may occur and allow the incisors to come together naturally.

In general, a frenectomy should be postponed until the eruption of the permanent canines unless there has been no measurable closure prior to canine eruption. This depends on total maxillary and mandibular arch development.

A premature frenectomy may be an unnecessary procedure and may complicate treatment procedures if the diastema does not close after the surgery. The frenectomy will produce scar tissue which can prevent the incisors from coming into contact either naturally or by orthodontic movement. The teeth should be brought together with an orthodontic appliance before surgery. If the teeth are moved together before surgery, retention of contact may be a problem prior to the eruption of the canines.

Elastics or rubber bands should never be looped around the teeth. The elastic may become lost subgingivally. Attach the elastic to an appliance!

Preventive and Interceptive Orthodontics

Preventive orthodontics is defined as any treatment which will allow the development of the occlusion so that orthodontic treatment is unnecessary. An example is the use of a space maintainer when there is a premature loss of a primary tooth. *Interceptive orthodontics* is defined as any treatment which corrects a developing malocclusion before it requires full orthodontic treatment. An example is the correction of an anterior crossbite with a simple appliance to avoid a loss in arch length as the occlusion develops. A comprehensive chapter on preventive and interceptive orthodontics has been written by Barber.[20]

Preservation of arch length is of prime importance when supervising the development of occlusion. Only the permanent molars exert a mesial component of force called the force of occlusion. The permanent molars also exert a strong force during eruption. The force of eruption is stronger in the mandibular arch because this force is needed to upright the tooth from its eruptive position. The mandibular molars erupt in a mesial and lingual direction while the maxillary molars face distally and buccally and swing mesially as they break through the mucosa into the oral cavity to exert their forces of occlusion. It is this force of occlusion which must be relieved during a period of premature tooth loss, hence the need for space maintenance.

Prior to initiating any preventive or interceptive orthodontic treatment, all diagnostic aids must be analyzed thoroughly to reach the correct diagnosis and establish the proper treatment plan. This means detailed analysis of study models and radiographs.

Space Maintenance

It should be remembered that space is not maintained for a single permanent tooth, but more properly, arch length is maintained since the individual primary teeth do not have the same mesiodistal diameters as their successors. Whenever space maintainers are thought to be indicated, a Moyer's mixed dentition analysis [21] should be performed to determine the presence of adequate arch length for the permanent teeth. If adequate arch length exists, a space regaining appliance or orthodontic referral is required.

Space maintainers, as such, are not necessary when one or two maxillary incisors are lost prematurely, because of the dissipation of the anterior component of force at about the canine eminence. They are indicated in the mandibular incisor region only if spacing is not evident or there is a tendency for the arch to collapse lingually.

Several types of space maintainers can be fabricated; however, only three types will be discussed:

1. *Loop types.* Band and loop or crown and loop space maintainers are probably the most commonly used but perhaps should not be (Fig. 20-26). They are designed for space maintenance when a single tooth in a quadrant is lost. When considering the sequence and pattern of eruption of the permanent teeth, the loop type of space maintainer is best employed (a) during the premature loss of the maxillary first primary molar only; (b) during the premature loss of the mandibular first primary molar prior to the eruption of the mandibular permanent incisors and first permanent molar; and (c) during the premature loss of the mandibular second primary molar after the eruption of the first permanent molar and prior to the eruption of the permanent incisors.

2. *Arch types.* These include the *fixed* and *semifixed lingual arch* and the *Nance holding arch* for single or multiple premature tooth loss. These are the most desirable types of space maintainers since they allow exfoliation and eruption to occur without regard to sequence or pattern. They also allow the erupting permanent teeth to shift in a mesial or distal direction during the development of the occlusion.

A lingual arch for the mandible is best anchored by bands on the first permanent molars with the arch wire contoured to ideal arch form in the anterior region. Since the incisor teeth tend to erupt lingually, very frequent observation is necessary if this appliance is placed prior to their eruption. The only contraindication to the

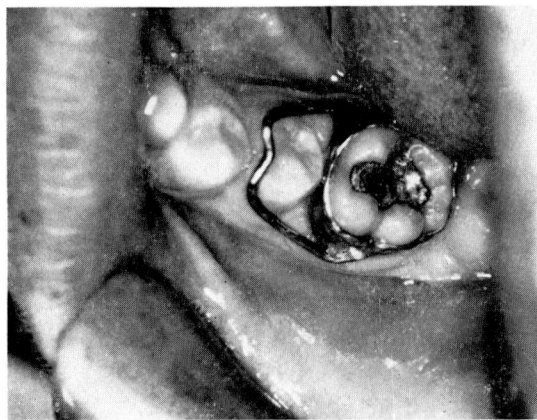

Figure 20-26. Band-loop space maintainer ready for removal. Note that the loop does not contact the erupting first premolar and the second premolar is impacted. Exfoliation of first primary molar allowed the first permanent molar and cemented space maintainer to move mesially. In addition the erupting second permanent molar was a contributing factor.

placement of a lingual arch is if there is inadequate arch length in an otherwise normally developing occlusion. Orthodontic consultation or space regaining is indicated.

The *Nance holding arch* is employed in the maxillary arch. It consists of bands on the anchor teeth (usually the first permanent molars although the second primary molars may also be used), a palatal arch wire (0.040 inches diameter) soldered to the two bands and a button or ribbon of acrylic over the center of the wire against the palatal vault for resistance. Again, the only contraindication is an inadequate arch length.

In cases where arch length is adequate but there is no excess, either or both of these appliances may be inserted to ensure that an adequate amount of arch length is maintained during the exfoliation of the primary teeth. There has been considerable discussion of the "leeway space" in pedodontics and orthodontics. Although it is true that the mesiodistal diameters of the primary molars and canines are greater than the premolars and permanent canines, the permanent incisors are larger than their primary predecessors. In general, the permanent mandibular incisors are slightly crowded and it is this crowding that is alleviated by the so-called leeway space.

3. *Removable acrylic types.* These include bilateral or unilateral acrylic space maintainers. In general, it is wise to construct fixed or semifixed types of space maintainers since these appliances rarely get lost or broken as do the removable acrylic type. However, when there is multiple tooth loss and the plane of occlusion and function are prime considerations, the removable acrylic types should be used. Other indications for the removable type are when the second primary molar is lost prematurely prior to the eruption of the first permanent molar and when there has been early *loss* of the first permanent molar. The distal surface of these space maintainers can be used as a guide for the eruption of the first permanent molar or second permanent molar. This is recommended in preference to the distal shoe appliance because damage may occur to either of the unerupted teeth (first molar and second premolar) and there is a possibility of introducing infection into the jaws with the distal shoe appliance.

Regaining Space

When inadequate arch length exists, space must be regained or an orthodontic referral is required. Several types of appliances may be used to regain space and each will perform its task as long as the principles and fundamentals of tooth movement are observed. A note of caution must be sounded with regard to the jack-screw types of space regainers. When a molar and a premolar are banded with a jack-screw between the two teeth to create space for an unerupted premolar, it is axiomatic that the premolar will move mesially more than the molar will move distally. This is simply because the molar provides more anchorage than the premolar. Space will be created but at the expense of the anterior region usually with the slipping of the canine contact.

Crossbites

Single tooth anterior crossbites are easily discovered, usually by the parent, and corrected when detected early. The acrylic inclined plane cemented to the teeth will usually correct an anterior crossbite within seven to fourteen days if there is sufficient space into which the tooth can move. If the appliance is to remain in place longer, close observation is needed to prevent permanent bite opening. Correction of single tooth crossbites is important to prevent loss in arch length and traumatic occlusion.

Multiple tooth anterior crossbites may be corrected with the acrylic inclined plane but careful diagnosis is needed since a patient with a developing class III malocclusion has the same appearance.

Single tooth posterior crossbites in the permanent dentition may be corrected with criss-cross elastics. Single tooth posterior crossbites in the primary dentition need not be corrected unless a midline deviation is present since the permanent successor does not necessarily erupt into the same position. The more common multiple tooth posterior crossbites are usually corrected with an expansion appliance. The same appliance can be used to correct the single tooth crossbites with midline deviation. Although removable appliances may be used, a fixed appliance such as the Adams expansion appliance ("W" appliance) works very efficiently. It may be used in those cases of both unilateral and bilateral crossbites. Reducing the incisal edge of the canine is not necessary and maintaining its height is sometimes helpful in retention. Overcorrection of the crossbite is probably the best method for gaining good retention.

Oral Habits

Thumbsucking will bring many children to the dentist for correction. The habit will produce an anterior open bite, protrusion of the maxillary anterior teeth and retrusion of the mandibular anterior teeth, and occasionally a posterior crossbite. All dentists agree that the habit should be discontinued at least prior to the eruption of the permanent incisors but there are differences in the general approach to the problem.

It is difficult to force a child to stop sucking his thumb unless he wants to stop. If the child is told about his thumb habit in a nonshameful manner with the dentist playing the role of helper, the child will usually express a willingness to give up the habit. If the child wants to give up the habit, almost any type of reminder will help the child, for example, a bandage, poor tasting substance or palatal crib. However, if the child does not want to give up his habit, rarely will a nonpunitive appliance eliminate the habit. Punitive appliances may stop the habit but psychiatrists are of the opinion that other psychological problems may develop. If the habit is eliminated the malocclusion caused by the thumbsucking will usually be self-correcting. An oral screen is of value in helping the child to stop bedtime thumbsucking.

TONGUE-THRUSTING AND TONGUE-RESTING. Tongue-thrusting and tongue-resting are far more difficult habits to correct since they involve retraining of the tongue musculature. The habit must be evaluated from the standpoint that it may possibly be physiologic. The tonsils may be enlarged forcing the tongue anteriorly thus causing a *relative* macroglossia. The malocclusion from tongue-thrusting is usually characterized by an anterior open bite with bimaxillary protrusion and occasionally a posterior crossbite. A tongue-thrusting habit may be associated with a thumbsucking habit. Treatment is difficult and consists of wearing a palatal tongue crib with concurrent myofunctional exercises assuming, of course, that there is no physiological basis for the habit.

LIP-BITING. The lip-biting habit is characterized by a slight anterior open bite, protrusion of the maxillary anterior teeth, retrusion of the mandibular anterior teeth and chapping of the lower lip. The habit may be corrected with the placement of a lip bumper. This appliance consists of bands with buccal tubes on the mandibular molars, a labial arch of 0.045 inches diameter and an acrylic shield in the anterior region. This appliance is similar to the Denholtz appliance for space regaining.

MOUTH-BREATHING. Mouth-breathing can be corrected with an oral screen. However, before it is placed, the dentist must examine the oropharynx to ascertain whether the child is breathing through his mouth because of enlarged tonsils and adenoids. A consultation with an otolaryngologist is helpful in determining whether the lymphoid tissue should be removed before instituting therapy. In many instances where the tonsils and adenoids are the etiologic factor in the mouth breathing, an oral screen will not be helpful unless the lymphoid tissue is removed.

Consultation

Consultation should be integrated into the treatment plan of the patient where indicated. Many of the dental specialties may be called upon for advice or treatment, or both. The physician may need to be consulted regarding some facets of the medical history (for example, "heart murmur").

Although many consultations may take place by telephone, it is wise to secure any advice in writing to avoid misinterpretation and also for it to become a permanent part of the patient's record.

REFERENCES

1. Ellis, R. G., and Davey, K.: *The Classification and Treatment of Injuries to the Teeth of Children*, 5th ed. Chicago, Year Book Medical Publishers, 1970.
2. Henning, F. R.: Reimplantation of luxated teeth. *Aust Dent J, 10*:306, 1965.
3. Ohman, A.: Healing and sensitivity to pain in young replanted human teeth. *Odontol Foren Tidskr*, 73:168, 1965.
4. Andreasen, J. O., and Hjorting-Hansen, E.: Replantation of teeth—I. *Acta Odontol Scand*, 24:263, 1966.
5. Anderson, A. W., Sharav, Y., and Massler, M.: Periodontal reattachment after tooth replantation. *Periodontics*, 6:161, 1968.
6. Shulman, L. B., Kalis, P., and Goldhaber, P.: Fluoride inhibition of tooth-replant root resorption in Cebus monkeys. *J Oral Ther Pharm*, 4:331, 1968.
7. Greulich, W. W., and Pyle, S. I.: *Radiographic Atlas of Skeletal Development of the Hand and Wrist*, 2nd ed. Stanford, Stanford University Press, 1959.
8. Sims, W.: The interpretation and use of Snyder tests and *Lactobacillus* counts. *JADA*, 80:1315, 1970.
9. Graykowski, S. A., Barile, M. F., and Stanley, H. R.: Periadenitis aphthae: clinical and histopathologic aspects of lesions in a patient and of lesions produced in rabbit skin. *JADA*, 69:118, 1964.
10. Bennett, I. C., and Law, D. B.: Incorporation of tetracycline in developing enamel and dentin in dogs. *J Dent Child*, 34:93, 1967.
11. Massler, M., Schour, I., and Poncher, H. G.: Developmental pattern of the child as reflected in the calcification pattern of the teeth. *Am J Dis Child*, 62:33, 1941.
12. Glenn, F. B.: A consecutive six-year study of the prevalence of congenitally missing teeth in private practice of two geographically separated areas. *J Dent Child*, 31: 269, 1964.
13. Sarnat, H., and Massler, M.: Microstructure of active and arrested dentinal caries. *J Dent Res*, 44:1389, 1965.
14. Frank, A. L.: Therapy for the divergent pulpless tooth by continued apical formation. *JADA*, 72:87, 1966.
15. Newbrun, E.: Sucrose, the arch criminal of dental caries. *J Dent Child*, 36:239, 1969.
16. Kimmelman, B., and Tussman, G. C.: Research in the designs of children's toothbrushes. *J Dent Child*, 27:60, 1960.
17. McDonald, R. E.: *Dentistry for the Child and Adolescent*. St. Louis, Mosby, 1969. p. 129.
18. Mack, E. S.: A restorative pedodontic prac-

tice without amalgam. *J Dent for Child*, 37:428, 1970.
19. Laswell, H. R., Welk, D. A., and Regenos, J. W.: Attachment of resin restorations to acid pretreated enamel. *JADA*, 82:558, 1971.
20. Barber, T. K.: Pedodontic orthodontics. In Goldman, H., *et al.* (Ed.): *Current Therapy in Dentistry* (vol. 3). St. Louis, Mosby, 1968, pp. 737–776.
21. Moyers, R. E.: *Handbook of Orthodontics for the Student and General Practitioner*, 2nd ed. Chicago, Year Book Medical Publishers, 1963.

Chapter 21

Diagnosis and Treatment Planning for Geriatric Patients

ARTHUR ELFENBAUM

AGE AND AGING

ELDERLY PEOPLE consult a dentist for the same reasons given by younger patients. They want relief from pain or discomfort; they need a minor or major rehabilitation of the masticatory mechanism; they seek to correlate a systemic disorder with an oral cause or effect; they are interested in oral cosmetics; or they request a checkup.

The so-called population explosion that characterizes the latter half of the twentieth century is a phenomenon that concerns dentistry in the same way that it affects any other occupation. Most dentists are aware that the number of elderly patients in their practices is gradually increasing. The observation conforms with the statistical reports that at the turn of the century there were three million people in the United States who were sixty-five years of age and over, and they constituted 3 percent of the total population. The arbitrary figure of sixty-five was foisted upon us by industry and commerce, but it is in no way related to the biologic or psychosocial maturity of people, and it is destined to determine our life and living for many years to come.

At this writing, which is only about one lifetime since the century began, we have almost twenty million people in our population who have reached and passed sixty-five years of age, which means that one in every ten of us is classified as elderly. It should also be noted that the span of life, now acknowledged to be seventy-two years, is not much more than the "threescore years and ten" that the Psalmist established as a lifetime, but life expectancy, considered to be seventy-two years at birth, decrees that the longer we live, the more years we may expect to see, although it is assumed that mortality has its limits.

A liberal overall view of the elderly ones among us reveals that there are millions of older individuals who are in comparatively good health and who do everything possible to preserve it. They eat and exercise with discretion, continue to follow their occupations and take an active part in the socioeconomic welfare of their communities. As subjects in gerontologic investigations, they are not given too much consideration, mainly because they do not complain. For them, aging is a stage in their development without any resemblance to disease. Having a modicum of poetry still left in our soul, we like to refer to them as *the hardy perennials in the garden of life.*

However, they do manifest some benign regressive aging changes that can be called senescent in the true sense of the word (Latin: *sen,* old; *escent,* growing). The changes are familiar ones, and we accept them as normal *for them*. It is not surprising that an old man becomes gray and somewhat bald. The aging woman dislikes her wrinkling skin, and she resorts to the use of cosmetic preparations to overcome it. Most elderly people are conditioned to use bifocal glasses to counteract presbyopia, and for their hearing loss (presbycusis), they submit to the use of appropriate devices. Their gait is slower, probably because of a fibrosis of the muscles, and there is a consequent incoordination in their actions. The loss of moisture, fat and elasticity from the soft tissues of their bodies and the reduction of their skeletal bone mass are associated with a reduction in height and weight, although some elderly indulge in food and fluids enough to enlarge the body's fat depots.

Psychologically, many oldsters notice their loss of immediate memory and their improved ability to recall remote incidents. When they find themselves at a loss to give a logical account of events in their past life, they often fabricate occurrences to make the story acceptable, but with no intention of telling untruths. The phenomenon may be associated with little strokes that occur in older people during sleep and with the known reduction with age in the quantity and quality of blood in the cerebral circulation. The consequent hypoxia may account for the death of a number of brain cells, and they are never replaced, but since we are normally endowed at birth with many millions of brain cells, the loss of a few thousand is not serious.

It so happens that all the cells, tissues and organs of the body do not show their senescence at the same time, or at the same rate, or in the same way in all people. As soon as an aging change becomes evident, some hardy elderly ones notice it and immediately adapt themselves to the altered situation. They even anticipate the changes, accept them as a challenge and overcome them, and the constant little victories stimulate them, keeping them young.

The hardy elderly also know about oral health. The everyday media of communication tell them about it. Their dentist probably gave them an occasional lecture on oral hygiene. In many schools, children are now being taught by their teachers or by a dental hygienist how to take care of their teeth. It also seems likely that children who drink fluoridated water during the years when their teeth are developing will, all other things being equal, have acceptably good dentitions in their advanced years, and they will not be willing to sacrifice salvageable teeth in their old age as their ancestors did in the early years of the present century. In the 1920's the theory of focal infection was so prevalent that infected teeth, actually or supposedly, were extracted in order to cure almost any kind of bodily ailment, and it was generally accepted that edentulousness was an inevitable concomitant of old age.

At the other end of the spectrum of aging changes, we find millions of old people who are generally described as senile. They are chronically ill and frequently incapacitated. They cannot withstand the everyday stresses of life that serve to stimulate their hardy counterparts, although being able to live implies the stimulation of beneficent stresses. In their case too, all their cells, tissues and organs do not age at the same time, or at the same rate, or in the same way, but they have lost the ability to adapt themselves to changing circumstances. In fact, they resist change, whether it involves food, housing or clothing. To pursue the horticultural metaphor that we applied to the hardy old people, we choose to refer to these disadvantaged ones as *the broken blossoms in the garden of life.*

If their aging is not a disease, they are vulnerable to many infirmities—heart disease, cancer, cerebrovascular accidents, hypertension, atherosclerosis, nutritional deficiencies, respiratory disorders, diabetes, arthritis, influenza and many others. It is no consolation to them that the same diseases occur among children, although in general, the pathoses are acute in character in children, but chronic in the elderly.

Many of the old and "broken" individuals also suffer from what is known as an organic brain syndrome, usually an involutionary phenomenon that is characterized by what is called second childhood in common parlance. It is a regression to a more elementary emotional state that hinders interpersonal communication. It should not be assumed that it affects only the indigent, nor should it be taken for granted that such patients are found only in domiciliary facilities. Only 5 percent of the total number of people in the United States who are in the sixty-five plus bracket are in institutions. That means that the others are in the community and go to the private offices of dentists and physicians for health service, or if they are housebound, the service must be brought to them.

The mouths of the "broken" people are often characterized by an insufficient and inefficient masticatory economy. Their food is usually of the soft, fluid and low residue kind that is generally conducive to constipation. The laxatives that they use to give them relief generally flush out the nutrients in the food. Mineral oil dissolves vitamins A, D, E and K, and as a result there may be evidences of vitamin deficiencies in the oral soft tissues and jawbones, or the tissues are not adequately nourished and cannot tolerate the presence of removable prostheses. The success of a dental prosthesis depends as much on the compatibility of the tissues that support it as on the technical perfection with which it was constructed.

Having mentioned the large population of elderly people at the two extremes of the spectrum of aging changes, we must not forget the many millions in the vast area between the two extremes. It will be found that they manifest every shade of health and illness, and since the mouth is an integral part of the body, the dentist will have to learn about the patient's general health before he can evaluate the oral health. The day has long passed when all oral problems were approached from a purely mechanical and cosmetic point of view. The modern dentist is the mouth physician who considers dentistry as a biologic science.

ESTABLISHING RAPPORT WITH THE ELDERLY

When an elderly patient consults the dentist, he should be greeted immediately. Many old people, irrespective of their socioeconomic situation, often feel lonely and unwanted, and to be alone in a small reception room for too long a time may initiate a claustrophobia. A momentary word of assurance by the assistant that the dentist will be available soon is enough to provide the needed comfort.

THE IMPORTANCE OF OBSERVATION IN GERIATRIC DENTISTRY

When the patient enters the operatory, the dentist should be on hand, not only to offer a word of greeting and a handshake but to observe the patient's constitution, posture, gait, complexion, and a thousand and one other signs that might have some implications in dentistry. A glance is usually adequate. The characteristic stoop of an elderly person's shoulders may indicate an osteoporosis of the spine, and if the jawbone is similarly affected, it should be taken for granted that resorption of the mandible will be a problem. The stooped posture, kyphosis, is usually accompanied by some protrusion of the lower jaw, which means that dentures will have to be constructed with an edge-to-edge occlusion.

When elderly people walk, they tend to shuffle their feet instead of alternately lifting them up and setting them down, often with a definite click, as they did when they were young. The muscles of mastication behave in much the same way as they age. Young people chop their food as they eat with an up-and-down motion, but the elderly make more use of a slow grinding motion, more with the posterior teeth, which would appear to justify the use of almost cuspless posterior teeth for fixed or removable prostheses.

An elderly patient's changed voice often provides a clue to some bodily aging changes. The pip-squeak voice of an old man is an indication that his vocal cords are calcified. The raspy voice of a smoker's throat is often a warning to look for a so-called leukoplakia or a cancerous lesion of the oral and oropharyngeal mucosa. The masculinized voice of an elderly woman is sometimes one of the signs that constitute the postmenopausal syndrome, a most difficult complex to treat. A nasality of the voice may be a clue to a maxillary sinusitis, often the cause of a toothache in the maxillary posterior teeth, the reason why the patient consulted the dentist, although the treatment belongs to the rhinologist.

As the patient walks from the doorway of the operatory to the dental chair, the pill-rolling fingers of parkinsonism or the gait of a hemiplegic should notify the dentist that removable prostheses will present a management problem for the patient. If a patient has the slap-foot ataxic gait of tabes dorsalis and complains of a sore in his mouth, the dentist should remember to don gloves before he touches the luetic oral tissues.

A patient who adopts the typical orthopnea position on the edge of the chair before he leans back is indicating that he may have a cardiac or pulmonary disturbance. The dentist must remember not to keep the patient in the chair too long and not to fatigue him. The patient probably has nitroglycerin tablets in his pocket, and he should place one under his tongue.

When the patient is seated, the dentist is able to make observations at closer range of the exposed parts of the body. If the dentist notices skin lesions on the face, such as a verruca (wart) or an epithelioma, or tophi on the helix of the ear (a possible clue to gout), he should remember to bring them to the attention of the patient's family. The ear of old people is usually more or less pale and thin because the blood supply is in general reduced in quantity in the later years, but if the ear is full-blooded, polycythemia should be suspected and precautions taken if exodontics has to be considered.

A plexus of venous capillaries in the cornea of the eye (bloodshot) may be an indication of a vitamin B complex deficiency, possibly due to alcoholism. The malnutrition is often evidenced by poor tolerance of the oral tissues. Edematous hands and ankles are possible clues to a cardiac failure, a serious consideration in the management of a dental patient. A severely enlarged arm may be the result of a radical resection of the axillary glands in an ipsilateral mastectomy.

A dentist does not have to know the fine distinction between a cerebrovascular accident due to trauma or that caused by a thrombus, but the resulting hemiplegia is a big problem in removable prosthodontics. A patient who hyperventilates loud and long may be severely disturbed emotionally and be restless during dental procedures.

EXAMINATION OF THE ORAL CAVITY

Following a survey of the mouth and the use of all appropriate additional diagnostic aids, a critical mouth examination should be made and recorded on a chart. The dentist is then ready to declare his final diagnosis and treatment plan.

Lesions of the Oral Mucosa in the Elderly

When the ecology of the mouth of elderly people is given serious study, it is no wonder that the tissues are subject to so many disorders. Furthermore, the mouth contains numerous areas of transitional tissues, and they are reputed to be vulnerable to pathoses because, although they have some of the characteristics of the adjacent tissues, they do not have their protective qualities. Examples are the junction of the firm masticatory mucosa of the gingiva with the delicate lining of the labial and buccal mucosa; where the papillated dorsum of the tongue meets the thin mucosa of its ventral surface; the separation of the hard and soft palates; and the vermilion border of the lip that does not have the hair of the skin or the mucous glands of the lip to protect it. Any lesion on these transitional areas must be given serious attention.

Among the hazards that affect the oral mucosa are the reduction in the flow of saliva, the reduced quantity and quality of the vascular supply, the loss of tone of the muscles of mastication and expression, the traumata inflicted by teeth and foods, the overall effects of the many drugs that the elderly consume and the oral manifestations of the many diseases and disorders to which odler people are subject.

Some of the pathoses that afflict the mucosa of older individuals are candidiasis, leukoplakia, desquamative gingivitis, recurrent aphthae and lichen planus. A great deal is now being said about the early detection of oral cancer, but it should be a routine procedure in every oral survey, irrespective of the patient's age. Special attention should be given to the base of the tongue by drawing it forward slightly and turning it from side to side. Cancer is a treacherous disease because it is frequently painless in the early stages. The lack of pain as a diagnostic symptom could end fatally. When pain becomes evident, it is almost too late.

The ventral surface of the tongue should also be examined for venous varicosities. They may indicate pulmonary or cardiac disease; more commonly, they are unassociated with disease and represent an age change.

In debilitating systemic diseases the tongue often becomes edematous, atonic and enlarged (macroglossia). In the construction of dentures for such patients, every device should be used to afford a little extra room for the tongue—omit all second molars, use premolars for the first molars, use an edge-to-edge occlusion, and set the posterior teeth off the ridges but keep the occlusion in balance.

One of the most difficult symptoms of which elderly patients complain (especially those in the postmenopausal period) is the painful, burning tongue (glossodynia). The discomfort is relentless. A dry mouth (xerostomia) aggravates it. For relief, the patient sucks on sweet hard candies incessantly. In appearance, the tongue shows all the evidences of atrophy. It begins with the atrophy of the filiform papillae which, as they droop and disappear, expose the reddish heads of the less numerous fungiform papillae, and when they too atrophy, the taste buds, having lost their natural protection, become confused in discriminating between sweet, salt, sour and bitter. The loss of the sweet taste seems to be most disturbing emotionally, and the afflicted person overindulges in sweet foods and liquids. The appetite is spoiled, dietary intake is inadequate, nutritional requirements are deficient, and digestion is disturbed. It is worth repeating that the consumption of soft, low residue foods leads to constipation, and laxatives are used liberally. Cathartics force the excretion of undigested food and its nutrients, and mineral oil dissolves out the oil-soluble vitamins (A, D, E and K), often with oral manifestations of vitamin deficiencies.

The tongue frequently shrinks in size, and its color resembles that of raw, red beef. If the patient has natural or artificial teeth, the hypersensitive tongue makes their edges feel sharp. The dentist is often blamed for poor service, and the patients visit the office repeatedly for adjustments. The fault, of course, is with the patient, but it takes the patience of a Job to convince the patient and the family that the patient needs sympathy, empathy, compassion and a nutritious diet for supportive treatment.

The causes of glossodynia are many and varied, but the most common are (a) vitamin B complex deficiency; (b) pernicious anemia; (c) hormonal imbalance; (d) emotional upsets; and (e) a combination of the four factors. If the dentist has the knowledge and wants to take the time, he can teach the patient and the family what to eat and why, but it takes several hours to dispense such information properly. He certainly cannot, and should not, prescribe medication for pernicious anemia or hormonal imbalance. Except for a few comforting words of advice and encouragement, the dentist cannot pretend to give a patient a psychotherapeutic treatment for an emotional disturbance. Unfortunately, the family physician is almost as badly handicapped as the dentist, but he must not tell the patient that the burning of the tongue is caused by an allergy to the plastic material in the dentures and that it should be changed to vulcanite.

However, the combined effort of an understanding physician and a sympathetic dentist can do much for an elderly patient with glossodynia who has lost the interpersonal relationship that once made him or her a social personality.

Age Changes in the Oral and Perioral Structures

It should be remembered that the mouth undergoes aging changes that parallel those that occur in the rest of the body, although they do not necessarily happen simultaneously. Occasionally one may see decalcified and severely carious teeth or advanced periodontal disease in the mouth of a healthy and hearty old person or an excellent dentition with perfect occlusion in an elderly patient with a recalcitrant systemic disease.

Aging changes are to be seen in every part in and around the mouth: the perioral structures, the occlusion, the individual teeth, the oral soft tissues, jawbones and saliva. However, it should be stressed that although all the diseases and disorders that are encountered in the oral tissues of the elderly do not have the same characteristics of the pathoses with the same names that occur in the mouths of younger people, in general, the same systemic diseases are of an acute character in the young and more chronic in the old. This may not be true in 100 percent of oral and systemic disorders, but it should serve as a working hypothesis.

The dentist is accustomed to seeing age changes in the perioral structures. The loss of moisture, fat and elasticity from the skin, the subcutaneous tissues and the muscles of the lips and cheeks render them less pliable than they used to be. The consequent wrinkling is characteristic, but the replacement fibrosis prevents the mouth from opening as wide as it could formerly. Hence, the question of restoring the vertical dimension in oral rehabilitation gives rise to a serious prosthodontic problem. Extremely debilitated patients whose mandibles hang low, because the force of gravity is greater than that exerted by the muscles of expression and mastication, cannot possibly determine where their physiologic rest position is. The flabbiness of their muscles cannot contribute to the effective retention of complete dentures. Consequently, the prognosis is in jeopardy, and it should be discussed with the patient's family to obviate misunderstandings.

Age Changes in the Teeth

The endemic mottling of the developing dental enamel in youngsters is attributed to the high content of fluorides in the local drinking water. It appears as white defects when the teeth erupt, but the whitish areas become yellowish as the surface is stained by foods and smoking and cannot be abraded or bleached. In elderly people the extrinsic fluorides in foods and fluids impart a yellowish discoloration to the dental enamel, even if the person does not smoke; the color is not spotty or patchy. The concentration of fluorides in the enamel decreases from the outer surface and inward toward the dentin.

The Cracked-Tooth Syndrome

It was mentioned above that calcifications in various parts of the body are concomitant with the aging process. There is increased calcification of the dentin with age which reduces its elasticity, causing vertical cracks to form in the enamel that stain yellow from food and more so from smoking. The dentin itself also becomes harder, but more brittle, and it is quite common to find that cusps snap off spontaneously, especially if bruxism is a factor. The so-called cracked tooth syndrome is becoming the subject of considerable study in geriatric dentistry.

The Role of Radiology in Geriatric Dentistry

Although radiology is only one of the aids to diagnosis in dentistry, it is important enough to be given extra emphasis, especially on the evaluation of the character of the bone as it is seen in the radiographic images. Large, loose images of the radiolucent marrow spaces with broken and irregular trabecular radioplaque lines can only mean that the bone is of poor quality, and the prognosis cannot be favorable for the success of periodontics or removable denture prosthodontics.

If the images of the alveolar lamina dura are poor or absent, and are not continued onto the crest of the alveolar bone, the character of the bone is not good, nor is it to be trusted if the trajectory lines of the mandible and those that give support to tipped teeth are indefinite. A dentist should be able to determine the radiographic appearance of bone almost at a glance. It is a most important factor in the determination of prognosis, and prognosis is at least as important as diagnosis.

TREATMENT PLANNING IN GERIATRIC DENTISTRY

For younger and self-reliant patients there may be some excuse for a reasonable dentist-patient discussion of a treatment plan and an estimated fee, but in gerodontics, the dentist should make all the decisions. A thorough clinical and roentgenographic evaluation of the patient's oral tissues should tell him how much rehabilitation can be tolerated. Consultation with the physician and family will help to make decisions. A responsible member of the family should be present for the declaration of the prognosis of the treatment and for case presentation. It may be necessary to explain that the prognosis of a treatment often depends on the response of the patient to it, rather than on the treatment itself. The patient's family should know that if the patient needs the treatment but does not want it (and that is not uncommon), there is no point in proceeding any further. In many cases, the only reason that the family wants to provide dentures for grandma is that the daughter is ashamed to introduce her toothless mother to her friends.

If the dentist feels sure that no matter how perfectly the dentures are constructed, they will have to be relined or remade within a few months after they are delivered, and if an additional fee will have to be made for the adjustment, he had better state all the facts before he begins the treatment. Any explanation for changes given after delivery, no matter how scientific it may be, can only be interpreted by the patient and the family as an alibi. When the patient's bodily and mental state and the condition of the oral tissues indicate a poor prognosis for prosthodontic rehabilitation, the dentist should have the courage to declare that he would plan to remove any possible focus of infection or any traumatogenic tooth and leave the patient edentulous, even if the fee is not a factor in the discussion. It would be incumbent, however, on the dentist to consult with the physician about proper nutritional support for the patient.

Restorative Dentistry in the Geriatric Patient

If dental restorations or abutments for fixed or removable partial dentures for the elderly involve the cusps, protection against the splitting of the tooth can be provided by the use of onlay-inlays (commonly called shoeing the cusps) or three-quarter crowns with as much as possible of the dentin being preserved.

If the teeth are abraded, the excessive area of the flat occlusal table is conducive to the fracture of a tooth, even by the reduced masticatory force that is normal in the aged. The force can be further reduced by beveling the occluso-axial angles, and by fashioning sluiceways to let ground food escape from between the flat occluding surfaces and into the mouth to form a bolus. A slight transverse bulge near the gingival edge of a cast crown will divert food away from the gingival free margin and prevent its irritation.

For fixed partial dentures the pontics should be narrowed buccolingually to reduce occlusal stress and also to afford the tongue a little extra room.

Teeth that are slightly mobile can be made more rigid by splinting, but only if the roentgenograms show that a promising prognosis can be predicted by the favorable character of the bone. In designing removable partial dentures, provision must be made for the equitable distribution of masticatory forces over all the teeth, natural and artificial. Other ideas for the preservation of the remaining natural teeth should be gathered from textbooks and articles on prosthodontics, but only those that are based on biologic principles should be adopted.

Cavity Preparation

When preparing cavities for restorations in the teeth of older patients, one should remember that secondary dentin increases the dimension between the floor of the cavity and the dental pulp. It may be true that sharp line angles in cavity preparations, sharp retention undercuts with inverted cone burs and pins to anchor restorations may cause fracture lines in dentin and lead eventually to longitudinal fractures of teeth. It must not be forgotten that the aging process in teeth accounts for the loss of moisture in the dentin, and the resulting dehydration is another factor in the fracture of cusps, crowns and roots. The thinning of cementum as age advances, although it continues to be deposited throughout life, may also involve a loss of the elasticity of the dental root.

Now that so many people are living to more advanced ages, we are beginning to see a new phenomenon in dental caries—an initial rampant form of caries in the teeth of people in their late seventies and after they have been caries-free for many years. When carious lesions occur in the elderly because of the decomposition of packed food particles, the progress of the decay is slow and chronic, and it extends gradually along the dentinoenamel junction, but when it occurs initially in the later years, it attacks any surface of the tooth, especially the exposed parts of the roots or the cementum surfaces inside periodontal pockets. The main cause of the destruction is the loss of the salivary flow in old age, resulting in xerostomia.

The reduction of the salivary flow is mostly in the serous, rather than the mucous component, and the resultant ropy saliva is conducive to the formation of plaque, the villain in dental caries and periodontal disease. The dryness of the mouth also interferes with the retention of dentures, and it makes the mucosa susceptible to infection and trauma and to various pathoses. The failure of the salivary flow may be due to atrophy of the salivary glands and replacement of the epithelial lining of the ducts by fibrous tissue.

The flow of saliva in xerostomia may sometimes be stimulated by the use of a sialogogue (pilocarpine, ammonium chloride), but increasing the water intake is often sufficient. The presence of ropy saliva in the mouth is a detriment in making impressions; it is conducive to the propagation of dental caries and mucositis and to the poor retention of dentures. Much of it can be removed before dental procedures.

Despite the extensive carious lesions just described, many of the teeth can be salvaged by excavating the decay, but without exposing the pulp. The cavity is then washed with hydrogen peroxide, irrigated with warm water, mopped with cotton pellets and gently dried with a slow stream of warm air. Calcium hydroxide paste is applied to the residual dentin and covered with a thin layer of ZOE, all sealed in with cement. A few weeks later, all the treatment material is removed. It will then be seen that what was soft dentin is now harder, presumably because it has absorbed calcium from the hydroxide material.

The alkalinity of the calcium hydroxide has neutralized the acidity of the carious dentin. Both the hydroxide and the ZOE have stimulated a deposition of secondary dentin, making it safer to excavate a little more dentin. It has been shown that in carious lesions, the deep layers do not harbor bacteria. Hence, the procedure now is to prepare the cavity to receive another layer of calcium hydroxide, the ZOE above it, then crown and bridge cement for a base, and amalgam for a restoration. The tooth is now salvaged and may give service for a long time. The practitioner should keep up with the literature to see if investigators recommend better methods and materials, but it should be evident that even rampant dental caries is not always an indication for the extraction of a tooth.

Periodontics in the Geriatric Patient

It is still true that after middle age, most teeth are lost because of periodontal disease, but new techniques are saving many teeth that in former years were sacrificed. Local and systemic factors are being studied, and dentists are learning that better results are obtained when the patient, as well as his periodontal problem, is treated, often with the cooperation of a physician. The patient may need nutritional and psychologic therapy in addition to the local instrumental, surgical and chemical treatment.

It will often be found that if the onset of the periodontal disease occurred in the younger years, and the disease has progressed, the treatment in the later years (if any of the teeth remain!) is complicated, and the prognosis is not favorable unless the patient and the practitioner give the condition their constant attention. If all the local and systemic causative and contributing factors are kept under control, the teeth and their periodontium may be preserved.

If the onset of the periodontal pathosis is a recent occurrence, probably because the patient's periodontium was able to tolerate the causative, contributing, exacerbating and precipitating factors for many years, the resulting pathosis takes on a chronic character. The gingiva is pale because of the hypovascularity that seems to be normal for elderly people, and it has a fibrotic appearance. Some investigators believe that the fibrosis is a vicarious form of inflammation, but without any of its usual signs. The pale tissue is firm, forming a cuff around the tooth and probably helping to hold it in place.

If, for some reason, the alveolar bone atrophies, the gingiva recedes simultaneously, the teeth are clean and firm, and in many instances the roentgenographic image of the alveolar bone shows no other abnormality except a reduction in mass. Occasionally it will be seen that the periodontal ligament space is narrower and the roots are slightly hypercementosed. Are these evidences that nature is trying to lock the teeth more firmly in place?

The loss of moisture and elasticity that is characteristic of aging tissues is also evident in the jawbones. This, together with the reduction in the quantity and quality of blood in the marrow, makes it necessary to use extra care in exodontics. Overmanipulation may lead to slow postsurgical healing, dry socket and fracture of the jawbone.

NUTRITION IN THE ELDERLY

There is every indication that the dentist and his auxiliary personnel will become concerned with the diet and nutrition of patients. The subject is vast and complicated, especially when it concerns elderly people whose food intake, grocery shopping, cooking and eating habits depend on the state of their health. Medical cooperation is essential in many cases, but in general, a well-balanced diet served in pleasant surroundings has more therapeutic value than we think. Without being faddist, it is safe to say that for a well-balanced meal, 25 percent of the calories should come from protein; 55, from non-refined carbohydrates; and 20 from fats, mostly polyunsaturated. An ample supply of water should be consumed every day if the physician approves of it, and he should also determine whether or not the protein intake will tax the patient's digestive and metabolic capacity.

CONCLUSION

To conclude this biologic approach to diagnosis in dentistry and treatment planning, the author wishes to leave the reader with a few maxims that he can use at the chair in his everyday practice, even if some of them have been mentioned in the foregoing text.

1. The mouth is an integral part of the body entity, and any disorder or anomaly in it may be correlated with an abnormality in any other part of the body—or mind.

2. A dental patient is not an articulator with legs.

3. The dentist must know the tissues into which and upon which he places his restorations and appliances, and he must have a deep understanding of the *total* patient of whom those tissues are only a part.

4. The success of dental treatment depends on the environment in which it has to function; prognosis is as important as diagnosis.

5. It often takes courage for a dentist to tell the family of an elderly person that the health of the patient and the oral tissues will not tolerate extensive and expensive rehabilitation, even if there is no question about the fee.

6. The best oral treatment for some elderly patients may be to remove all possible sources of infection, traumatogenic factors and useless poor teeth, and leave the patient edentulous, but provision must be made for the patient to receive an adequate and nutritious diet.

7. The dentist must consider himself to be the mouth physician, and believe that his prosthetic treatments are therapeutic devices as important to the patient's health as any mechanical appliance planned by a medical physician.

8. Although a dental prosthesis is constructed in a laboratory by a technician and transferred by the dentist from a plaster model to the patient's mouth, the architectural planning and preparation are the products of one who is versed in basic biologic science.

9. Geriatric dentistry means much more than making more complete dentures for more old people.

10. A dentist's fee should be based on what he knows as well as on what he does.

Author's Index

Abrams, A., 195
Ackerman, L. V., 46, 84
Adler, P., 105
Aduss, H., v, 219
Alban, A., 105
Alexander, A. G., 105
Allen, A. C., 45
Allström, R., 105
American Cancer Society, 123
American Dental Association, 107, 108
Anderson, A. W., v, 271, 297
Anderson, D. J., 165
Andreasen, J. D., 45
Andreasen, J. O., 297
Ante, I. H., 175, 185
Apfel, H., 270
Armitage, J. E., 270
Armstrong, D., 89
Arnim, S. S., 165
A. R. P. A. Internationale, 165
Ash, M. A., 185
Ash, M. M., 139, 166
Ayres, W. W., 46

Baastad, K. L., 107
Baboolal, R., 105
Backer, M. H., 46
Baer, P. N., 109
Bahn, A. N., 106
Baker, E., 108
Barber, T. K., 293, 298
Barile, M. F., 106, 107, 108, 297
Barnes, S. S., 46
Barton, P. R., 270
Barton, R. E., 185
Bass, C. C., 165
Bassett, R. W., 185
Batsakis, J. G., 46
Beckham, L. C., 165
Bender, I. B., 191, 196, 204
Benenson, A. S., 105
Bennett, I. C., 297
Berglund, S. E., 106
Berkenbilt, D. A., 106
Beutner, E. J., 107

Beveridge, E. E., v, 186, 204
Beyron, H., 139
Beyron, H. L., 165
Bibby, B. G., 106, 107
Bickley, H. C., 106
Blacklow, R. S., 89
Boggs, D. R., 46
Bowers, G., 145, 164
Brauer, J. C., 185
Brecker, S. C., 180, 185
Brewer, H. E., 106
Bromberg, L. K., 46
Brooke, R. I., v, 65
Brophy, D., 46
Brown, E. M., 106
Brown, L. R., 106
Burket, L. W., 46
Burlakow, P., v, 21, 46
Burnett, G. W., 106
Butcher, E. O., 164
Byrd, B. L., 204

Cahn, J., 89
Cahn, L. R., 46
Cameron, G., 192, 204
Cameron, J. M., 46
Cancellaro, L. A., 164
Candell, A., 106
Cannon, A. B., 46
Casey, K. L., 89
Cauley, E. P., 45
Charbeneau, L. C., 185
Charpentier, J., 89
Chauncey, H. H., 109
Chayes, C., 140
Chercheue, R., 185
Churchill, H. R., 46
Clark, R. L., 46
Cogswell, W. W., 165
Cohen, D. W., 139, 165
Cohen, L., v, ix, xi, 3, 46, 85, 87, 89, 110, 111, 112, 114
Cohn-Stock, G., 270
Cooke, B. E. D., 46
Crabb, H. S. M., 45

Crissey, J., 198, 204
Critchley, P., 106
Crosby, R. G., 108
Curzon, M. E. J., 106
Cutcher, J. L., 64

Dahlgren, S. E., 84
Dameshek, W., 46
Darling, A. I., 45
Davey, K., 297
Davies, R. M., 106, 108
Davis, B. D., 106
Delaney, A. J., 46
de Stoppelaar, J. D., 106
Devine, K. D., 217
Dick, H. M., 106
Dirks, O. B., 106
Dito, W. R., 46
Dlabow, N. H., 108
Dodds, T. C., 108
Doerr, R. E., 185
Domokos, A., xiii
Dowdle, W. R., 106
Drinnan, A. J., v, 65
Duell, R., 198, 204
Duell, R. C., 106
Dulbecco, R., 106
Dummett, C. O., 164
Duncan, G. G., 46

Edgerton, 213
Egyedi, P., 270
Eisen, H. N., 106
Elfenbaum, A., v, 299
Ellis, R. G., 297
Engel, L., 106
Englert, R. J., 46
Ensing, H., 185
Ericsson, Y., 108

Fenner, F., 106
Fischman, S. L., v, 65
Fisher, A. K., 45
Foote, F. W., 46
Forrest, S. P., 204
Francis, T. C., 106, 108
Frank, A. L., 274, 287, 297
Frankel, M. A., 106
Frazell, E. L., 46
Freese, A. S., 139
Frostell, G., 106

Gallios, J. A., 289
Gardner, A. F., ix
Gelb, A. F., 106
Genco, R. J., 106
Gerhard, R. J., v, 6, 19, 167, 185, 205, 218

Gerrold, F. P., 123
Gibbons, R. J., 106, 107
Gilmore, E., 106
Gilmore, H. W., 185
Ginsberg, H. S., 106
Gitlin, B. N., 166
Gjermo, P., 107
Glavind, K., 108
Glenn, F. B., 297
Glickman, I., 165
Goldberg, M., 198, 204
Goldhaber, P., 297
Goldman, H. M., 46, 84, 107, 108, 139, 165, 204, 298
Goodale, R. H., 118
Gorlin, R. J., 84, 107
Gottlieb, B., 164
Graf, H., 107, 165, 166
Graykowski, E. A., 106, 107, 108, 297
Greene, G. W., 270
Greene, R., 164
Greulich, W. W., 297
Grossman, L. I., 270
Guichet, N. F., 139

Haenszel, W., 46
Harris, C. A., 238, 270
Harwell, R., 106
Hawkins, G. R., 109
Hayes, M. L., 107
Hayward, J. R., 270
Helm, S., 237
Hendron, J. A., 165
Henle, G., 107
Henle, W., 107
Henning, F. R., 297
Hennon, D. K., 107
Henstell, H. H., 46
Herzog, H., 165
Hinds, E. C., 270
Hine, M. K., 45, 84, 108
Hjorting-Hansen, E., 297
Hoffman, G. M., 165
Horsfall, F. L., 107
Howell, F. V., 204
Howell, R. N., 198, 204
Huffman, R., 185
Hutter, R. V. P., 123
Hyman, G. A., 109

Ingle, J. I., 189, 191, 192, 193, 194, 204
Ingraham, R., 185
Ingraham, R. Q., 107

Jankelson, B., 165
Jans, R. B., 46
Jenkins, G. N., 107
Jensen, S. B., 106, 108
Jonck, L. M., 270

Jones, J. C., 84
Jones, W. A., 84
Jordan, H. V., 108

Kalis, P., 297
Kay, L. W., 107
Keele, C. A., 89
Kennett, S., v, 238
Kenny, G. E., 106
Kerr, D. A., 45, 185
Keyes, P. H., 107
Kilian, M., 108
Kimmelman, B., 297
King, W. J., 108
Klingsberg, J., 164
Kole, H., 261, 270
Kopel, H. M., 198, 204
Koper, A., 217
Koser, R., 185
Krogh-Paulsen, W., 165
Krol, A., 217
Kruger, G. O., 270
Kupczak, L. J., 108
Kutscher, A. H., 109

Lambson, G. O., 106
Lane, C. W., 46
Laney, W. R., 210, 217
Lang, L. A., 107
Lang, R. L., 185
Laskin, D. M., 217
Laswell, H. R., 298
Law, D. B., 297
Lawson, B. F., 191, 204
Leach, S. A., 107
Lee, R. H., vi, 207
Lee, W. B., 107
Lehner, T., 107
Lever, W. F., 45
Levy, B. M., 45, 84, 108
Lewis, A. B., 45
Elvin-Lewis, M., vi, 90
Lilly, E. S., 84
Lilly, G. E., 64
Lim, R. K. S., 89
Lind, P. O., 84
Lindbom, A., 84
Linkow, L., 185
Lipke, D., 165
Litt, M., 46
Lobiz, W. C., 46
Loe, H., 106, 107, 108, 109
Looby, T. P., 46
Losee, F. L., 107

Macapanpan, I. C., 165
MacBryde, C. M., 89
MacIntosh, R. B., 270

Mack, E. S., 297
MacKenzie, W. R., 107
Madden, R. M., 106
Malone, W. F., vi, 6, 19, 167, 185, 205
Manly, R. S., 165
Mantel, N., 109
Marci, F., 106
Marlette, R. H., 84
Martensson, R., 84
Massler, M., 166, 297
McCarthy, P. L., 204
McDonald, R. E., 204, 297
McElroy, D. L., 185
McGrew, E. A., 46
McNamana, T. F., 109
Medak, H., vi, 21, 46, 119
Meldenhall, R., 204
Melzack, R., 89
Mergenhagen, S. E., 107, 108
Merrill, S. S., 106
Microbiological Associates, Inc., 108
Millard, H. D., 185
Miller, H. P., 46
Mitchell, D., 191, 204
Mitchell, D. F., 107, 165
Moffatt, T. W., 46
Montgomery, H., 45
Mook, W. H., 46
Morganelli, J. L., 185
Morris, M. L., 157, 165
Moyer, R. E., 294, 298
Mrklas, L., 108
Muhlemann, H., 165
Muhlemann, H. P., 165
Muhler, J. C., 106, 107
Mullaney, T., 198, 204
Myers, G. E., 185

Nabers, C. L., 165
Nadler, S. C., 165
Nahmias, A. J., 106
Natiella, J. R., 270
Natkin, E., 192, 204
Newbrun, E., 297
Nisengard, R. J., 107
Nizel, A. E., 218, 289
Nolte, W. A., 108

Obwegeser, H. L., 248, 251, 255, 270
Ochsenbein, C., 165
O'Donnell, L. J., 109
Ohman, A., 297
Old, J. S., 46
Oppenheim, J. J., 108
Orban, B., 164, 204
Ore, D. E., vi, 271, 289
Oringer, M. J., 185
Ozimek, J. T., vi, 6, 19, 167, 205

Pasqual, H. N., 46
Pauls, F., 106
Pendelton, E. C., 218
Persico, D., xiii
Phillips, R. W., 185
Platt, D., 108
Poncher, H. G., 297
Porter, Z. C., vi, 141
Posselt, U., 139, 165
Powell, R. N., 105
Preiskel, H. W., 185
Prinz, H., 45
Pritchard, J., 165
Pritchard, J. F., 147, 165
Prophet, A. S., 105
Pruzansky, S., vi, 219
Pyle, S. I., 297

Ramadan, A. B. E., 147, 165
Ramfjord, S., 153, 165
Ramfjord, S. P., 139
Rashid, P. J., 45
Ravel, R., 118
Ray, H. G., 165
Rayne, J., 270
Regato, J. A., 46
Regenos, J. W., 298
Renstrup, G., 165
Richards, A. G., 64
Riethe, P., 108
Riley, D. P., 204
Ritchey, B., 192, 204
Rizzo, A. A., 108
Robbins, S. L., 108
Robinson, H. C., 45
Rölla, B., 107
Rothaar, R. E., 107
Roworthy, R. H., 218
Ruben, M. P., 108
Russell, W. O., 46

Sabrodsky, S., 108
Sandler, H. C., 121, 123
Santos, H. A., 165
Sarnat, B. G., 140
Sarnat, H., 297
Scavizzi, F., 106
Scheman, P., 139
Scherp, H. W., 106
Schiott, C. R., 106, 107, 108
Schmaman, A., 84
Schour, I., 297
Schulman, S. M., 108
Schultz, L. C., 185
Schuyler, C., 140
Schuyler, C. H., 165
Schwartz, L., 140

Schwartz, W. R., xiii
Segal, N. A., 46
Seligman, S. J., 106
Seltzer, S., 191, 196, 204
Selvig, K. A., 108
Seward, G. R., vi, 47, 64
Shafer, W. G., 45, 84, 108
Sharav, Y., 297
Sharry, J. J., 217
Sheft, D. J., 108
Shimkin, M. H., 46
Shklar, G., 204
Shore, N. A., 140
Shrago, G., 108
Shulman, L. B., 297
Sibley, L., 165
Silness, J., 108
Simon, B. I., 108
Sims, W., 108, 277, 297
Skach, M., 108
Skinner, E. W., 185
Smith, I., 84
Smith, W. A., 166
Smulow, J. B., 165
Snyderman, R., 108
Solow, B., 237
Sommerfeld, R. M., vi, 207
Soulairac, A., 89
Spear, G. R., 165
Spies, T. D., 46
Stafne, E. C., 46
Standish, S., 107
Stanley, H. R., 108, 297
Stanley, Jr., H. R., 107
Steinberg, A. I., 108
Steiner, M. S., 64
Stewart, S., 108
Stookey, G. K., 106, 107
Strand, C., 46
Sturdevant, C. M., 185
Sundstrom, F., 108
Swain, R. H. A., 108

Taichman, N. S., 108
Tamm, I., 107
Taylor, J., 195
Taylor, J. A., 107
Tempel, T. R., 108
Thaller, J. L., 165
Theilade, E., 109
Thoma, K. H., 46, 270
Thomas, H. G., 107
Tiecke, R. W., 45, 46
Tocchini, J. J., 185
Toller, P. A., 59, 64
Trott, J. R., 106
Turetsky, S., 165
Turlington, E. G., 217

Tussman, G. C., 297
Tylman, S. D., 185

Updegrave, W. J., 64
Urbanek, V. E., vi, 124
U. S. Public Health Service, 84, 218

van Houte, J., 106
Vogel, A., 165
Volpe, A. R., 108
Von Der Fehr, F. R., 108, 109

Wall, P. D., 89
Wantulok, J. C., 196
Warner-Lambert Pharmaceutical Co., 107
Wassmund, M., 259, 270
Way, E. L., 89
Weed, L. L., 237
Weinberg, L. A., 165
Weinmann, J. P., 165
Weinmann, K., 108

Weiss, R. S., 46
Welk, D. A., 298
Wheelock, M. C., 46
White, D. O., 106
Widman, F. K., 118
Williams, J. E., 107
Wilson, W. H., 185
Winer, R. A., 109
Winter, G. B., xiii, 278, 279, 280, 281, 282
Wolff, H. G., 86, 89
Woods, W. B., 106
Woodworth, J. V., vi, 8, 17

Yurhstas, A., 165

Zander, H. A., 165
Zegarelli, E. V., 109
Zinsser, H., 109
Ziontz, M., 204
Zipkin, I., 109
Ziskin, D. E., 45
Zucas, S. A., 109

Subject Index

Accra, Ghana, caries rate, 92
Actinomycosis, 100, 203
   salivary glands, 38
Adenoameloblastoma, 70
Adenoma
   canalicular, 40
   oxyphilic, 40
   pleomorphic, 39
   sebaceous cell, 40
Adrenal gland, diseases of, 12–13
Agranulocytosis, 44
   following thiouracil drugs, 12
Allbright's syndrome, 78
Allergic reaction, 26
   contact, 40
   erythema multiforme, 26
   oral manifestations of, 40–41
Alveolectomy, 239, 243
Ameloblastoma, 69–70
   histology, 70
   radiography, 70
Amelogenesis imperfecta, 179, 280–281
American Academy of Oral Pathology, 120
American Lecture Series in Dentistry, vii–viii
Anaphylaxis
   localized, 91
   penicillin, 9, 40–41
Anatomy, morbid, of lesions, radiography of, 56–58
Anemia(s)
   classification of, 111
   diagnostic tests of, 110–112
   hypochromic, 43
   manifestations, 4, 13, 43, 304
   pernicious
      manifestations of, 4, 13, 43
      glossodynia, 303–304
   sickle cell, 43, 111
Ankylosis, 274, 282–283
   in transplantation, 268
Antibiotic therapy
   candidiasis, 99
   hairy tongue, 32
   respiratory infection, 14
Anticoagulant therapy, and drug interactions, 10–11

Anticonvulsant therapy, in epilepsy, 15–16
Aphthae, 102–105
   in children, 278–279
Apertognathia, 261
Apical scar, 67
Arthritis
   in Reiter's disease, 26
   rheumatoid, 10, 28
      aphthous ulcers, 102–103
      Sjögren's syndrome, 38
      temporomandibular joint, 15
Aspiration, of fluid-filled cavity, 59
Aspirin
   burn, 42
   contraindicated, 13
   reaction to, 4, 40
Asthma, attack during dental therapy, 14

Behcet's disease, 26
Biopsy, methods of, 122–123
Blood
   chemistry
      blood urea nitrogen, 114
      cholesterol, 115
      creatinine, 114–115
      glucose, 115
      uric acid, 115
   clotting
      function, tests, 113
      mechanism (Diagram), 114
   coagulation, physiology of, 114
   conditions affecting
      red cells, 110–112
      white cells, 112
   dyscrasias
      diuretics produce, 11
      endodontic therapy in, 202–203
      oral manifestations of, 43–45
      treatment of, 13
   enzymes, levels, 116, 117
   platelet function, tests of, 113–114
   values
      red cells (Table), 111
      white cells (Table), 112
   vessels, tumors of, 30–31

Bone
  abnormalities, 239–245
  alveolar, removal, 239, 243
  changes, in elderly, 305
  cysts
    latent, 69
    solitary, 68–69
    traumatic, 196
  dento-alveolar surgery, 263–265
  diseases of, 71–78
    blood enzyme levels, 117
  enostosis, exostosis, distinguished from osteoma, 81–82
  exostosis, distinguished from fibrous hypertrophy, 243
  graft, 157, 184–185
  loss, 147–148, 153, 154–155
  radiography of, in elderly, 305
  sheets of, radiography, 58
Bone marrow depression
  epilepsy, 16
  hematologic diseases, 13
  respiratory disease, 14
  rheumatic disorders, 15
Boxers, neuroma, injury of, 31

Calculus(i)
  deposition of, in diabetics, 12
  salivary, sialography of, 61
Cancer, responsibility for detection, 13, 21, 35, 119, 303
Candidiasis, 99–100
Canker sores, 102–105
Carcinoma
  adeno-, 36, 40
  adenoidcystic, 39–40
    histology, 40
  basal cell, 36
  of bronchus, 5
  epidermoid, 39
    false diagnosis of, 31
  erythroplakia, 34
  intraoral, survival rate, 35
  laryngeal, 14
  of maxillary antrum, 243
  mucoepidermoid, 39
  renal cell, 195–196
  squamous cell, 24, 35–36, 195–196
  transitional cell, 37
Cardiovascular disease, 10–11
  See also Heart Disease
Caries
  activity tests, 92–93, 277
  control, 94–95, 170–172
    in children, 287–291
    in elderly, 307–308
  emergency treatment, 169–170, 271–272
  epidemiology of, 92

Caries (*Continued*)
  etiology, 92–93
  laboratory diagnosis, 93–94
  microbiology of, 92–93
  radiography of, 49
  restorative materials, 172–174
    for children, 292–293
Case presentation, principles of, 205–206
Casts, dental
  in children, 276–277
  facial deformities, surgery for, 253
  occlusion, 167–168, 253
  orthodontics, 236
  preprosthetic, 209
Cavity, fluid-filled, aspiration and radiography of, 59
Cellulitis,
  pain of, 88
  in periapical disease, 95
Cementoma, 70
  radiography of, 70, 195
Cephalometric radiography, 62–63
  facial deformities, surgery for, 252–253
  in orthodontics, 235
Cephaloridine, contraindicated in genitourinary disease, 16
Chart, charting, of oral cavity, 6, 19, 145–147
Cheilitis, 99, 213
Cheilosis, 41
Chemotherapy, 13
Cherubism, 79–80
  histology, 80
  radiography, 80
Chin correction, 262–263
Christmas disease, 113
Collagen diseases, 28–29
  histology, 28
Color coding, in diagnostic record, 20
Contact allergies, 40
Corticosteroid therapy
  adrenal insufficiency, 12
  candidiasis, 99
  infection management, 201
  pemphigus vulgaris, 25
Corticotomy, 264–265
Cortisone, 9–10, 12
Crepitus, in children, 234
Curettage, in pocket elimination, 159
Cyto-Kit, 120–121
Cyst
  dentigerous, 67–68
  follicular, 195–196
  hemorrhagic, 68–69
  latent bone, 69
  with odontoma, 70–71
  radicular, 66–67
    histology, 66–67
  radiography of, 59, 66, 68, 69, 71
  residual, 67

Cyst (*Continued*)
   solitary bone, 68–69
   traumatic, 68–69
   traumatic bone, 196
Cytology, oral, 120–121
   classification of findings, 121

Dental history
   See History (case)
Dentinogenesis imperfecta, 179, 280
Dento-alveolar surgery, 263–265
Dentures
   causes of failure, 175–176
   construction for elderly, 303
   diagnostic aids, 208–209
   difficulty in wearing
     osteoradionecrosis, 73
     pernicious anemia, 13
     sore mouth, 99
     vitamin B complex deficiency, 41
   ill-fitting
     epulis fissuratum, 23, 211, 245–246
     papillary hyperplasia, 24
       histology, 24
     tissue treatment for, 211–212
   occlusal dimension, 132, 177–179
   oral conditions, ideal, 209–210, 238
Dermal lesions, oral manifestations of, 24–28
Diabetes
   endodontic therapy, 201–202
   periodontal disease, 12, 117
   treatment of, 11–12, 41
   urinalysis for, 115–116
Diagnosis
   decisions of, 186–188
   principles of, 6
   treatment as, 189–190
Diet
   caries, effect on, 92
   children
     analysis, 287–291
     intake diary, 288
     nutritional analysis, 290–291
     recommendations, 289, 290–291
     sweet-intake analysis, 290–291
   of edentulous patients, 211
   of elderly, 304, 308–309
Dilantin
   allergic reaction, 41
   hyperplasia, 144, 279
Drug(s)
   case history, 9–10
   interactions, 9, 11
   reactions
     asthma, 14
     and endodontic therapy, 200–201

Drug(s) (*Continued*)
     erythema multiforme related to, 26
     hayfever, 14
   See also individual names of drugs and therapy
       programs
Dry socket, 71, 308
   histology, 71
   radiography, 71
Dyskeratosis, with papillomatosis, 24
Dysplasia
   fibrous, 78–79, 117
     histology, 79
     radiography, 78–79
     enlarged maxillary tuberosity, 243
   radiography of, 56–58

Ear diseases, pain of, 88
Education, patient, enlisting cooperation, 7, 136, 158, 205–206
Emphysema, 14
Enamel
   dentigerous cyst, 67
   invagination, 192
Endocarditis, bacterial subacute
   clubbing of fingers, 5
   prophylaxis, 10
Endocrine disorders, 11–13, 117–118
   See also individual names
Endodontic therapy
   manifesto of, 199
   periodontics, 156–157
   prerequisites for, 186–190
   systemic disorders, 200–203
Epilepsy, 15–16
   Dilantin hyperplasia in children, 279
Epulis fissuratum, 23, 211
   malignant transformation of, 34–35
   surgical removal, 245–246
     preprosthetic, 210
Erythema, in contact allergy, 40
Erythema multiforme, 26
   distinguished from acute herpetic gingivostomatitis, 279
Erythroblastosis fetalis, 280
Erythroplakia, 34
   histology, 34
Eskimos, torus palatinus in, 244
Examination
   in edentulous patients, 207–209
   pathologic, need for, 119
   in periodontics, 141–152
   radiographic, 47
   sequence, procedures, 4, 6, 7, 19–20, 21, 186–188
Eyes
   diseases, pain of, 88
   mucocutaneous syndromes, 26

Face
  deformities of, surgery for, 251–267
  fractures, radiography of, 63–64
  pain of, 87–89
Federation Dentaire Internationale, 19
Fibrinoid necrosis, in collagen diseases, 28
Fibroma, 29–30
  ossifying, 80
    histology, 80
    radiography, 48, 56, 80
Fibro-osseous lesions, 78–81
Fibrosarcoma, of mesenchymal lesions, 37
Fibrosis, submucous, malignant transformation of, 34
Fischer's angle, 178
Fluoride
  caries control, 94–95, 288, 291–292
  color change of teeth, 305
    in children, 280
  gel composition, 74n
  radiation therapy, application prior to, 213
Foreign bodies, buried, radiographic localization of, 54–56, 57, 62
Frenectomy
  in orthodontics, 220, 231, 278, 293
  "Z" plasty method, 246–247

Gastrointestinal diseases, treatment of, 13–14
Gate control theory of pain, 85
General Electric Panoramic, 56
Genioplasty, 262–263
Genitourinary diseases, treatment of, 16, 26
Gentamicin sulfate, contraindicated in genitourinary disease, 16
Geriatric
  broken blossoms, 300
  hardy perennials, 299
  population, 299
Gingiva
  hemorrhages, in thrombocytopenic purpura, 45
  hyperplasia, 144–145
    in leukemia, 44
  hypertrophy, from anticonvulsants, 16
  rubella vaccination, disturbances following, 279
  surgery, 161–162
Gingivitis
  in diabetics, 12, 41
  in hypertrophy, hyperplasia, 23
  microbiology of, 90–91, 96–99
  streptococcal, 279
  ulcerative, acute necrotizing, incidence, etiology, 96–97
Glomerulonephritis, 16
Glossary of Prosthodontic Terms, 126
Glossitis
  ankyloglossia, 278
  migrating, 22
  in pernicious anemia, 13
  rhomboid, median, 22

Glossopyrosis, in pernicious anemia, 13
Gonorrhea, oral effects of, 98
Grafts
  bone, 157
  mucosal, 248
  ridge, 249–250
  skin, 248, 251
Granuloma
  dental, 65–66
    histology, 66
    radiography, 66
  development, 95
  eosinophilic, 76–77
  giant cell
    radiography, 48, 56, 75
    reparative, 74–75
  pyogenicum, 23
  salivary glands, effect on, 38

Hand-Schuller-Christian disease, 76
Headache, pathophysiology, diagnostic features, 86–87
Heart diseases
  treatment of, 4, 5, 10–11, 15, 201–202
  valve replacement, treatment of, 10
Hemangioendothelioma, 31
Hemangioma, 30–31
  histology, 30–31
Hemangiopericytoma, 37
Hematologic diseases, 13
Hemophilia, 13
  endodontic therapy, 202
  partial thromboplastin time, 113
Hepatitis, treatment of, 14
Hepatocellular disease, 14
Herpes
  infections, 100–102, 279
  labialis, distinguished from chancre of lip, 5
  simplex, 100–101
  zoster, 101
Histiocytosis X, 76–77
History (case)
  dental, 6, 7, 141–143
  medical, 6, 7, 8–18, 141, 219–220
  See also Diet, children, *and* Questionnaire
Hodgkin's disease, lymphadenopathy in, 5
Hyperkeratosis
  defined, 32
  lesions, 32–35
  with lichen planus, 24
Hyperparathyroidism, 16, 75–76, 117
  histology, 75–76
  radiography, 75
Hyperplasia, 22–24
  Dilantin, 144, 279
  of gingiva, 144–145
  unilateral, 261–262
Hypertension, treatment of, 11

Hyperthyroidism,
  symptoms, 4–5
  tests for, 116–117
  treatment of, 12
Hypertrophy, 22–24
  fibrous, distinguished from exostosis, 243
Hypoplasia
  of enamel, 281
  and erythroblastosis fetalis, 280
Hypotension, drug interactions in, 11, 15
Hypothyroidism
  tests for, 118
  treatment of, 12

I.R.M., caries control medication, 169–170
Implantology, 184–185
India, submucous fibrosis, 34
Injury, oral manifestations of, 41–43
  traumatic, in children, 272–275
Intermaxillary opening, reduced, relief of pulpal pain, 202

Jaundice
  symptoms, 4
  treatment, 14
Jaw
  diseases
    bone, inflammatory, 71–74
    fibro-osseous lesions, 78–81
    nonodontogenic neoplasms, 81–83
    odontogenic lesions, 65–71
  fractured, radiography of, 56, 63–64

Keratotic lesions, 32–34
  histology, 33, 34

Laxatives, as cause of vitamin deficiencies, 304
Letterer-Siwe disease, 76
Leukemia, 44–45
  chemotherapy, 13
  endodontic therapy, 202–203
  mucogingival line, 144
Leukoedema, 33
Leukokeratosis, 33
Leukopenia, 44
  antiarrhythmic agents produce, 11
Leukoplakia
  candidal, 34
    histology, 34
  clinical, so-called, 32
  "mild," 33
  nonreversible, 33
    histology, 33
    malignancy of, 34
Lichen planus
  erosive, 24
    cytologic smear, 120
    malignancy, 34

Lichen planus (*Continued*)
  forms of, 24
  histology, 24
Lip
  biting, in children, 296–297
  chancre of, distinguished from herpes labialis, 5
  solar keratosis of, 34
Lipiodol ®, 60
Lipofibroma, 29–30
Lipoma, 29
Liposarcoma, of mesenchymal lesions, 37
Liver, diseases of, 14
  one-stage prothrombin time, 113
Lupus erythematosus, 28
Lymphadenopathy, cervical, 5
Lymphangioma, 31
Lymphoepithelial lesion, benign, 40
Lymphoepithelioma, 36–37
Lymphoma, treatment of, 13
  lymphadenopathy, 5
Lymphomatosum, papillary cystadenoma, 39

Malignancy. See Carcinoma, *and individual names of tumors*
Mandible
  apertognathia, 261
  asymmetry, 261–262
  bone cavity, lingual lesion, 69
    radiography, 69
  changes, due to kidney stones, 16
  fractures, radiography of, 56, 63–64
  genioplasty, 262–263, 265
  loss of, 214–215
  micrognathia, 260
  movements, parafunctional, 125–126, 149, 151
  prognathism, 252, 253–259, 263–264
  prosthodontics, 209–210, 250–251
Masticatory pain-dysfunction
  syndrome, 126–134
  clinical features, 128–131
  etiology (chart), 127
  occlusal factors, 126–128
  psychogenic factors, 128
  treatment, 131–134
Maxilla
  fractures, radiography of, 56, 63–64
  loss of, 214
  prognathism, 259
  prosthodontics, 209–210, 251
  protrusion, 264
  retrognathism, 260–261
  submucosal vestibuloplasty, 247–248
Maxillary tuberosity
  denture fitting, 208, 243–244
  tuberoplasty, 248–249, 251
Medical history. See History (case)
Melanoameloblastoma, 70
Melanoma, 37

Menopause
  hypertrophy, hyperplasia during, 23
  post-, 303
Menstruation
  hypertrophy, hyperplasia during, 23
  ulcer, recurrent aphthous, 103
Metabolic diseases, 41
  See also individual names.
Microbial disease, oral manifestations (Table), 104
Micrognathia, 260
Moniliasis, 99–100
  in denture wearers, 40
Mononucleosis, infectious, 101–102
  petechiae in, 4
Morphea, 29
Mouth-breathing
  in children, 296–297
  gingivitis, 144
Moyer's mixed dentition analysis, 294
Mucocele, 42
Mucocutaneous syndromes, 26
Mucosa, oral
  infections of, 96–99
  lesions, in elderly, 303–305
  metastases to, 37
Multiple sclerosis, 16
Mumps, 38
Muscle
  activity, parafunctional, psychogenic conditions for, 128
  attachments, abnormal, 246–247
  tissue, tumors of, 31
Myeloma, multiple, 77–78
Mylohyoid ridge, removal, 239
Myoblastoma, granular cell, 31
Myxofibroma, 29

Neoplasms, radiography of, 56–58, 83, 195–196
Nervous tissue, tumors of, 31–32
Neuralgias, facial, pain of, 88–89
Neurofibroma, 31
Neurofibromatosis, 4, 31–32
Neurological problems, 15–16
Neuroma, 31
Neutropenia, 91
Nevus, 26–28
  flammeus, 31
  nonpigmented, 26–27
    histology, 27
  pigmented, 27–28
    histology, 27–28
    malignant transformation of, 34, 35
Nikolsky's sign, in pemphigus vulgaris, 25
Nose, diseases, pain of, 88
Number system, of tooth designation, 19

Occlusal analysis
  diagnostic casts, 167–168, 236

Occlusal analysis (*Continued*)
  functional, 134–139, 148–151
  need for, 20, 192–193
Occlusion
  crossbite, 231, 296–297
  dento-alveolar surgery, 263–265
  disharmony, 231
    causes of, 126–128
  in elderly, 304–305
  equilibration, 159–160, 163, 178
  facial deformities and, 251–267
  interocclusal appliances, 131–135
  prosthodontics, 176–180
Odontoma, 70–71
  radiography of, 56, 71
Orthopantomogram, 56
Ostectomy, body
  for mandibular prognathism, 255
  premaxillary (Wassmund), 259
Osteitis,
  condensing, 72–73
  sclerosing, 191
Osteogenic sarcoma, 82–83
  radiography, 83
Osteoma, 81–82
Osteomalacia, 117
Osteomyelitis, 71–73
  chronic sclerosing, 72–73
    histology, 73
    radiography, 72–73
  with periapical disease, 95
  suppurative, 72
Osteoporosis, periapical, 192
Osteoradionecrosis, 73–74
  histology, 73
  prevention, 73–74
  radiography of, 73
Osteotomy, subsigmoid (subcondylar)
  for apertognathia, 261
  for mandibular micrognathia, 260
  for mandibular prognathism, 255–258

Pachyderma oralis, 33
Paget's disease, 80–81, 116, 117
  histology, 81
  incidence, 48
  maxillary tuberosities, 243
  radiography, 81
Pain
  carious, in children, 271–272
  chief dental complaint, 7, 271–272
  discrimination of, 196–197
  facial, 87–89
  gate control theory of, 85
  headache, 86–87
  physiology of, 85–86
  syndromes, 3
  threshold of, 4, 197

Palate
  cleft,
    bite plates for, 132–133
    prosthodontics for, 215–217
    radiographic investigation of, 59–60
  papillomatosis of, 24, 34, 35
    histology, 24
Panorex, 56
Papanicolaou smear, for epidermoid carcinoma, 39
Papilloma, 29
Parakeratosis, with lichen planus, 24
Parkinson's disease, 4
Parotitis
  epidemic, 38
  following thiouracil drugs, 12
  postoperative, acute, 38
Particles, in oral tissue, radiography of, 57–58
Passavant's ridge, 217
Pemphigoid, mucous membrane, benign, 26
Pemphigus vulgaris, 25–26
  histology, 25–26
  surgical procedures, 203
Penicillin, reaction to, 9, 14, 40–41
Periadenitis mucosa necrotica recurrens, 102–103
  Behcet's disease resembles, 26
Periapical bone, radiographic examination of, 50–51
Periapical disease, conditions which resemble, 194–195
Periapical infections, microbiology of, 95–96
Periarteritis nodosa, 28
Pericoronitis, pain of, 88
Periodontium
  assessment of, 144–145, 187–188
    pockets in, 145–147
    radiographic, 52, 141, 152–153
    recording, 20
    screening test, 51
  disease of
    in diabetics, 12, 41
    microbiology of, 90–91
  in gerodontics, 308
  pain of, 3, 87
  pockets, 145–147, 149–150
  prosthesis, 181–182
  surgery, 161–164
  systemic disease and, 153–154
Peutz-Jeghers syndrome, 4
Photographs, 235–236, 168
Plaque
  caries and, 92–93
  periodontal disease and, 90–91, 158
Plasma proteins, 110
Polycythemia, 112
  cyanosis resulting from, 4
  vera, 43–44

Port-wine stain, 31
Pregnancy
  dental surgery contraindicated, 201
  gingival hyperplasia, 144
  hypertrophy, hyperplasia during, 23
  proliferations, 23
Pro-Banthine ®, contraindicated with respiratory disease, 14
Procaine, allergic reaction to, 40
Prognathism, surgical corrections for
  mandibular, 253–259, 263–264
  maxillary, 259
Prosthodontics
  bone quality, and success of, in elderly, 305
  fixed
    classification, 180–181
    causes of failure, 174–176, 179–180
    occlusal factors, 132, 176–179, 180
    preprosthetic surgery, 209–210, 238–251
    removable, classification, 180–181
    following radiation therapy, 212–214
    tooth supported, 182–183
Pruritus, in contact allergies, 40
Psychogenic aspects of oral disease
  allergies, alleged, and, 200–201
  bruxism and, 125
  in children, 283, 296
  in denture wearing, 210
  in elderly, 299–301
  in endodontics, 186–187, 200
  gingivitis and, 96
  masticatory pain-dysfunction syndrome and, 128
  in pulp testing, 196–197
Puberty
  gingival hyperplasia during, 144
  hypertrophy, hyperplasia during, 23
  proliferations, 23
Pulmonary infections, treatment of, 14
Pulp
  capping
    direct, 285
    indirect, 283–285
  hyperemia of, pain of, 87
  infection, 95–96
  pulpectomy, 287
  pulpotomy, 286–287
Pulpitis
  chronic, 191–192
    radiography, 191–192
  emergency treatment, 169–170
  granuloma, 65–66
  histological diagnosis, 95
  pain of, 3, 87, 191
Pulp testing
  in children, 277
  with granuloma, 65
  interpretation, 198
  modalities, 197–198, 277

Pulp testing (*Continued*)
  requisites, 197
  temporary non-response, 266, 277
Purpura
  symptoms, 4
  thrombocytopenic, 45

Questionnaire
  medical history, 8–9
  samples of
    adult dental patients, 17–18
    dental habit, 142
    dental history, 143
    food intake diary, 288

Radiation therapy, 38, 43
  candidiasis following, 99
  osteoradionecrosis, 73
    prevention of, 73–74
  prosthodontics following, 212–214
  removal of teeth prior to, 74, 199–200, 213
  sialectasis, 60
Radiograph, radiography
  air-contrast, 59
  bite wing, 47, 48, 49, 51
  Bosworth's method, 54–55
  cephalometric, 62–63
  chest, 48
  Ciesynsky technique, 51
  Clark's parallax method, 54–55
  contrast, 59–60
  film types, 49
    examination of, 48–49
    holders, 50–51
  in gerodontics, 305
  interpretation, 48–49
  intraoral x-ray source method, 52
  long-cone method, 50–51
  markers, 62
  in orthodontics, 234
  parallax method, 54–55
  parallel film method, 50–51
  in pedodontics, 275–276
  periapical techniques, 47, 50–51
  Richard's tube head, 50, 51
  rotational tomography, 52, 56–58
    machines for, 56
  rule of isometry, 51
  screening tests, 48
  sialography, 60–62
  stereoscopy, 55–56
  surveys, 167
  triangulation techniques, 54
  views at right angles method, 54
  views, selection of, 47–48
Ranula, floor of mouth, 42–43
Receptor organs, 85
Reiter's syndrome, 26

Replantation, of teeth, 184–185, 267–270
  avulsed, in children, 275
Respiratory disease, 14
  cyanosis and, 4
Restorative materials, 172–174
  in children, 292–293
Reticulo-endothelial system disorders, 76
  reticulum cell sarcoma, 37
Retrognathia, 260–261
Rhabdomyosarcoma, 37
Rheumatic disorders
  endocarditis, bacterial, and, 10
  treatment of, 11, 15
Rickets, 117
Ridge, and prosthodontics
  alveolar, 239–243
  atrophic, 247–250
  grafting, 249–250
  irregular, 239–243
  mouth, lower floor of, 249
  mylohyoid, 239, 250
Rinn film holder, 50–51
Roentgencephalometry
  in gerodontics, 306, 308
  in orthodontics, 234–235
Roots
  defects, 187, 189
  fractures, 274
  radiographic examination of, 50–51
  removal, buccal window technique, 239
  resorption, in periapical disease, 95
Root canal cultures, 95–96
Rotograph, 56
Rubella vaccination, gingival disturbance following, 279

Sagittal split (Obwegeser)
  for apertognathia, 261
  for mandibular micrognathia, 260
  for mandibular prognathia, 255–258
Salicylates
  contraindicated, with anticoagulant therapy, 11
  for rheumatic disorders, 15
Salivary ducts, 59, 60–62
Salivary glands
  lesions of, 37–40
  mucocele, 42
  radiation effects, 38, 60, 213
  sialectasis, 60
  sialography, 60–62
Scleroderma, 28–29
Screening tests, 48
  for periodontal disease, 51
Scurvy, 4, 117
Sebaceous cell adenoma, 40
Senescence, 299–302
Serum sickness, penicillin, 9, 40–41

Sialectasis, sialography of, 60
Sialography, 60–62
Sinus
   infected, and toothache, 14, 302
   sinusitis, pain of, 88
   tracks, radiography of, 59
Sjögren's syndrome, 38
   sialography of, 60–61
Skin, tints, pigmentation, diseases associated with, 4
Solar keratosis of the lip, 34
Southeast Asia, submucous fibrosis, 34
Space maintainers, types and usage, 294–295
Speech,
   appliance, for cleft palate, 217
   in orthodontic diagnosis, 220, 234
Splints
   Hawley type, 160–161
   occlusal, 133–134
      double full, 161
      full, 161
   palatal bite plates, 132–133
   in periodontal treatment, 181–182
   teeth, mobile, in elderly, 306–307
   temporary, 157–158
Stabe film holders, 50–51
Stevens-Johnson syndrome, 26
Stomatitis
   aphthous, 102–105
   hemorrhagic, 26
   herpetic, 116
   herpetic gingivostomatitis, acute, 100–101
      in children, 279
   nicotinic, 23–24
   Vincent's 96–97
Stomatognathic system, 124–126
Surgery in children, 283, 293
Syphilis, 97–98
   congenital, 97
   lymphadenopathy, 5
   oral mucosa, infections in, 97–98

Temporomandibular joint dysfunction. See Masticatory pain-dysfunction syndrome.
Tests
   anemia, diagnostic, 110–112
   biopsy, 122–123
   bleeding time, 113
   blood
      cell levels
         red, 110–111
         white, 112
      whole, clotting time, 113
   clot retraction, 113–114
   cytological, 120–121
   Dextrostix, 115
   Kirby-Bauer, 96
   Labstix, 115

Tests (*Continued*)
   partial thromboplastin time, 113
   platelet count, 112–113
   prothrombin time, one-stage, 113
   Schilling test, 111–112
   Sickledex, 111
   thyroid disease, 117–118
   tourniquet, 113
Tetracycline, contraindicated in children under eight, 275, 280
   in genitourinary disease, 16
Thiouracil therapy, 12
Thrush, 99–100
Thumbsucking, 234, 296
Tissue
   conditioning, for dentures, nonsurgical, 210–212
   integrity, for dentures, 207–208
   sheets of, radiography, 57
   soft, abnormalities, 29–32, 169, 245–247
      in children, 277–279
   soft, malignant lesions, 34–37
Toller's aspiratory needle, 59
Tongue
   ankloglossia, 278
   coating, from antacids, 13
   geographic, 22
   glossitis, rhomboid, median, 22
   glossodynia, in elderly, 303–304
   hairy, 32
   macroglossia, in elderly, 303
   reduction, 261
   thrust habit, 152, 296
Tooth, teeth
   ankylosed, 282–283, 293
   clenching, 125, 149, 151
   color change, from fluorides, 305
   congenital absence of, 281–282
   cracked-tooth syndrome, 192, 305
   dentigerous cyst, 67–68
   designation, 19–20
   displacement, due to injury, 274–275
   endodontics, decision factors, 187–188
   eruption hematoma, 278
   fractured, 189, 192, 272–274
   hereditary defects, 280
   implantology, 184–185
   mobility, 147, 157–158
   replantation, 267–270, 275
   sensitive, in diabetics, 12
   stains, 280
   unerupted, radiographic localization of, 54–56
Torus
   mandibularis, 82
      interference with dentures, 244–245
   palatinus, 82
      interference with dentures, 244
   removal, for dentures, 208

Transplantation of teeth, 267–270
Trauma
  loss of oral anatomy, 214–215
  to oral tissue, 41–43
  to teeth, 170
    in children, 272–275
Treatment, sequence of, for restorative dentistry, 171–172
Trench mouth, 96–97
Tuberculosis, 98–99
  lymphadenopathy, 5
  salivary glands, 38
  treatment of, 14
Tuberoplasty, 248–249
Tuberosity, maxillary. See Maxillary tuberosity.
Tumor, odontogenic, classification of, 69
Two-Digit System, of tooth designation, 19–20

Ulcers, recurrent aphthous, 102–105
Uremia, 16
Urethritis, in Reiter's disease, 26

Varicella, 101
Vestibuloplasty
  secondary epithelialization, 248, 251
  skin graft, 248, 251
  submucosal, 247–248, 251
Vincent's infection, 96–97

Warthin's tumor, 39
White lesions, 32

Xerostomia
  in elderly, 303–304
    and caries, 307
  radiation therapy and, 43, 213
Xylocaine ®, allergic reaction to, 40